Trauma Certified Registered Nurse (TCRN®) Examination Review

Kendra Menzies Kent, MS, RN-BC, CCRN, CNRN, SCRN, TCRN, is the nursing director of the Marcus Neuroscience Institute at Boca Raton Regional Hospital in south Florida. She is a highly experienced critical care trauma nurse and an accomplished instructor, with multiple specialty certifications in critical care and extensive clinical experience in a majority of critical care specialty areas. Ms. Kent is also an educational consultant for Med-Ed Seminars in Charlotte, North Carolina, and a speaker for Health and Sciences Television Network (HSTN) and HSTN videos. Ms. Kent has edited or contributed to *Decision-Making in Medical Surgical Nursing, Evaluation Process: Competency-Based Orientation, Expert 10-Minute Physical Examination Expert Rapid Response, AACN Neuroscience Orientation PowerPoint for Traumatic Brain Injury, Critical Care Essentials,* and *CCRN Review Q&A.* She is the author of *Adult CCRN Certification Review: Think in Questions, Learn by Rationale* for Springer Publishing Company.

To my wonderful husband, Robby, and to my parents,
Sid and Judy, for all the love and support they have given me.

I also gratefully acknowledge the work of Sarah Miller,
who contributed to the review questions and rationales.

Contents

Introduction

Welcome to the journey toward certification. This book was written to help guide the pathway of the journey. It is written in a question/answer format to encourage you to think in questions when studying for the examination. When you study, I encourage you to ask yourself, "What questions about this particular topic could appear on the certification exam? What would be a good question?" This prepares you for questions; you are not just attempting to memorize content for the certification examination.

The book provides multiple-choice questions similar to the questions that are found on the Trauma Certified Registered Nurse (TCRN®) examination. These questions allow the nurse to practice taking an examination and will assist the nurse with determining areas that require further study prior to taking the TCRN examination. The answers and rationale, including some test-taking skills, are provided for every question, further preparing the nurse for the real examination.

WHY CERTIFICATION?

The most important reason for becoming certified is to do it for yourself. Certification is viewed as a mark of excellence in an area of specialty. It can be seen as an achievement and qualification by peers, physicians, health care institutes, and patients/families. Becoming certified takes dedication to trauma nursing and demonstrates a level of competency. The TCRN examination is developed to verify knowledge in trauma nursing.

Box I.1 Reasons to Become Certified

Validate your knowledge of trauma to your hospital and peers
Validate your knowledge of trauma to the patients
Validate your knowledge of trauma to the physician
Promote continuing excellence in the nursing profession
Demonstrate competency
Promote self-confidence
Encourage continuing education
Hospital credentialing
Monetary benefit (from some hospitals)

TCRN EXAMINATION INFORMATION

The TCRN examination was developed by the Board of Certification in Emergency Nursing (BCEN) and incorporates care of a trauma patient, from prevention and injury to rehabilitation. The examination covers all ages: pediatrics through geriatrics. The examination follows the test plan developed by the BCEN and the test is developed and reviewed by experts in trauma nursing. The *TCRN Application Handbook* can be accessed from the BCEN's website (www.bcencertifications.org). The examination application can be completed online. The TCRN is a 4-year certification for trauma nurses.

EXAMINATION

The TCRN examination is 150 scored multiple-choice questions, with 25 unscored questions that will not count for or against you. Those 25 questions are included as "tests" for use in future examinations. You will not know which questions count, so complete all 175 questions as if they all do. The test is not arranged per any body system but is randomized. You may have one question on chest trauma and the next one may be on spinal cord injury. The time allowed to complete the examination is 3 hours.

To be eligible to take the TCRN examination one must be a licensed RN: 2 years of practice, at an average of 1,000 practice hours per year, across the trauma continuum are recommend. *Trauma practice* is defined as providing direct patient care, supervision, education, and advocacy for patients and their families; 20 to 30 hours of trauma-specific coursework across the trauma continuum is recommended.

The TCRN examination is offered year-round as a computer-based test (CBT) through Pearson's VUE testing centers. Once BCEN receives the application, applicants may schedule an appointment on Pearson's VUE website to sit for the examination. Immediate test results with score breakdown are available. Following successful completion of the examination, a certificate will be sent in the mail within 3 to 4 weeks.

Renewal of your TCRN certification can be achieved through continuing education (CE) or retaking the examination. The CE requirement is 100 hours. Of the 100 hours of CE, 50 must be from an accredited source and 75 must be within the clinical category. For more details on renewal, use the BCEN's website for recertification and understanding CE.

EXAMINATION REVIEW

This TCRN examination review is a blueprint for the examination content. Each major body system is divided into subheadings and topics.

Box I.2 TCRN Examination Review

Clinical Practice: Head and Neck	29	A. Neurologic trauma
		  1. Traumatic brain injuries
		  2. Spinal injuries
		B. Maxillofacial and neck trauma
		  1. Facial fractures
		  2. Ocular trauma
		  3. Neck trauma

Clinical Practice: Trunk	36	A. Thoracic trauma
		  1. Chest wall injuries
		  2. Pulmonary injuries
		B. Cardiac injuries
		  1. Great vessel injuries
		C. Abdominal trauma
		  1. Hollow organ injuries
		  2. Solid organ injuries
		  3. Diaphragmatic injuries
		  4. Retroperitoneal injuries

(continued)

Box I.2 TCRN Examination Review (*continued*)

		D. Genitourinary trauma
		E. Obstetrical trauma (pregnant patients)
Clinical Practice: Extremity and Wound	25	A. Musculoskeletal trauma
		1. Vertebral injuries
		2. Pelvic injuries
		3. Compartment syndrome
		4. Amputations
		5. Extremity fractures
		6. Soft-tissue injuries
		B. Surface and burn trauma
		1. Chemical burns
		2. Electrical burns
		3. Thermal burns
		4. Inhalation injuries
Clinical Practice: Special Considerations	22	A. Psychosocial issues related to trauma
		B. Shock
		1. Hypovolemic
		2. Obstructive (e.g., tamponade, tension, pneumothorax)
		3. Distributive (e.g., neurogenic, septic)
		4. Cardiogenic
		C. SIRS and MODS
Continuum of Care	21	A. Injury prevention
		B. Prehospital care
		C. Patient safety (e.g., fall prevention)
		D. Patient transfer
		1. Intrafacility (within a facility, across departments)
		2. Interfacility (from one facility to another)
		E. Forensic issues
		1. Evidence collection
		2. Chain of custody
		F. End-of-life issues
		1. Organ/tissue donation
		2. Advance directives
		3. Family presence
		4. Palliative care
		G. Rehabilitation (discharge planning)
Professional Issues	17	A. Trauma quality management
		1. Performance improvement
		2. Outcomes follow-up and feedback (e.g., referring facilities, EMS)
		3. Evidence-based practice
		4. Research
		5. Mortality/morbidity reviews
		B. Staff safety (e.g., standard precautions, workplace violence)
		C. Disaster management (i.e., preparedness, mitigation, response, and recovery)

(*continued*)

Box I.2 TCRN Examination Review (*continued*)

D. Critical incident stress management
E. Regulations and standards
    1. HIPAA
    2. EMTALA
    3. Designation/verification (e.g., trauma center/trauma systems)
F. Education and outreach for interprofessional trauma teams and the public
G. Trauma registry (e.g., data collection)
H. Ethical issues

EMS, emergency medical services; EMTALA, Emergency Medical Treatment and Active Labor Act; HIPAA, Health Insurance Portability and Accountability Act; MODS, multiple organ dysfunction syndrome; SIRS, systemic inflammatory response syndrome; TCRN, trauma certified registered nurse.

For clinical practice categories, the nursing process will be distributed as follows:

Assessment	18%
Analysis	31%
Implementation	31%
Evaluation	20%
Recall	21%
Application	61%
Analysis	18%

The following are testable nursing tasks on the examination:

I. Assessment
    A. Establish mechanism of injury
    B. Assess, intervene, and stabilize patients with immediate life-threatening conditions
    C. Assess pain
    D. Assess for adverse drug and blood reactions
    E. Obtain complete patient history
    F. Obtain a complete physical evaluation
    G. Use Glasgow Coma Scale (GCS) to evaluate patient status
    H. Assist with focused abdominal sonography for trauma (FAST) examination
    I. Calculate burn surface area
    J. Assessment not otherwise specified
II. Analysis
    A. Provide appropriate response to diagnostic test results
    B. Prepare equipment that might be needed by the team
    C. Identify the need for diagnostic tests
    D. Determine the plan of care
    E. Identify desired patient outcomes
    F. Determine the need to transfer to a higher level of care
    G. Determine the need for emotional or psychosocial support
    H. Analysis not otherwise specified

III. Implementation
    A. Incorporate age-specific needs for the patient population served
    B. Respond with decisiveness and clarity to unexpected events
    C. Demonstrate knowledge of pharmacology
    D. Assist with or perform the following procedures:
        1. Chest tube insertion
        2. Arterial line insertion
        3. Central line insertion
        4. Compartment syndrome monitoring devices:
           a. Abdominal
           b. Extremity
        5. Doppler
        6. End-tidal CO_2
        7. Temperature-control devices (e.g., warming and cooling)
        8. Pelvic stabilizer
        9. Immobilization devices
      10. Tourniquets
      11. Surgical airway insertion
      12. Intraosseous needles
      13. Intracranial pressure (ICP) monitoring devices
      14. Infusers:
           a. Autotransfusion
           b. Fluid
           c. Blood and blood products
      15. Needle decompression
      16. Fluid resuscitation:
           a. Burn fluid resuscitation
           b. Hypertonic solution
           c. Permissive hypotension
           d. Massive transfusion protocol (MTP)
      17. Pericardiocentesis
      18. Bedside open thoracotomy
    E. Manage patients who have had the following procedures:
        1. Chest tube insertion
        2. Arterial line insertion
        3. Central line insertion
        4. Compartment syndrome monitoring devices:
           a. Abdominal
           b. Extremity
        5. End-tidal CO_2
        6. Temperature control devices (e.g., warming and cooling)
        7. Pelvic stabilizer
        8. Immobilization devices
        9. Tourniquets
      10. Surgical airway
      11. Intraosseous needles
      12. ICP monitoring devices
      13. Infusers:
           a. Fluid
           b. Blood and blood products

       14. Needle decompression

       15. Fluid resuscitation:

          a. Burn fluid resuscitation

          b. Hypertonic solution

          c. Permissive hypotension

          d. MTP

       16. Pericardiocentesis

   F. Manage patients' pain relief by providing:

       1. Pharmacologic interventions

       2. Nonpharmacologic interventions

   G. Manage patient sedation and analgesia

   H. Manage tension pneumothorax

   I. Manage burn resuscitation

   J. Manage increased abdominal pressure

   K. Provide complex wound management (e.g., ostomies, drains, wound vacuum-assisted closure [VAC], open abdomen)

   L. Implementation not otherwise specified

IV. Evaluation

   A. Evaluate patients' response to interventions

   B. Monitor patient status and report findings to the team

   C. Adapt the plan of care as indicated

   D. Evaluation not otherwise specified

V. Continuum of care

   A. Monitor or evaluate for opportunities for program or system improvement

   B. Ensure proper placement of patients

   C. Restore patient to optimal health

   D. Collect, analyze, and use data:

       1. To improve patient outcomes

       2. For benchmarking

       3. To decrease incidence of trauma

   E. Coordinate the multidisciplinary plan of care

   F. Continuum of care not otherwise specified

VI. Professional issues

   A. Adhere to regulatory requirements related to:

       1. Infectious diseases

       2. Hazardous materials

       3. Verification/designation

       4. Confidentiality

   B. Follow standards of practice

   C. Involve family in:

       1. Patient care

       2. Teaching/discharging planning

   D. Recognize need for social/protective service consults

   E. Provide information to patient and family regarding community resources

   F. Address language and cultural barriers

   G. Participate in and promote lifelong learning related to new developments and clinical advances

H. Act as an advocate (e.g., for patients, families, and colleagues) related to ethical, legal, and psychosocial issues
I. Provide trauma patients and their families with psychosocial support
J. Assess methods continuously to improve patient outcomes
K. Assist in maintaining the performance improvement programs
L. Participate in multidisciplinary rounds
M. Professional issues not otherwise specified

PREPARATION

Be positive! Avoid any negative thoughts about passing the examination. These can result in a self-fulfilling prophecy. Set the test date and then establish a realistic schedule for preparing for the examination. Set your priorities: Study those areas you are less familiar with first. Look at the percentage devoted to each body system and establish timelines based on the percentage of questions pertaining to that topic. Know your best method of study—by yourself or in study groups—and follow that method. Flash cards, practice questions, review courses, study books in outline format, and study books in narrative format are available to assist you. Practice your test questions within a set time limit to familiarize yourself with the time limitations. Allow 2 minutes or less per question (remember, the rule is 50 questions per hour).

When using the practice test questions to study, determine several things when reviewing the answers and rationale. Analyze why you missed the question: Did you just not know the content? Go back and restudy the relevant section. Did you misread the question? Did you misread the answers? Did you miss an important element in the question or scenario? Was there a clue based on age, timeline, or symptoms you missed?

DAY OF THE TEST

Eat a healthy meal and limit the amount of liquids you drink (to avoid the need for breaks) before the examination. Remember, restroom breaks are allowed but the testing time does not stop!

Do not try to cram immediately before the test; this will increase your anxiety level. After the examination, make plans to do something special for yourself.

Know how to get to the testing site before the day of your scheduled exam. Plan your route and know how long it will take to get there at the time of day you are scheduled to take the examination. Running late and feeling hurried will increase your anxiety and can poorly affect your test-taking skills. Plus, if you are more than 15 minutes late, they will not let you in to take the examination.

Bring your letter of approval and two forms of identification (one picture ID). You cannot bring anything into the testing room, so leave everything in the car or at home (they will usually have a locker you can put personal items in during the examination).

If you need some assistance with computer-based testing, you are allowed to do a tutorial on the computer before you start your examination. The test time begins once you start the first question of the actual examination. Leaving the testing site without authorization results in an automatic voiding of the test. You will only be allowed 3 hours from the time the test is started.

Results of the examination will be presented onsite at the completion of your examination following a test evaluation.

TEST-TAKING SKILLS

Frequently, the difference between pass and fail depends on test-taking skills. An important reminder: Do not read into the question; take the question and information provided at face value. Answer all questions; do not leave any questions blank. A blank answer will be counted against you. Answering the question, even if it is an "educated" guess, will give you a one out of four chance of being correct.

Key words are important phrases or words used to focus attention on what the question is specifically asking. Examples include *always, earliest, first, on admission, best, least, immediately,* and *initial.*

> ▶ **HINT:** If the question asks for the "best" response, this is an indication that all answers are probably correct and you will have to determine the best answer for that particular scenario.

Eliminate incorrect options first. Sometimes you will immediately see an answer that is incorrect. Mark through it to narrow down your options and improve your odds. Frequently, you can narrow the choices down to two that are more correct than others.

> ▶ **HINT:** Eliminating incorrect options often gives a 50/50 chance for an educated guess of the correct answer.

Avoid those answers with words such as "always" or "never." There is rarely a time in the medical field that you will always or never do a particular action. If three of the four answers are similar, choose the answer that does not sound similar.

Do not change answers unless you are absolutely certain. You can "bookmark" a question that you are not sure about to return to it at the end of the test. Sometimes you will feel more comfortable with the question after you come back to it.

> ▶ **HINT:** First impressions are usually good! Do not take too much time on any one question.

Do not let it worry you if you do not know all the answers. Take a deep breath and keep going. Rejoice in those answers you know and find easy!

> ▶ **HINT:** You really are not supposed to know all the answers.

Do not try to establish patterns, such as using "two As in a row" for answers.

If there is a long scenario with large amounts of data, read the question first, then read the scenario, then reread the question. Sometimes erroneous data will be included that is not required to answer the question. Too much time may be spent trying to comprehend the whole scenario and trying to work through all of the information and data can be time consuming.

▶ **HINT:** Do not forget to reread the question to make sure you read it correctly the first time.

Read all answers before you make a choice; there may be more than one correct answer but one will be the better answer to the question.

▶ **HINT:** Do not answer the first one that appears to be correct. Choose the most correct answer.

Read the question carefully and answer only the question asked. Do not read into the question or think that you require more information/data to answer the question.

▶ **HINT:** The question will provide you with all the information needed to correctly answer it.

Time-frame questions are frequently used on the test. Use the time frame to assist with making the correct choice. Example: Which complication of subarachnoid hemorrhage is seen 7 to 10 days after the bleed?

▶ **HINT:** All answers may be correct but only one will occur more commonly during the time frame provided in the question.

Questions may be worded using the lead-in, "What is the gold standard?" This is not asking what is the most common routine, but which is the most reliable and accurate.

Scenarios: Read the patient's description word for word. Read the question, then formulate your answer. Read the answer options and choose the one closest to your answer. Reread the question after answering to ensure that you understood the question correctly.

▶ **HINT:** Once the question is answered, you are done. Move on to the next question. Do not second-guess yourself.

Look for answers that facilitate the patient. Facilitative words include *nurture, aid, support, reinforce, encourage,* and *assist.*

Part I

Clinical Practice: Head and Neck

Neurological Trauma

TRAUMATIC BRAIN INJURY

MECHANISM OF INJURY

■ *What is the most common blunt mechanism of injury that causes traumatic brain injury (TBI)?*

■ **Motor vehicle collision (MVC)**

An MVC is one of the most common mechanisms of injury that results in traumatic brain injury. The injury can range from mild to severe TBI. A fall is the most common mechanism of TBI in pediatric patients younger than the age of 12 years. Most adolescent TBI results from an MVC, sports injuries, and assault (Box 1.1).

> ▶ **HINT:** A major component of prevention of TBI in MVC is the proper use of seat belts and car seats.

Box 1.1 Common Causes of Blunt TBI

Motor vehicle collision
Motor pedestrian injury
Fall
Sports-related injury
War injuries
Domestic violence

TBI, traumatic brain injury.

■ *What is it called when a moving object impacts a stationary head?*

■ **Acceleration injury**

Blunt trauma to the head is described based on the mechanism of injury. The term *acceleration injury* indicates a moving object, such as a baseball bat, impacting the head. Deceleration injury is when the head is moving and strikes a stationary object, such as in MVC when the head hits the windshield.

> ▶ **HINT:** When you accelerate, you put something into motion. So, when an object hits one's head, it causes the head to accelerate, or move. This is an acceleration injury.

■ *What is it called when a brain injury occurs without any impact to the head itself?*

■ **Indirect injury**

An indirect injury occurs when the brain moves in the cranial vault following an acceleration–deceleration without the head impacting an object. A direct injury is an impact to the head, either through an acceleration, deceleration, or acceleration–deceleration mechanism.

> ▶ **HINT:** There are bony protrusions in the skull; when the brain moves against these rough edges it causes injury, even without a direct impact to the head.

■ *Following a gunshot to the head, the bullet is found within the cranial vault. What type of injury is this?*

■ **Penetrating injury**

Penetrating injury with a gunshot wound indicates that the bullet entered the cranial vault but did not exit it. The bullet remains in the skull. Perforating injury is when the bullet enters and exits the cranium. Penetrating injuries to the brain also include stab wounds through the cranium or penetrating stab wounds to the face, which can enter the cranium. Tangential injury occurs when the bullet glances off the skull; these types of injuries may have a lower mortality rate.

> ▶ **HINT:** In some penetrating injuries to the skull, the bullet is left in the cranium and not retrieved because it is located in an area of the eloquent brain. Retained bullet or skull fragments have not been found to significantly increase infection risk.

■ *Following an impact to the head, an injury to the brain occurs on the opposite side of the impact. What is this injury called?*

■ **Contre-coup injury**

A coup injury occurs at the area of impact and a contre-coup injury is brain injury that occurs on the opposite side of the impact. Coup–contre-coup injuries are commonly associated with epidural and subdural hematomas.

> ▶ **HINT:** The mechanism of injury that most commonly causes a coup–contre-coup injury is an impact to the lateral side of the skull.

■ *What type of injury results in diffuse axonal injury (DAI) to the brain?*

■ **Rotational injury**

Rotational injury, such as in vehicle rollover, can result in shearing of the brain tissue. This type of injury is called *diffuse axonal injury*. Presence of DAI indicates a poorer functional outcome of the TBI patient.

> ▶ **HINT:** Decreased level of consciousness that is out of proportion to CT scan findings is indicative of DAI.

■ *What type of injury causes chronic traumatic encephalopathy?*

■ **Repetitive injuries**

Repetitive TBIs that trigger progressive degeneration of brain tissue result in chronic traumatic encephalopathy (CTE). The injuries frequently are mild traumatic brain injuries (MTBI) related to contact sports injuries.

> ▶ **HINT:** CTE may also be found in veterans of war and victims of domestic violence.

■ **What patient population is most likely to present with a chronic subdural hematoma (SDH)?**

■ **Elderly**

Elderly patients are likely to present with chronic SDH. Other patient populations include alcoholics and dementia patients. Chronic SDHs tend to hemorrhage slowly. These patients have cortical atrophy, which allows for more blood volume to accumulate before an increase in intracranial pressure (ICP) occurs (Box 1.2).

> ▶ **HINT:** Chronic SDH patients are frequently misdiagnosed initially as suffering "old age" or stroke.

Box 1.2 Classifications of SDH

Acute SDH	Onset within 24 hours after injury
Subacute SDH	Onset within 24–48 hours after injury
Chronic SDH	Onset days to weeks after injury

SDH, subdural hematoma.

■ **Secondary injuries include cerebral edema. What is the cerebral edema caused by ischemic or hypoxic insult following a TBI called?**

■ **Cytotoxic edema**

Cytotoxic edema causes intracellular swelling and is a result of hypoxia or anoxic injuries. Vasogenic cerebral edema is a swelling or extra fluid in the interstitial space and is a result of trauma to the tissue. TBI will have a combination of both cytotoxic and vasogenic edema. Following a brain trauma, there is a loss of autoregulation in the areas of injury. Cerebral blood flow is shunted away from the uninjured areas of the brain to the areas of injury. This causes a "steal phenomenon" and results in hypoxia in uninjured areas of the brain.

> ▶ **HINT:** Mannitol is used to treat cerebral edema and pulls fluid from the interstitial space. It is most effective with managing vasogenic edema.

■ **What is the anatomical difference in pediatric patients that makes them more likely to experience a brain injury with a trauma?**

■ **The head is larger in proportion to the body**

The head of a child is larger in proportion to the rest of his or her body and the stability of the neck and ligaments is not fully developed. This makes the child susceptible to TBI in an MVC.

> ▶ **HINT:** Once the child is no longer in a car seat, the child typically places the shoulder harness behind him or her as it does not fit appropriately. This increases the likelihood of TBI.

■ *What is the triad of symptoms typically seen in shaken baby syndrome (SBS)?*

■ **Subdural hematoma, retinal hemorrhage, and cerebral edema**

SBS is a result of a violent shaking of the child. This is also called *abusive head trauma*. The head may or may not have contacted an object but the movement of the brain contents causes a shearing effect. The result is typically bilateral SDH and DAI. The injury is often fatal and can cause lifelong severe neurological disabilities.

> ▶ **HINT:** Retinal hemorrhages have a characteristic pattern for SBS and are used frequently to assist with the diagnosis of SBS (Box 1.3).

Box 1.3 Signs of TBI Caused by Child Abuse

Injuries that cannot be explained by the reported trauma
Associated long-bone fractures
Associated cervical injuries
Poor hygiene
Bruises at varying stages of healing
Multiple complex skull fractures with reported single-impact history

TBI, traumatic brain injury.

TRAUMATIC INJURIES

■ *What type of fracture is a displaced comminuted fracture of the skull?*

■ **Depressed skull fracture**

A depressed skull fracture is a comminuted fracture that is displaced into the meninges and brain tissue. This injury is commonly associated with epidural, subdural, and parenchymal hematomas. A linear skull fracture has a nondisplaced fracture line.

> ▶ **HINT:** The displacement of bony pieces into the meninges causes the tearing of meningeal vessels and the development of epidural and subdural hematomas.

■ *A patient develops cerebrospinal fluid (CSF) leak following a blow to the side of the head. What type of fracture does this patient have?*

■ **Basilar skull fracture**

Basilar skull fractures may result in CSF leaks from ears (otorrhea) or from the nose (rhinorrhea). The base of the skull is divided into the anterior, middle, and posterior skull base or fossa. Fractures may occur anywhere throughout the skull bases, but the anterior fossa is the most common area for basilar skull fractures.

> ▶ **HINT:** A blow to the side of the head causes the basilar skull to buckle, resulting in fracture lines along the basilar skull.

■ *What is an area of the brain parenchyma with hemorrhage following TBI called?*

■ **Contusion**

Contusions are areas of parenchymal hemorrhage that result from acceleration/decelera-tion and blunt impact. Contusions may initially appear as several areas of small hemor-rhages, but these can increase and combine into a larger hematoma. Approximately one third of the contusions will expand in 24 hours.

> ▶ **HINT:** Initial CT scan following TBI may not show the contusion. Frequently, follow-up CT scans in 24 hours are obtained to identify the contusion or deter-mine the increase in size of the contusion.

■ *Is an epidural hematoma (EDH) most commonly caused by laceration of an artery or of bridging veins?*

■ **Artery**

Laceration of an artery is the most common cause of EDH. The most common artery involved in EDH is the middle meningeal artery. Laceration of veins may also result in bleeding in the epidural space but is less common than arterial involvement. Tearing of bridging veins will hemorrhage into the subdural space (venous sinuses are located in sub-dural space) causing subdural hematoma.

> ▶ **HINT:** An EDH typically expands rapidly as a result of being an arterial hemor-rhage; SDH may be a slower hemorrhage because of its venous involvement.

■ *Tearing of pial veins will cause bleeding following a trauma. Where is the hemorrhage located?*

■ **Subarachnoid space**

Tearing of small pial veins cause bleeding into the subarachnoid space and is called *suba-rachnoid hemorrhage (SAH)*. SAH may also involve blood in the ventricles but isolated ven-tricular hemorrhage following trauma is unusual.

> ▶ **HINT:** SAH following trauma does not usually result in vasospasms as does SAH following aneurysm rupture.

■ *What are the two secondary injuries that have the greatest effect on neurological outcomes following TBI?*

■ **Hypotension and hypoxia**

Secondary injuries are those neurological injuries that occur to the brain after the initial trauma. It has been found that hypotension and hypoxia are the two most important deter-minants of neurological outcomes (Box 1.4).

> ▶ **HINT:** Priority of care for managing TBI patients is airway/breathing to improve oxygenation and resuscitation to reestablish perfusion to prevent fur-ther neurological injury.

[handwritten notes:]
EDH = artery
SDH = vein
Trauma SAH = vein
Aneurysm SAH = artery

Box 1.4 Secondary Injuries

Systemic Secondary Injuries	Intracranial Secondary Injuries
Hypotension	Increased ICP
Hypoxia	Cerebral edema
Anemia	Expanding mass lesions (hematomas)
Hypercapnia	Hydrocephalus
Hypocapnia	CNS infections
Hyperthermia	Seizures
Hyperglycemia	Brain ischemia
Electrolyte abnormalities	
Acid–base abnormalities	

CNS, central nervous system; ICP, intracranial pressure.

ASSESSMENT/DIAGNOSIS

■ *A patient develops bilateral periorbital ecchymosis following traumatic injury to the head. What is the cause of the ecchymosis?*

■ **Basilar skull fracture**

Patients with basilar skull fracture may develop periorbital ecchymosis (raccoon eyes) and bruising on the mastoid process called *Battle's sign.*

▶ **HINT:** Raccoon eyes and Battle's sign may not appear immediately following a trauma and typically develop later following injury.

■ *What is the best method to test drainage from the nose for the presence of CSF?*

■ **Halo test**

The halo test is used to determine the presence of CSF in drainage from the nose (rhinorrhea) or from the ears (otorrhea). To perform a halo test, dab the drainage onto gauze and look for a yellow ring surrounding the drainage. This is a positive halo and indicates presence of CSF.

▶ **HINT:** The halo test is more reliable than testing the drainage for glucose because drainage may contain blood, which also has glucose. A glucose test for CSF has more false positives.

■ *What lab test may be used to improve the accuracy of the diagnosis for CSF in drainage?*

■ **Beta-2 transferrin**

A halo ring test can cause false positives so the gold standard (most diagnostic) is the lab testing of the drainage for CSF. Beta-2 transferrin is a variant of transferrin and is used as an endogenous marker for CSF in other bodily fluids.

▶ **HINT:** Beta-2 transferrin has been called *CSF-specific transferrin* because it is highly specific for CSF.

■ *What diagnostic study is considered the gold standard for identifying skull-base fractures?*

■ **CT scan**

High-resolution CT scan of the head is considered the gold standard to identify skull-base fractures. Differentiation between suture lines and fracture is required to assure an accurate diagnosis.

> ▶ **HINT:** Clinical findings may be used to assist with diagnosis of basilar skull fracture if unable to visualize fracture on head CT scan.

■ *Diagnostic CT scan of the brain found air present in the cranium and basilar skull fracture. What is the air in the cranium called?*

■ **Pneumocephalus**

Pneumocephalus is a complication of basilar skull fracture and may be identified on brain CT scan. Air enters through the fracture into the cranium. Management of pneumocephlaus may be with oxygen administration.

> ▶ **HINT:** Pneumocephalus can become a tension pneumocephalus with a resulting elevation of ICP.

■ *An MTBI may be defined by the Glasgow Coma Scale (GSC). What GCS would indicate minor brain injury?*

■ **GCS 13 to 15**

MTBI (used to be called a *concussion*) is often classified as a GCS between 13 and 15 (Box 1.5). The patient does not have to experience a loss of consciousness to have a traumatic brain injury. MTBI can be graded on severity (Box 1.6).

Box 1.5 Diagnosis of MTBI

GCS between 13 and 15
Temporary loss of consciousness
Posttraumatic amnesia for less than 24 hours
Transient neurological abnormalities
Transient confusion

GCS, Glasgow Coma Scale; MTBI, mild traumatic brain injury.

> ▶ **HINT:** To be diagnosed as MTBI, neurological abnormalities must not be the result of alcohol, drugs, or caused by other injuries.

Box 1.6 GCS Classification Severity TBI

GCS 13 to 15	Mild traumatic brain injury
GCS 9 to 12	Moderate traumatic brain injury
GCS 3 to 8	Severe traumatic brain injury

GCS, Glasgow Coma Scale; TBI, traumatic brain injury.

> ▶ **HINT:** Limitations of using the GCS to determine the severity of neurological injury is in intubated and aphasic patients.

■ *A patient presents with an altered level of consciousness following a head trauma. What is the best diagnostic procedure used to identify skull and brain injuries initially?*

■ **Noncontrast CT scan**

Noncontrast CT scan is useful in the immediate posttraumatic period to identify intracranial pathology that would indicate the need for immediate surgical management. Noncontrast CT scan is used to identify skull fractures, hematomas, contusions, mass effects, presence of foreign objects, and the presence of cerebral edema (Box 1.7).

> ▶ **HINT:** Pediatric patients with a GCS greater than 15 may be candidates for a noncontrast CT scan.

Box 1.7 Indications for Noncontrast CT Scan TBI

Suspect loss of consciousness or posttraumatic amnesia if one of the following is present: Vomiting, age older than 60 years, headache, drug or alcohol intoxication, deficits in short-term memory, GCS < 15, focal neurological deficit
Signs of basilar skull fracture
Posttraumatic seizures
Presence of coagulopathy
Dangerous mechanism of injury (i.e., ejection from vehicle)

GCS, Glasgow Coma Scale; TBI, traumatic brain injury.

■ *What is the most sensitive indicator of an increased ICP?*

■ **Change in the level of consciousness (LOC)**

A change in LOC is a sensitive indicator for neurological deterioration and an increase in ICP. When performing neurological assessments, it is very important to assess for LOC (Box 1.8).

> ▶ **HINT:** A change in LOC can include both a change in alertness and a change in orientation.

Box 1.8 Symptoms of Neurological Deterioration

Decreased level of alertness
Development of confusion or disorientation
Unequal pupils and change in pupillary response
Dilated pupil(s) or constricted pupils
Vision changes
Vomiting
Seizures
Worsening headache
Changes in respiratory patterns
Cushing's triad

> ▶ **HINT:** Cushing's triad (increased systolic pressure, widened pulse pressure, and bradycardia) are signs of impending herniation but are late signs of an increased ICP.

■ *What is the most commonly used diagnosis of DAI?*

■ **Clinical diagnosis**

Clinical diagnosis reveals a poor neurological status and a decreased level of consciousness that are out of proportion with the injury observed on CT scan. DAI involves microscopic injuries, therefore is not seen as large changes on diagnostic studies such as a CT scan. CT imaging may demonstrate small punctate foci of hemorrhage but this is not found in all cases of DAI.

> ▶ **HINT:** It may be several days before the diagnosis of DAI is made because of the delay in CT presentation of contusions.

■ *A patient presents to the emergency room following a fall off a ladder. The family reports some altered loss of consciousness after the fall. What should be included in the nurse's admission history?*

■ **Duration and severity of altered LOC**

A reported altered LOC requires more information from those who observed the injury. This includes the duration of the altered mentation, degree of altered LOC, other neurological symptoms experienced, and mechanism of injury.

> ▶ **HINT:** The observer of the traumatic event is a better historian than the person who experienced altered LOC. Patients typically cannot recall the event, deny the loss of consciousness, or are not really aware of how long they were unconscious.

■ *What question may the trauma nurse use to evaluate the presence of retrograde amnesia following a TBI ?*

■ **"What was the last event before your injury that you remember?"**

Retrograde amnesia is the loss of memory before the traumatic event. It is commonly determined by asking the patient about the last thing he or she remembers before the traumatic event. Posttraumatic amnesia is the loss of memory from the time of unconsciousness until the first memory after the event. Antegrade amnesia is the inability to create new memory after the event. An example of antegrade amnesia is when a person is unable to remember anything that happened the rest of the day despite being conscious.

> ▶ **HINT:** "What is the first thing you remember after the event?" is a question used to evaluate posttraumatic amnesia.

■ *A rapidly expanding EDH following a severe TBI can result in an uncal herniation. Which pupil will dilate following uncal herniation?*

■ **Ipsilateral**

Uncal herniation is a lateral displacement and herniation of brain tissue caused by a unilateral expanding mass. The pupil affected by the herniation is the ipsilateral pupil. It will dilate and become nonreactive. SDH may also be a rapidly expanding mass and can cause uncal herniation with dilated ipsilateral pupil.

> ▶ **HINT:** Dilated pupil is caused by the injury or stretch of cranial nerve (CN) III (oculomotor). CNs do not cross (except CN IV), so symptoms are ipsilateral.

■ *Which of the hematomas following TBI has the classic presentation of a lucid period?*

■ **EDH**

EDH has a classic presentation of a period of lucidity. The patient may have been unconscious initially, experiences a period of being awake, then loses consciousness again.

▶ **HINT:** Not all EDHs experience this classical presentation but of all the hematomas, EDH is the one that is most likely to.

■ *What complication of abdominal trauma can increase ICP and worsen neurological outcomes?*

■ **Abdominal compartment syndrome (ACS)**

ACS is a complication of abdominal trauma. It causes an increase in abdominal pressure that results in a decrease in venous drainage from the brain. This elevates the intracerebral blood volume and ICP. Increased pressure in the thoracic cavity can have the same effect as ACS. Multisystem trauma patients with combination abdominal or thoracic trauma with brain injury should be assessed for the presence of ACS; treatment should be initiated to lower abdominal and thoracic pressures.

▶ **HINT:** ACS can be measured and monitored with bladder pressure readings.

■ *What is a commonly used assessment tool to measure the deficit in cognitive functioning following a TBI?*

■ **Ranchos Los Amigos Scale**

The Ranchos Los Amigos Scale is used to measure a deficit in cognitive function. The tool is frequently used to determine the patient's level of cognitive functioning for rehabilitation capabilities and prognosis following TBI. The scale is divided into eight stages (or 10 stages in the revised version) ranging from appropriate to coma.

▶ **HINT:** Level VI on the revised score is the point at which the patient requires moderate assistance (versus maximal assistance) and is the point that benefits greatly from rehabilitation.

MEDICAL/SURGICAL INTERVENTIONS

■ *What is the primary management of a depressed skull fracture?*

■ **Surgical debridement**

Following a depressed skull fracture, surgical debridement is used to remove the bony pieces that cause damage to the meninges and brain tissue. This is followed later by cranioplasty to replace the portion of the debrided skull.

▶ **HINT:** The use of cranioplasty to repair the skull defect also serves a cosmetic purpose.

■ *What is the prehospital and emergency room priority of care for severe traumatic brain injured patients?*

■ **To check airway and breathing**

Hypoxia and hypotension are secondary injuries that will worsen neurological outcomes. The prehospital goals are to initiate treatment to prevent secondary injuries. This includes obtaining and maintaining airway and breathing to prevent hypoxia and initiating fluid resuscitation to prevent hypotension and hypoperfusion. Care should also be taken to secure the cervical spine as cervical spine injuries are commonly associated with head trauma.

> ▶ HINT: Intubation is considered in patients with GCS of less than or equal to 8.

■ *What are the mean arterial pressure (MAP) and the PaO$_2$ goals for TBI?*

■ **MAP and PaO$_2$ greater than 80 mmHg**

Systemic hypoxia is an independent predictor of increased morbidity and mortality. A single episode of hypotension (blood pressure less than 90 mmHg) is associated with worsening outcomes. Maintaining an MAP greater than 80 mmHg in severe traumatic brain-injured patients (GCS less than 8) will improve brain perfusion. If GCS is more than 8, then MAP is maintained greater than 70 mmHg. Oxygenation goal is to maintain PaO$_2$ between 80 and 120 mmHg and arterial saturation greater than 92% to prevent secondary hypoxic injuries.

> ▶ HINT: Goal in managing severe TBI is to optimize cerebral blood flow while minimizing cerebral edema and ICP.

■ *An ICP monitor was placed in the trauma intensive care unit (ICU) to monitor a patient with severe traumatic brain injury. What should be the goal for the cerebral perfusion pressure (CPP)?*

■ **Maintain pressure greater than 60 mmHg**

CPP is a measurement used at the bedside to estimate cerebral blood flow (CBF). The CPP is calculated when the patient has an ICP monitor and the goal is to maintain greater than 60 mmHg to improve CBF (Box 1.9). The ICP should be maintained at less than 20 mmHg. If CPP is less than 60 mmHg following adequate fluid resuscitation, a vasoconstrictor may be administered to increase MAP. CPP more than 70 mmHg is not recommended because of the risk of volume overload and acute respiratory distress syndrome (ARDS).

> ▶ HINT: To improve CPP, increase MAP and reduce the ICP. The focus of interventions is on both sides: the driving force (MAP) and the opposing force (ICP) (Box 1.10).

Box 1.9 Calculation of CPP

MAP – ICP = CPP

CPP, cerebral perfusion pressure; ICP, intracranial pressure; MAP, mean arterial pressure.

Box 1.10 Indications for ICP Monitor

GCS < 8
Abnormal brain CT scan includes:
   Hemorrhage
   Contusions
   Swelling
   Herniation
   Compressed basal cisterns
Normal brain CT scan and two or more of the following:
   Age older than 40 years
   Unilateral or bilateral motor posturing
   Systemic hypotension
Patient will not be examined for a prolonged period of time

GCS, Glasgow Coma Scale; ICP, intracranial pressure.

> ▶ **HINT:** Infants and young children may tolerate increased pressure better because of open sutures and fontanelles, but they can still experience increased ICP and may require ICP monitoring similar to adults.

■ *What is the osmotic diuretic used to treat cerebral edema and lower ICP?*

■ **Mannitol**

Mannitol is an osmotic diuretic that is used to increase serum osmolality, creating a pull of fluid from the extravascular to intravascular space. This lowers cerebral edema and ICP. While administering mannitol, care should be taken to avoid hypovolemia (because of the diuresis) and hypotension. Fluid resuscitation may be required to prevent hypovolemia. Serum osmolality and sodium levels need to be obtained at least every 6 hours with hyperosmolar therapy.

> ▶ **HINT:** Hold administration of mannitol if serum osmolality is greater than 320 mOsm/L.

■ *What is the potential adverse effect of administering hypertonic saline to lower cerebral edema?*

■ **Central pontine myelinolysis (CPM)**

Hypertonic saline (3%, 7.5%, 23%) may also be used to increase serum osmolality instead of mannitol (Box 1.11). The highest risk for causing CPM is in hyponatremic patients. If the patient has a normal serum Na^+ (sodium) level, the chance of causing CPM when using 3% saline in appropriate dosages is rare. Monitor serum Na^+ levels while administering hypertonic saline and hold if Na^+ levels are greater than 160 mEq/L (Box 1.12).

> ▶ **HINT:** Avoid administering hypertonic saline in patients who are hyponatremic. Mannitol would be the better answer in that situation.

Box 1.11 Hyperosmolar Therapy

3% Saline	100 mL intravenous every 2 hours as needed
Mannitol	0.25–1 g/kg intravenous every 6 hours

Box 1.12 Adverse Effects of Hyperosmolar Therapy

Mannitol	Hypertonic Saline
Rebound phenomenon	Rebound phenomenon
Hyperosmolar state	Central pontine myelinolysis
Dehydration	Hypernatremia
Acute renal failure	Worsening pulmonary edema

■ *Sustained hyperventilation with hypocarbia and respiratory alkalosis can cause what harmful effects in a traumatic brain-injured patient?*

■ **Reduced CBF**

PaCO$_2$ is a potent cerebral vasodilator. If the PaCO$_2$ is decreased because hyperventilation and hypocarbia occur, this causes cerebral vasoconstriction, reduced CBF, and a decrease in ICP. Sustained or aggressive hyperventilation is not recommended because of its effect on CBF, even though it can lower ICP. The PaCO$_2$ goal is 35 to 45 mmHg (maintaining on the lower side of normal if ICP is elevated).

> ▶ **HINT:** When a patient suddenly loses consciousness because of a rapidly elevating ICP, the trauma nurse may hyperventilate for a short period to lower the ICP until definitive management of the patient can occur.

■ *A patient is admitted to the ICU after craniotomy to remove acute SDH. The bone is left out and will be replaced at a later date. What is this called?*

■ **Bone flap**

A bone flap is removed during the craniotomy and not replaced to allow for more room for the brain to swell. This is called *decompressive surgery*. Patients still can herniate through the bone flap, causing strangulation of brain tissue, and will still need to be treated for an increase in ICP. A hemicraniectomy may also be performed to allow a greater amount of decompression.

> ▶ **HINT:** The trauma nurse should assesses the bone flap for tension or any bulging, indicating an increase in ICP.

■ *What is the temperature goal when caring for a severe TBI patient?*

■ **Between 36°C and 37°C**

Elevated body temperatures have adverse effects on TBI patients and normothermia should be maintained. Even though non-brain-injured patients' fever is allowed to increase body temperatures to the range of 38.3°C to 38.5°C, the brain may begin to experience injury at a temperature greater than 37°C. Fever increases brain metabolism, elevates levels of proinflammatory cytokines, and may increase ICP. Hypothermia has also been found to worsen outcomes in traumatic brain-injured patients and should be avoided unless there is refractory elevated ICP.

> ▶ **HINT:** Remember neurological patients are also at risk for central neurogenic fever and can elevate body temperatures rapidly and severely.

■ *Which type of IV fluid is most commonly used to maintain fluid volume in a TBI patient?*

■ **Normal saline (NS)**

NS is an isotonic crystalloid commonly used to resuscitate and maintain fluid volume in a TBI patient. NS may also be used initially to correct hyponatremia (Na^+ less than 140 mEq/L).

▶ **HINT:** Avoid dextrose in the intravenous (IV) fluids because hyperglycemia is considered a secondary injury and can worsen neurological outcomes.

■ *Sedation and analgesia may be provided to control agitation and pain following TBI. What adverse effect should be monitored closely to prevent secondary brain injuries?*

■ **Hypotension**

Analgesia and sedation can lower the ICP and facilitate mechanical ventilation but may cause vasodilation with hypotension and decreased CBF. Hypotension is a secondary injury that may worsen neurological outcomes. Close monitoring of blood pressure (BP) is required when administering analgesics and sedatives. Analgesia and sedation may also affect respiratory functions and should be used cautiously to prevent respiratory depression and hypoxia, unless mechanically ventilated.

▶ **HINT:** Sedation also involves the potential loss of an accurate neurological assessment.

■ *How long should the seizure prophylaxis be continued following a severe TBI?*

■ **For 7 days**

Seizure prophylaxis is recommended for 7 days following a severe TBI. If the patient has not had a seizure within 7 days following the trauma, the antiepileptic drug may be discontinued. Seizure prophylaxis is not recommended in mild to moderate traumatic brain-injured patients.

▶ **HINT:** Continuous electroencephalogram (EEG) monitoring may be used to identify nonconvulsive seizures in TBI patients not waking up following the trauma.

■ *When would a barbiturate coma be considered following a severe TBI?*

■ **When there is persistent elevation in ICP**

Inducing a barbiturate coma is not the first-line treatment to manage an increased ICP, but may be used if the ICP is refractory despite tier-one interventions (i.e., osmolar therapy) (Box 1.13). Continuous EEG monitoring is frequently used to titrate the barbiturate therapy by burst suppression.

▶ **HINT:** Monitor hemodynamics of a patient in a barbiturate coma because of the adverse effect of myocardial depression.

Box 1.13 Potential Treatments for Refractory Increased ICP

Barbiturate coma
Decompressive craniotomy
Mild hyperventilation ($PaCO_2$ 30–34 mmHg)
Mild hypothermia (33°C–35°C)
Neuromuscular blocking agents

ICP, intracranial pressure.

▶ **HINT:** Corticosteroids are not recommended in managing cerebral edema or increased ICP in TBI patients.

NURSING INTERVENTIONS

■ *A gastric tube is required in a patient with TBI. What type of gastric tube should be placed?*

■ **Orogastric tube (OGT)**

An OGT is the preferred gastric tube in patients with TBI with a potential risk of having basilar skull fracture. Nasogastric tube placement can result in the tube entering the brain through the cribriform fracture in basilar skull fractures. The cribriform plate is located in the anterior fossa or skull base.

▶ **HINT:** Never place any nasal tube following facial or head injury because of the risk of brain cannulation.

■ *Where is the gauze placed in patients with rhinorrhea?*

■ **Taped under the nose**

Frequently, gauze is taped under the nose to absorb the drainage. This allows for the estimation of the amount of drainage or CSF leak that is occurring.

▶ **HINT:** Never pack the nose with gauze in patients with rhinorrhea. This can increase the risk of meningitis.

■ *Following a basilar skull fracture with a known CSF leak, at what level should the head of the bed (HOB) be placed?*

■ **Greater than 30 degrees**

The HOB should be elevated greater than 30 degrees in patients with a known CSF leak. Conservative treatment is usually recommended for basilar fractures and CSF leaks, which include strict bed rest; elevated HOB; no coughing, sneezing, and straining. Antibiotic prophylaxis is not recommended following a basilar skull fracture and CSF leak.

▶ **HINT:** Instruct the patient with a CSF leak not to forcefully blow his or her nose.

■ *A patient is being discharged home from the emergency department following an MTBI while playing football. What is the most appropriate recommendation on when the patient can return to playing football?*

■ **Once the patient is symptom-free**

Current guidelines recommend a graduated increase in the level of activity for the athlete progressing from the initial stage of "light exercise" toward "full contact" activity, once the athlete is completely symptom-free at rest. This is to prevent a secondary impact syndrome, which can result in death and repetitive injuries.

▶ **HINT:** Second-impact syndrome can occur with a second impact within hours to weeks of the initial TBI.

■ *A patient with a TBI should be placed in what position to lower the ICP?*
■ **Elevate the HOB**

Elevating the HOB by 30 degrees facilitates venous drainage, lowers blood volume in the cranium, thereby lowering the ICP. Laying the HOB flat will increase an ICP. Also maintain the neck in a neutral position to avoid jugular vein constriction.

> ▶ **HINT:** Maintain an elevated HOB in TBI patients unless contraindicated by other injuries.

■ *A severe traumatic brain-injured patient in the ICU develops a temperature of 39°C. What nursing intervention should be performed to lower the body temperature?*
■ **Apply a cooling blanket**

Elevated body temperatures should be managed quickly in brain-injured patients to prevent secondary brain injury. Applying a cooling blanket to lower the body temperature is a nursing intervention that may be used. Other methods to lower the body temperature may include administering antipyretic medications, controlling of room temperature, and intravascular cooling (Box 1.14). The goal is to maintain a normothermic body temperature.

> ▶ **HINT:** Shivering can also increase metabolism and should be treated if it occurs during cooling of the patient.

Box 1.14 Other Interventions for TBI Patient

Appropriate and early nutrition
Venous thrombosis prophylaxis
Stress ulcer prophylaxis
Early mobility
Prevent infections
Treat hyperglycemia (> 180 mg/dL)
Prevent skin breakdown

TBI, traumatic brain injury.

COMPLICATIONS

■ *Following a depressed skull fracture, the patient develops fever and elevated white blood cell (WBC) counts. What would be the potential complication of the depressed skull fracture?*
■ **Meningitis**

CNS infections, such as meningitis, are potential complications following a depressed and basilar skull fracture.

> ▶ **HINT:** Signs of an infection are elevated fever and WBC count; meningitis is the infection associated with depressed skull fracture.

■ *Which CN may be injured by a basilar skull fracture if patient presents with asymmetrical facial expressions?*

■ **Facial (CN VII)**

CN injuries can be associated with basilar skull fractures. CN I (olfactory or sense of smell) can be affected if the cribriform plate is fractured. CN II (optic) injury can result in unilateral blindness and dilated pupil. The facial nerve (CN VII) is more commonly damaged with middle fossa and temporal bone injury.

▶ **HINT:** CN injuries can occur with skull fractures and facial fractures.

■ *A head CT scan of a trauma patient finds intracerebral hemorrhage. What medication therapy would the trauma nurse suspect the patient to be taking?*

■ **Anticoagulation or antiplatelet therapy**

Anticoagulation and antiplatelet therapy are the common therapies that result in intracerebral hemorrhage and may occur following any trauma. Reversal of the bleeding complications is considered a priority and may include administering a reversal agent if there is an antidote for the medication. Correct the coagulopathy with prothrombin complex concentrates (PCC) in life-threatening bleeds. Other blood products may include fresh frozen plasma (FFP) and cryoprecipitate.

▶ **HINT:** If the patient was on antiplatelet therapy, administer platelets.

■ *Repetitive MTBIs in contact sports can result in what complication?*

■ **Chronic traumatic encephalopathy (CTE)**

CTE is a complication of repetitive brain trauma frequently seen with players of contact sports (Box 1.15). This used to be called *punch drunk* in boxing. These repetitive injuries result in deposit of tau proteins in the cortex resulting in degeneration and atrophy of the brain similar to that seen in cortical dementia.

▶ **HINT:** The pathophysiology of CTE is similar to Alzheimer's disorder and Parkinson's disease, but this is a preventable dementia.

Box 1.15 Symptoms of CTE

Memory loss
Depression
Suicidal thoughts and suicide
Aggressive behavior
Tremors
Ataxia (gait abnormality)
Slowed movements
Speech abnormalities
Confusion

CTE, chronic traumatic encephalopathy.

■ *A patient presents to the clinic with frequent headaches and states he had a concussion about 2 months ago. What is the cause of the headaches?*

■ **Posttraumatic headaches**

Posttraumatic headaches develop in about 30% to 40% of patients following MTBI. The headaches may increase during periods of stress, tension, or activity (Box 1.16).

> ▶ **HINT:** Management of posttraumatic headache is similar to benign headaches and includes abortive treatments with triptans.

Box 1.16 Complications of MTBI

Headaches
Posttraumatic stress disorder
Fatigue, exhaustion
Sleep disturbances
Posture and balance issues
Memory problems
Seizures

MTBI, mild traumatic brain injury.

■ *What is the brain's ability to reorganize neural pathways called?*

■ **Plasticity**

Plasticity is the ability of the brain's neural pathways to reorganize based on stimulation, new experiences, and new learning. Pediatric brains have greatest plasticity but adult brains can reorganize neural pathways to learn and improve one's recovery. Engaging in activities helps the brain develop new pathways.

> ▶ **HINT:** The brain is most susceptible to plasticity early after a trauma, so rehabilitation begins on admission.

■ *How many months following the TBI does the neurological improvement begin to slow down?*

■ **At about 6 months**

The greatest improvements following TBI occur within the first 6 months then begin to slow down with minimal improvement after 1 year.

> ▶ **HINT:** Inform the family that it may take up to 1 year after the injury to have an understanding of the degree of physical recovery achieved; however, psychological recovery may take even longer.

SPINAL CORD INJURY

MECHANISM OF INJURY

■ *A hyperflexion injury may result in rupture of which ligament?*

■ **Posterior longitudinal ligament**

Hyperflexion injury occurs when the spine is flexed beyond the normal range of motion. An example is a head-on MVC. The head continues forward with sufficient speed and force for the chin to touch the chest. The stretch occurs posteriorly, causing the rupture, or tearing, of the posterior ligaments. The anterior vertebral body may be involved in a compression or wedge fracture. This injury may result in subluxation and/or disk herniation. A pediatric patient is at high risk for this mechanism of injury because of the laxity of longitudinal ligaments.

> ▶ **HINT:** A "lipstick sign" is when the trauma victim has lipstick on her shirt, which can indicate a hyperflexion injury.

■ *A patient is diagnosed with cervical injury following a rear-end MVC. What is the most likely mechanism for the spinal injury?*

■ **Hyperextension**

Hyperextension injuries occur when the spine is moved into an extreme hyperextension position. The stretch of the spine is now occurring anteriorly, so the anterior longitudinal ligament would be the most likely ligament to be injured. The posterior vertebral body is at highest risk for fractures. Subluxation and herniated disks may also occur with this mechanism of injury. Extreme hyperextension can cause compression injury from the ligamentum flavum, resulting in cord contusion and hypoxia.

> ▶ **HINT:** Whiplash is commonly caused by hyperextension mechanism of injury.

■ *Axial loading or vertical compression mechanisms result in what type of vertebral fracture?*

■ **Burst fractures**

Axial loading is force applied vertically through the spine, causing increased pressure and vertebral burst fractures. Bone and disk matter are sent in all directions, including into the spinal canal, causing cord injury. This is commonly seen with diving injuries.

> ▶ **HINT:** Burst fractures are considered unstable even with intact ligaments because of the risk of bony pieces impinging on or penetrating the spinal cord.

■ *Side impact MVC can result in which type of mechanism of injury to the spinal column?*

■ **Rotational**

Rotational injuries occur with a twisting motion of the spine. Lateral flexion of the spine, along with axial rotation, is the mechanism for injury that causes rupture of posterior longitudinal ligament, dislocation of facets, and vertebral compression fractures.

▶ **HINT:** The most common cause for rotational injury is side-impact MVC with unrestrained occupant.

■ *What type of trauma is most likely to result in a distraction injury to the cervical spine?*

■ **Hangings**

Distraction injuries occur when the spine comes to a sudden stop while weight and momentum of body continue to pull, causing tearing and laceration of the spinal cord.

▶ **HINT:** Another trauma that has been associated with distraction mechanism of injury is bungee-cord jumping.

■ *Following a gunshot wound, the bullet is found to travel near the spinal cord but did not transverse through the cord. The injury to the spinal cord would be caused by what mechanism?*

■ **Concussion**

Concussive forces from the velocity of the bullet can cause injury to tissue without direct contact with the tissue. Penetrating cord injuries are caused by gunshot wounds and stab wounds. Gunshot injuries can penetrate the spinal cord and may be of high or low velocity. Low-velocity injuries may not be associated with bony fractures.

▶ **HINT:** Avoid MRI if bullet fragments are present within the spinal cord or cord canal because of the effects of the magnet.

■ *Trauma to the spinal column resulting in burst fractures may cause cord injury through which mechanism?*

■ **Direct compression**

Primary injuries are those that occur as a result of the initial traumatic injury. This includes tissue destruction (lacerations, avulsions), compression (bony fragments, hematomas), and ischemia (damage or impingement of spinal arteries). Spinal cord injuries can occur without radiographic evidence of vertebral fractures or dislocations. Secondary injuries are those injuries to the spinal cord that result in further injury and neurological deficits after the initial trauma (Box 1.17).

▶ **HINT:** Level of function may be one or two levels above the level of injury as a result of secondary injuries that worsen neurological function.

Box 1.17 Secondary Injuries to Spinal Cord

Ischemia/hypoperfusion
Vasogenic edema
Release oxygen free radicals
Acid–base imbalances
Inflammation
Hemorrhage/hematomas
Obstruction CSF flow

CSF, cerebrospinal fluid.

TRAUMATIC INJURIES

■ *Which of the types of odontoid fractures is considered to be a stable fracture?*

■ **Type I**

Odontoid (also called *the dens*) is the bony structure of C2 that comes up anteriorly into the ring of C1 and allows for rotational movement of the neck. Fractures of the odontoid are classified into types I, II, and III, based on where the fracture occurred on the odontoid bone (Box 1.18). This is also used to describe stability and guides the treatment of the fracture. Type I is considered the most stable of the odontoid fractures. Instability of odontoid fractures is caused either from cord compression or penetration of bony fragment or ligament disruption between the odontoid process and the anterior aspect of C1.

> ▶ **HINT:** Type II odontoid fractures are the most common and are considered the most unstable of the odontoid fractures.

Box 1.18 Types of Odontoid Fractures

Type I	Tip of odontoid bone above transverse ligament
Type II	Base of odontoid between transverse ligament and body of axis
Type III	Bone extend into the vertebral body

> ▶ **HINT:** Another less common odontoid fracture is the vertical fracture through the odontoid and axis body.

■ *What is the bilateral fracture of the ring of C2 with or without subluxation called?*

■ **Hangman's fracture**

Hangman's fracture (also called *traumatic spondylolisthesis*) is the bilateral fracture through the neural arch of C2. This injury may or may not be associated with anterior subluxation. Even though it is called Hangman's fracture, it is less likely to be seen with hangings. It is most commonly associated with falls and MVCs. Hanging typically causes fracture-dislocation of C2 and complete disruption of ligaments between C2 and C3. The burst fracture of the ring of C1 is called *Jefferson's fracture*.

> ▶ **HINT:** Often associated with other spine pathologies, including osteoarthritis, and may be seen in elderly patients.

■ *Which type of cervical injury commonly results in death at the scene of an MVC?*

■ **Atlanto–occipital dislocation**

Atlanto dislocation (also called *internal decapitation*) is the avulsion of the atlas (C1) from the occiput and is usually fatal or results in prehospital cardiopulmonary arrest. The severe disruption of ligaments allows the cranium to move out of alignment of the spine. There are cases of patients presenting without neurological injury who commonly complain of the sensation that their "head is falling off."

> ▶ **HINT:** Atlanto–occipital dislocation is more common in the pediatric population than in adults.

■ *What is the instability between C1 and C2 that results in excessive movement between these two joints called?*

■ **Atlantoaxial instability**

Atlas (C1) and axis (C2) instability may result from a cervical trauma and commonly involves injury to the transverse ligament or odontoid process. Injury severity varies from subluxation to dislocation.

> ▶ **HINT:** Congenital disorders may increase the risk of atlantoaxial instability as a result of ligament laxity. Down syndrome is an example.

■ *A patient presents with a total loss of motor and sensory function below the level of injury. What is this type of injury called?*

■ **Complete cord injury**

There is some degree of correlation between the level of function and level of radiographic injury, but this is not always consistent. The neurological level of injury (NLI) is the most caudal spinal cord level at which the normal motor/sensory function persists following spinal cord injury.

> ▶ **HINT:** An incomplete cord injury may initially appear functionally as a complete cord due to inflammation and edema in the cord.

■ *A football player presents with motor impairment greater in the upper extremities than the lower extremities following a traumatic injury. What is this incomplete injury called?*

■ **Central cord syndrome**

This spinal cord injury occurs in the central portion of the cord and is characterized by greater involvement of the upper extremity than the lower, especially the hands. The upper extremity axons are located in the central portion of the spinal cord and the axons that control the lower extremity movement are located laterally in the cord. This incomplete cord syndrome is frequently caused by a hyperextension injury or a fall. There is often a gradual return to function with the lower extremities returning first, followed by the upper, and finger movement returns last with the hand being the most common site of residual motor weakness. Urinary retention and sensory abnormalities vary with the severity of injury.

> ▶ **HINT:** Key to recognizing this syndrome is weakness in the upper extremities with less weakness in the lower extremities.

■ *What is typically spared in a patient with an anterior cord syndrome following a traumatic injury?*

■ **Vibratory sensation and proprioception**

Anterior cord syndrome is characterized by immediate onset of complete motor paralysis and loss of pain and temperature with preservation of posterior column of sensation (includes vibration sense, position sense, deep pressure, two-point discrimination, and light touch). The anterior horn of the spinal cord contains the lower motor neurons (LMN) and signs of LMN involvement include flaccid paralysis, atrophy of muscles, and areflexia. These are frequently associated with anterior cord syndromes. These are caused by the occlusion/compression mechanism of injury (i.e., traumatic herniated or dislocated disk, presence of bone fragments, or epidural hematoma) or infarcted spinal cord in the areas supplied by the anterior spinal artery.

> ▶ **HINT:** This is the worst prognosis of the incomplete injuries, with only 10% to 20% recovery of motor function.

■ *In Brown–Sequard syndrome, there is an ipsilateral loss of what function?*

■ **Motor function**

Brown–Sequard syndrome is a hemisection of the spinal cord that results in the ipsilateral loss of motor function and contralateral loss of pain and temperature. It is often seen with penetrating injuries but may also be seen with epidural hematomas and a traumatically herniated cervical disk.

> ▶ **HINT:** This syndrome has the best prognosis with a 90% recovery of ambulation, sensation, and bowel/bladder function if the injury was caused by compression.

■ *When the lumbosacral spinal nerves roots are damaged at level of L1 to L5, the syndrome is called?*

■ **Cauda equina syndrome**

Cauda equina syndrome (CES) is caused by damage to the lumbosacral nerve roots within the spinal canal at the level of L1 to L5. The cauda equina (CE) is a bundle of nerves distal to conus medullaris. *Cauda equina* is Latin for *horse's tail* and the nerve roots are called this because of the resemblance. CES results in areflexic bladder and bowel, and lower extremity paralysis. It is a peripheral nerve injury and so is considered to be an LMN lesion. The syndrome has variable motor and sensory losses. The prognosis of the recovery of motor function is good.

> ▶ **HINT:** A common sensory abnormality is called *saddle anesthesia* in which there is a paresthesia in the perineal region.

ASSESSMENT/DIAGNOSIS

■ *A lateral plain radiograph can be used to diagnose what type of injury?*

■ **Bony or vertebral fractures**

A lateral x-ray is used to visualize bony abnormalities and fractures. Ligament injuries are not identified on plain radiographs unless the spinal column is out of alignment. Flexion/extension x-rays may be obtained on an awake, cooperative patient without distracting injuries. MRI is the more definitive radiographic study used to identify ligament injuries.

> ▶ **HINT:** A patient with normal lateral cervical spine x-rays who complains of pain in the neck region should remain in cervical immobilization until flexion/extension views or MRI is obtained.

■ *While obtaining lateral radiographs of the cervical spine, what is most likely to interfere with visualization of the lower cervical vertebrae?*

■ **Shoulders**

Visualization from the occiput to T1 is required on lateral cervical x-ray to clear the presence of bony fractures. The shoulders frequently interfere with the ability to visualize C7 and the top of T1 in lateral C-spine radiographs. Obtaining a lateral x-ray in the swimmer's view can assist with identifying C7 and T1 vertebral bodies. Swimmer's view with a lateral x-ray involves downward traction on one arm and upward traction on the other with the x-ray beam aimed through the axilla of abducted arm.

▶ HINT: The trauma nurse can retract downward on both arms equally to pull the shoulders out of the way to improve visualization of the cervical spine.

■ *Which radiographic view is used to determine the height and alignment of vertebral bodies?*

■ **Anterior–posterior (AP)**

The AP view allows visualization of the vertebral bodies and determination of the height and alignment of the vertebral bodies.

▶ HINT: AP view with open-mouth techniques is the odontoid view and is used to recognize odontoid fractures.

■ *Which radiographic study can distinguish between spinal cord hemorrhage and vasogenic edema?*

■ **MRI**

An MRI is the gold standard for radiographic study of the spinal cord. It is able to distinguish between ischemic injury, edema, and hemorrhage within the cord.

▶ HINT: MRI is also considered the gold standard for recognizing spinal ligament injuries.

■ *What is the purpose of magnetic resonance angiography (MRA) following a blunt trauma to the cervical region?*

■ **Evaluate vertebral arteries**

A complication of a blunt trauma or flexion/extension injury to the neck may result in vertebral or carotid artery injuries. Arterial dissections are injuries associated with cervical fractures and spinal cord injuries.

▶ HINT: Altered mentation or neurological changes may indicate vertebral or carotid injury.

■ *The presence of sacral sparing following a traumatic spinal cord injury indicates what type of injury?*

■ **Incomplete injury**

Anal contraction with stimulation or ability to feel pinprick or touch around the anus is called *anal sparing* and indicates incomplete injury. This is a phenomenon of sensation in the sacral region even though sensation is absent in the thoracic and lumbar areas. Sacral fibers may be more protected from compression injury thus sparing the sacral dermatomes.

▶ HINT: Assessing for sacral sparing assists in determining an incomplete injury from a complete injury.

■ *Sensory assessment of cervical regions is tested through how many cervical levels?*

■ **C8**

There are seven cervical vertebrae and eight paired cervical nerve roots. Sensory assessment of the cervical region is tested through C8. The cervical region is the only portion of the spinal column that has a greater number of paired nerve roots than vertebrae.

> ▶ **HINT:** Sensory assessment is performed using dermatome levels in spinal cord–injured patients, whereas motor assessment is performed using myotome levels.

■ *Motor evaluation of the patient assesses which spinal cord tract?*

■ **Corticospinal**

The corticospinal tract controls voluntary movement assessed with motor evaluation. The spinothalamic tract controls pain and temperature and is assessed by pinprick, light touch, and temperature. The posterior column of the spinal cord is responsible for proprioception and stereognosis. Proprioception is the ability to know where the body and extremities are in space. Stereognosis is the ability to perceive or understand an object by sense of touch.

> ▶ **HINT:** The first part of the word identifies where the spinal tract originates and second part identifies where it terminates.

■ *What does the Modified Barthel Index (MBI) tool measure?*

■ **Functional outcomes**

The MBI is a functional outcome tool that may be used to assess the deficits associated with spinal cord injuries. The Functional Independence Measure (FIM) tool is another tool recommended to assess the deficits associated with spinal cord injuries.

> ▶ **HINT:** Acute spinal cord assessment may be done with American Spinal Injury Association (ASIA) scores, which utilize a motor index score, sensory index score, and functional outcome score.

MEDICAL/SURGICAL INTERVENTIONS

■ *What is the primary prehospital intervention utilized to prevent further injury to the spinal cord?*

■ **Immobilization**

The initial goal when caring for a trauma patient at the scene is to limit motion of a potentially injured spine and prevent further neurological involvement. A combination of a rigid cervical collar and supportive blocks on a backboard with straps is commonly used to stabilize the spine in the prehospital setting. The "neutral" position with the chin in midline position without hyperextension is recommended for spine immobilization.

> ▶ **HINT:** The use of rigid collars and spinal stabilization can increase intracranial pressure, increase the risk of skin breakdown, and aspiration.

■ *What is the primary management of a patient with burst fractures of cervical vertebrae?*

■ **Surgical cord decompression**

Burst fractures may require surgical removal of bone to achieve cord decompression. Bony pieces may compress the spinal cord and cause neurological injury. This injury requires surgical management; closed reduction with cervical traction is not recommended on burst fractures.

> ▶ **HINT:** Immobilization of the spinal column is important to prevent further injury to the spinal cord from bony pieces.

■ *What nonsurgical treatment is used on a patient with cervical subluxation and significant narrowing of the spinal column?*

■ **Cervical traction**

Cervical facet dislocation or subluxation can cause cord compression and may require closed reduction with cervical traction. Early closed reduction of traumatic cervical fractures with subluxation or narrowing of the spinal canal improves neurological outcomes. A halo vest may be used to stabilize cervical fractures externally, especially odontoid fractures.

> ▶ **HINT:** The inability to reduce a subluxation with external traction and weights may indicate locked facet.

■ *What is the primary treatment for neurogenic shock?*

■ **Fluid administration**

The complication of a neurogenic shock is systemic vasodilation with hypotension. Fluid resuscitation is the treatment of choice to correct the hypotension. If fluids do not improve the BP and perfusion, vasopressors may be initiated. The goal is to maintain the mean arterial pressure between 85 and 90 mmHg to increase perfusion and improve neurological outcomes. The bradycardia associated with neurogenic shock does not typically require treatment but if symptomatic, an external pacemaker may be placed.

> ▶ **HINT:** Neurogenic shock is classified as a distributive shock.

NURSING INTERVENTIONS

■ *What respiratory parameter should be closely monitored in a spontaneously breathing acute spinal cord injured patient?*

■ **Forced vital capacity (FVC) and/or negative inspiratory force (NIF)**

Respiratory parameters to monitor in a patient with a spinal cord injury to determine the ability to ventilate include FVC and NIF. The FVC is the forced maximal breath in followed by the maximal breath out. NIF is the ability to generate enough negative pressure in the chest to allow for inspiration. The FVC and NIF are used to evaluate the respiratory muscles and their ability to generate an adequate breath.

> ▶ **HINT:** These parameters are commonly used to evaluate a person's ability to breathe spontaneously and effectively.

■ *When should a bowel regimen begin following an acute spinal cord injury?*

■ **On admission**

When an acute spinal cord–injured patient is admitted, the bowel regimen should be ordered and initiated. A bowel regimen includes a suppository with finger stimulation timed appropriately for a once-a-day bowel movement. Timing of daily suppository for bowel training should be scheduled in acute care to facilitate rehabilitation and daily routines once the patient is discharged. A spinal cord injury above T12 may have reflex or spastic bowel, whereas a spinal cord injury below the T12 level may be hyporeflexic with a flaccid bowel.

> ▶ **HINT:** The bowel regimen should only be discontinued with severe diarrhea.

■ *A patient is able to void spontaneously following an acute spinal cord injury. What should the nurse assess for following the void?*

■ **Postvoid residuals**

If a patient with spinal cord injury is able to void spontaneously, use a bladder scan to assess for residual postvoiding. If greater than 200 to 300 mL, straight catheterization is recommended even if spontaneously voiding. Bladder training is the removal of the indwelling bladder catheter and intermittent catheterization used in the presence of urinary retention.

> ▶ **HINT:** Bladder training is initiated as soon as the patient is on the maintenance fluids or oral intake.

■ *What may be used to prevent postural hypotension in a spinal cord–injured patient when getting out of bed?*

■ **Abdominal binder**

Postural hypotension is a common complication following a spinal cord injury. Position changing should be performed slowly to avoid syncope or near-syncope. Applying compressive hose or leg wraps and abdominal binders to patients with spinal cord injuries prior to getting them out of bed can help prevent orthostatic hypotension.

> ▶ **HINT:** Maintain adequate fluid volume to assist with management of orthostatic hypotension.

■ *A patient is readmitted from rehabilitation following a cervical spinal cord injury. The patient suddenly develops hypertension with a BP of 210/120 mmHg. What would be the nurse's priority of care?*

■ **Find the source of stimulation and remove it**

Priority of care with a hypertensive spinal cord–injured patient resulting from autonomic hyperreflexia is to find the source of obnoxious stimulation and remove it. The trauma nurse should elevate the head of the bed to lower the pressure and assess the patient for the cause of the autonomic hyperreflexia (Box 1.19). Once the source is identified and removed, the patient's hypertension should resolve.

> ▶ **HINT:** Antihypertensives should not be the priority or first choice to manage the hypertension associated with autonomic hyperreflexia (AH) because once the source is removed, the patient will become hypotensive.

Box 1.19 Sources of AH and Nursing Interventions

Potential Sources	Nursing Interventions
Urinary retention	Bladder scan and intermittent catheterization
Restrictive clothing	Loosen or remove clothing
Pressure sores	Reposition off of pressure scores
Fecal impaction	Remove fecal impaction

AH, autonomic hyperreflexia.

COMPLICATIONS

▪ *At what level of spinal injury is the diaphragm affected, which, if a complete injury, requires ventilatory support?*

▪ **Fourth cervical level**

The C4 level innervates the diaphragm. A patient with a cervical injury to the spinal cord at the C4 level or higher loses innervation to the diaphragm and usually requires intubation and mechanical ventilation. Cervical injuries at the six or seventh cervical level (C6 and C7) may still require intubation and ventilation, at least in the acute period as a result of cord edema.

> ▶ **HINT:** Airway and breathing are the priorities of care in cervical spinal injuries.

▪ *The lack of ability to internally regulate temperature following a spinal cord injury is called?*

▪ **Poikliothermia**

Loss of thermoregulatory function occurs in cord injuries above the thoracolumbar outflow because of loss of sympathetic nervous system (SNS) stimulation. Poikliothermia is the lack of internal regulation of the body temperature, which occurs after a spinal cord–injury. Spinal cord–injured patients are unable to vasoconstrict and shiver to conserve heat or sweat to dissipate heat.

> ▶ **HINT:** Nursing interventions for spinal cord–injured patients include controlling the body temperature through external interventions.

▪ *What is the loss of motor and reflexes below the level of injury called?*

▪ **Spinal shock**

Spinal shock is the loss of reflexes, and motor function below the level of injury. Spinal shock occurs immediately after the injury and typically resolves within 2 to 16 weeks.

▶ **HINT:** Two of the reflexes routinely assessed in spinal cord–injured patients include anocutaneous and bulbocavernosous reflex.

■ *During neurogenic shock, what is the most common dysrhythmia?*

■ **Sinus bradycardia**

Neurogenic shock is caused by the interruption of descending sympathetic fibers in the thoracic and cervical cord producing vasodilation below the level of injury and hypotension. At the cervical level, complete injury interrupts sympathetic outflow to the heart, but the parasympathetic outflow remains intact via the vagus nerve causing bradycardia in neurogenic shock.

▶ **HINT:** Neurogenic shock is associated with symptoms of hypotension and bradycardia, whereas spinal shock is the loss of motor function and reflexes.

■ *What is the hypertensive crisis that can occur in patients following a spinal cord injury?*

■ **Autonomic hyperreflexia**

A spinal cord injury with lesions above T6 may exhibit signs of autonomic hyperreflexia. Autonomic hyperreflexia occurs with an obnoxious stimulation below the level of injury followed by life-threatening hypertension. Some of the potential causes of autonomic hyperreflexia include bladder distension, catheterization, urinary tract infection, testicular torsion, pressure sores, and fecal impaction.

▶ **HINT:** Autonomic hyperreflexia is not an early complication and only occurs after spinal shock has resolved.

■ *What electrolyte abnormality may commonly occur in a paraplegic patient as a result of prolonged non-weight-bearing?*

■ **Hypercalcemia**

Non-weight-bearing status for prolonged period of time allows calcium to move from bone to serum, thus increasing calcium levels. This is a long-term complication and may require administration of calcitonin.

▶ **HINT:** Hypercalcemia can cause vasoconstriction and hypertension.

■ *What is the level of innervation for the spinal cord patients to be able to feed themselves independently?*

■ **C5 through C7**

The fifth cervical level innervates the biceps, allowing for flexion of the elbow, whereas the seventh cervical level innervates the triceps, allowing the elbow to extend. The flexion and extension of the arm allows patients to be able to feed themselves, even if the required utensils need to be strapped to the hands.

▶ **HINT:** Flexing the wrist and spreading the fingers occurs at the C8 and T1 level of innervation and allows for fine motor control. This allows for greater independent activities of daily living (ADL).

■ *What is the level of innervation in which a paraplegic is able to push him- or herself a wheelchair?*

■ **Level of C6**

The level of C6 innervation is considered to be the level at which spinal cord–injured patients are able to perform ADL such as feeding, grooming, dressing, and pushing a wheelchair.

▶ **HINT:** This is the level of function, not necessarily the actual level of injury.

Questions

1. A patient with a ventriculostomy is now presenting with an increased intracranial pressure (ICP) reading of 18 mmHg. The priority nursing intervention for the management of this patient should be:

   A. Increase the head of bed (HOB) to 30 to 45 degrees
   B. Get an order for D₅NS fluids
   C. Decrease the HOB to 20 degrees
   D. Administer mannitol immediately

2. A patient was in an automobile accident and struck a tree, the airbag did not deploy, and the driver was not restrained. The patient has a contusion on the forehead from the steering wheel at the site of impact. This injury can be best described as:

   A. Contrecoup
   B. Accelerated injury
   C. Subluxation
   D. Coup

3. A patient presents with periorbital ecchymosis and drainage from the nares. This patient has a Glascow Coma Scale (GCS) of 9. Which of the following would *not* be an appropriate treatment modality for this patient?

   A. Frequent level of consciousness (LOC) and pupillary assessments
   B. Administer antibiotics as ordered
   C. Wrap eyes with gauze and pack nasal drainage
   D. Place nasal drainage on gauze to assess for a "halo sign"

4. After brain injury, cerebral blood flow frequently decreases to an ischemic level. To prevent further neuronal death, cerebral blood flow of well-oxygenated blood must be restored. Which of the following interferes with cerebral blood flow?

   A. Increasing the mean arterial pressure (MAP)
   B. Increasing intracranial pressure (ICP)
   C. Decreasing ICP
   D. Increasing systolic blood pressure (SBP)

5. A patient's MRI results just revealed an uncal herniation. The nurse will expect the patient to present with:

   A. Ipsilateral pupil dilation and motor weakness
   B. Conscious, lethargic, but oriented
   C. Ipsilateral pupil dilation and contralateral motor weakness
   D. A Glasgow Coma Scale (GCS) of 12

6. All of the following are presenting symptoms of a midbrain injury except:

   A. Resting tremor
   B. Respiratory insufficiency
   C. Abnormal pupil shape
   D. Loss of pupillary reaction

7. Mr. Jones has been admitted with a traumatic brain injury after a boating accident. His spouse is at bedside and reports that "he just is not himself today." The nurse educates the spouse about the injury sustained. Which of the following is *not* an acceptable response?

A. A behavioral characteristic of traumatic brain injury is the loss of control of one's emotions.

B. A behavioral characteristic of traumatic brain injury is combativeness.

C. A behavioral characteristic of traumatic brain injury is paranoia and fear.

D. A behavioral characteristic of traumatic brain injury is abusiveness.

8. The patient sustained a sudden blow to the head. CT of the brain is normal, pupils are equal and brisk, but the patient has an altered level of consciousness (LOC) and a low Glasgow Coma Scale (GCS). These are all characteristics of:

A. Diffuse injury

B. Traumatic subdural hematoma

C. Epidural hematoma

D. Subdural hematoma

9. After a brain injury with an increased intracranial pressure (ICP), a central nervous system (CNS) ischemic response can be activated called *Cushing's triad*. Which of the following depicts Cushing's triad?

A. Increased diastolic pressure, widened pulse pressure, bradycardia, and respiratory insufficiency

B. Increased systolic pressure, widened pulse pressure, bradycardia, and respiratory insufficiency

C. Increased systolic pressure, widened pulse pressure, tachycardia, and respiratory insufficiency

D. Increased diastolic pressure, widened pulse pressure, tachycardia, and respiratory insufficiency

10. A 45-year-old patient with an old spinal cord injury who is paraplegic presents with restlessness, anxiety, and complaining of a pounding headache with a pain rating of 8/10. Her blood pressure is 170/94 mmHg, heart rate is 60 beats per minute, and respiratory rate is 18 breaths per minute and regular. On assessment, the nurse notes perfuse forehead diaphoresis. Given the findings, the nurse suspects:

A. Spinal shock

B. Autonomic dysreflexia

C. Neurogenic shock

D. Distributive shock

11. While taking care of a spinal cord–injured patient, the physician orders immobilization with a RotoRest bed, bladder scanning every 6 hours with intermittent catheterization if reading is greater than 400 cc of urine, pulmonary toileting every 6 hours, and an abdominal binder. The nurse can advocate for the patient by also implementing:

A. The use of a halo vest

B. Enhancing the "quad cough" every 6 hours

C. Stimulating the rectum to encourage regular bowel movements

D. Changing position quickly and frequently

12. A 27-year-old female suffered a spinal cord injury. She is extremely upset because she is a newlywed and is not able to get pregnant and have children as her husband and she had planned. Which of the following responses would be the best response by the nurse when counseling the patient and her husband?

    A. Because of the disruption in the autonomic nervous system, she is not going to have a period anymore, therefore the ability to conceive is not possible.
    B. I know this is disappointing, but you are lucky to be alive and adoption is always an option.
    C. You might still be able to get pregnant but you won't be able to deliver vaginally, you will have to have a cesarean section (C-section) delivery.
    D. Pregnancy and a normal delivery are still possible; encourage her to talk with her physician about potential risks.

13. The autonomic nervous system controls involuntary vital functions and is divided into two subdivisions: parasympathetic and sympathetic. Which of the following is a result of parasympathetic stimulation in regard to respiratory function?

    A. Bronchial constriction
    B. Increased respiratory rate
    C. Bronchial dilation
    D. Pulmonary vascular constriction

14. A spinal cord injury results from multiple modalities of injury. When a patient has spinal cord edema and there is a possibility of necrosis from the spinal cord being compressed, this is a result of:

    A. Spinal cord concussion
    B. Spinal cord contusion
    C. Spinal cord transection
    D. Spinal cord ischemia

15. A patient has a spinal cord injury. After review of the case, the physician classifies the injury as a stable vertebral fracture. Which of the following descriptions does not describe evidence of spinal stability?

    A. Ligamentous integrity damage
    B. No injury to the spinal cord
    C. Angulation from normal loading is not probable
    D. Potential for displacement is minimal

16. A 6-year-old boy was climbing a tree and fell. His parents brought him to the emergency room for evaluation. The boy was moving his limbs, had no deformities, and had a hematoma on his buttocks. All of the radiographic studies were negative for fracture. The next morning, the patient was not moving his legs. What is the most probable injury sustained?

    A. Spinal cord injury
    B. Compressed nerve
    C. Spinal lesion
    D. Lumbar hematoma

17. On palpation of pulses in a shock patient, the findings differ when assessing a neurogenic shock patient versus a hypovolemic shock patient. What are the differences?

    A. Pulses are rapid and strong in hypovolemic shock
    B. Pulses are slow and strong in neurogenic shock
    C. Pulses are slow and weak in a neurogenic shock patient
    D. Pulses are rapid and strong in neurogenic shock

18. A patient in neurogenic shock displays distinctive skin temperature qualities to palpation versus patients who are experiencing hypovolemic shock. The difference is:

    A. Skin is warm and dry in neurogenic shock patients
    B. Skin is cool and moist in neurogenic shock patients
    C. Skin is cool and dry in hypovolemic shock patients
    D. Skin is warm and moist in hypovolemic shock patients

19. There are 31 pairs of spinal nerves. When a patient sustains a spinal injury, the dermatome is used to test sensation associated with spinal nerve injuries. All of these landmarks aid in the evaluation and utilization of the dermatome except which of the following?

    A. Dermatome cervicle-5 pairs with anatomical landmark of the top of the shoulders
    B. Dermatome T4 pairs with the anatomical landmark of the nipple line
    C. Dermatome T10 pairs with the anatomical landmark of the umbilicus
    D. Dermatome lumbar-1 pairs with the great toe

20. When accurately assessing sensory function of a spinal cord–injured patient, the nurse should:

    A. Begin at the level of no feeling and proceed to the area of feeling
    B. Begin at the top of the shoulders and progress to the big toes
    C. Begin at the level of feeling and proceed to the area of no feeling
    D. Begin at the big toe and progress to the top of the shoulders

21. A patient comes in with a vertebral injury after a motor vehicle collision with projection from the vehicle. The patient was stabilized and taken for radiographic studies of the spine. After the x-ray scan comes back, C7 to T1 is not visualized. What should the nurse except to be ordered next?

    A. Chest x-ray
    B. MRI of the cervical spine
    C. CT of the cervical spine
    D. MRI of the neck

22. The nurse is educating the family of a spinal cord–injured patient on why the monitoring of blood pressure in these types of injuries is very important. Which of the following is the best answer to explain the purpose of closely monitoring the blood pressure?

    A. Hypotension frequently occurs in spinal injury patients because blood vessels above the level of injury vasodilate and blood pools to the lower extremities.
    B. Hypertension frequently occurs in spinal injury patients because blood vessels above the level of injury vasoconstrict and blood pools to central circulation
    C. Hypotension frequently occurs in spinal injury patients because blood vessels below the level of injury vasodilate and blood pools to the lower extremities.
    D. Hypertension frequently occurs in spinal injury patients because blood vessels below the level of injury vasoconstrict and blood pools to central circulation.

23. Restlessness and agitation in spinal injury patients are frequently witnessed behaviors because of neurological involvement or because of the constraints in mobility and positioning. Patients are at increased risk for injury related to this altered mentation. All of the following are proper interventions and outcomes for these patients except:

    A. Administration of an ordered sedative
    B. Administration of methyl prednisone as ordered
    C. Education and reinforcement on the importance of immobility
    D. Administration of a short-acting paralytic as ordered if patient is being ventilated

24. A 17-year-old wrestler injured his head. He lost consciousness briefly, regained it, but was dizzy and complained of a headache. He was treated in the emergency department for a concussion, and education was provided to the patient and caregiver regarding not to have any contact sport activity until cleared as an outpatient by neurology. The young man played football 2 weeks later, was tackled, and didn't get up. The paramedic team initiated resuscitative measures, but when he arrived in the emergency room, he had no pulse and was not breathing. What injury should the nurse suspect?

    A. Sudden cardiac arrest
    B. Second-impact syndrome
    C. Concussion
    D. Double-impact injury

25. Which of the following is misinformation regarding the education delivered to a patient who suffered a minor head injury and is being cleared for discharge?

    A. Place ice packs to the head for 15 to 20 minutes every hour to decrease pain and swelling.
    B. Have someone wake you at different times during the night and ask you your name and phone number.
    C. Do not take ibuprofen because it can cause stomach bleeding and renal problems.
    D. Rest for the first 24 hours. Do not play contact sports or do activities that may result in a blow to the head until all symptoms have resolved.

26. Obvious complications for a patient with a spinal cord injury include deep vein thrombosis and pressure ulcers. What other intervention would be part of the ongoing monitoring for a patient with a spinal cord injury?

    A. Routine electrolyte monitoring
    B. Placing a urinary catheter
    C. Screening for acute abdomen
    D. Both A and C

27. Spinal cord–injured patients are at a high risk of having altered presentations of acute abdominal processes and frequently suffer from gastroparesis, paralytic ileus, constipation, and colitis. Which of the following has the least effect on the gastrointestinal system of spinal cord–injured patients?

    A. Central nervous system (CNS)
    B. Peripheral nervous system (PNS)
    C. Autonomic nervous system (ANS)
    D. Enteric nervous system (ENS)

28. A spinal cord–injured patient in the intensive care unit was just assessed by his physician. The physician placed orders for dantrolene sodium (Dantrium) to be added to the medication regimen. The patient asks the nurse what this treatment is for, the best response would be:

    A. This is an antispasmolytic agent that aids in preventing spasticity and muscle stiffness.
    B. This is given to reduce damage to nerve cells and decrease inflammation near the site of injury.
    C. This medication blocks or delays the reuptake of the neurotransmitters serotonin and norepinephrine by the presynaptic nerves. This increases the levels of these two neurotransmitters in the synapse and tends to elevate mood.
    D. This is indicated for neuropathic pain associated with spinal cord injury because interactions with descending noradrenergic and serotonergic pathways originating from the brain stem appear to reduce neuropathic pain transmission from the spinal cord.

29. A patient with a traumatic brain injury is now being treated with therapeutic hypothermia. What are some expected complications from this therapy?

    A. Shivering and hypercoagulation
    B. Diuresis and shivering
    C. Hypercoagulation and arrhythmias
    D. Arrhythmias and oliguria

30. A case of mild traumatic brain injury is an occurrence of injury to the brain that can result from a blunt trauma. Which of the following is the most accurate description of symptoms of a mild head injury?

    A. Continual confusion, unconsciousness, or seizure activity after brain injury
    B. A pattern of unconsciousness, consciousness, followed again by unconsciousness
    C. Infants and young children present with irritability, lethargy, or vomiting following brain injury
    D. Headache, dizziness, irritability, fatigue, or poor concentration are reported after brain injury

31. If there is a suspected mild brain injury, what would be the most reliable method of detection?

    A. PET
    B. CT of the brain
    C. Neuropsychological assessment
    D. MRI

32. A patient suffered a mild brain injury in a motor vehicle collision. The patient is currently experiencing poor attention span and fatigue, which is affecting the patient's job as an architect. What is indicated for this patient to achieve optimum care?

    A. Recommend the patient make an appointment with a psychiatrist
    B. Encourage the patient to seek rehabilitation and perform exercises
    C. Notify the neurologist of the persistent symptoms for a reevaluation of injury
    D. Notify the neurologist for need of further medication management

33. On assessment of a patient with suspected brain injury, all of the following would be pertinent questions to ask while obtaining a history except:

    A. Have any drugs or alcohol been used?
    B. Does the patient currently smoke tobacco products?
    C. Does the patient have a history of seizures?
    D. Was there any loss of consciousness after the injury?

34. What sign and symptom do a linear skull fracture, depressed skull fracture, and basilar skull fracture have in common?

    A. Headache
    B. Possible open fracture
    C. Palpable depression
    D. Periorbital ecchymosis

35. The nurse receives a patient with a suspected brain injury. A Glasgow Coma Scale (GCS) assessment is warranted. The patient's eyes opened and arms withdrew when cuticle pressure was applied. The patient had no verbal response but gasped when trying to say his name. The nurse did note a gasp when the patient was trying to follow commands. What would be this patient's GCS?

    A. 6
    B. 7
    C. 8
    D. 9

36. A patient comes into the emergency room after a concrete block fell on his head at a construction site. The patient's skull is indented and is actively bleeding from a laceration at the site. The patient is lethargic and mumbling that he has a severe headache. The patient is breathing 18 breaths per minute with an oxygen saturation of 98% on a nonrebreather mask, the current blood pressure is 108/66 mmHg, and the pulse rate is 110 beats per minute. What is the nurse's first priority to treat this patient?

    A. Prepare to intubate the patient
    B. Apply direct pressure to the bleeding site
    C. Assess the patient's pupils
    D. Start two large-bore intravenous sites

37. A patient was in a motor vehicle collision and presents with a positive lipstick sign. The cervical spine images identify a C4 fracture, subluxation, and compression fracture of anterior vertebrae. This is most likely because of:

    A. Hyperflexion
    B. Hyperextension
    C. Vertical compression
    D. Odontoid fracture

38. What best describes Jefferson's fracture?

    A. A fracture of the anterior and posterior arch of C1 without cord damage
    B. Bilateral fracture through arch C2
    C. Avulsion of C1 from the occipital bone
    D. A fracture of the dens

39. Ms. Smith came to the hospital with a spinal cord injury yesterday. The nurse in the intensive care unit (ICU) performs her morning assessment; the findings reveal that there is a complete absence of motor and sensory function below the level of the injury. The patient's presentation is reflective of her diagnosis of:

A. Central cord syndrome
B. Complete cord injury
C. Posterior cord injury
D. Necrosis of the spinal cord postinjury

40. A patient had a traumatic herniated disk and has subsequently been diagnosed with anterior cord syndrome. The patient has complete motor paralysis, loss of painful stimuli, and sense of temperature. The patient can feel light touch and notices position changes (proprioception). The patient asks whether this is a "good sign" of improvement. The best possible nurse response would be:

A. This is to be expected with your diagnosis, therefore you unfortunately can never move your legs again.
B. Yes, this is great progression and maybe you can move your legs today.
C. This is expected with your type of injury. Let's see whether you also feel vibration and deep pressure.
D. Yes, patients with your diagnosis always return to full ambulatory functioning.

41. All are characteristics of poikliothermia except:

A. It occurs in injuries above thoracolumbar outflow of the sympathetic nervous system
B. It lacks internal regulation of body temperature
C. There is an absence of vasoconstriction
D. Excessive shivering in order to conserve heat

42. The nurse notes that the patient frequently asks the same questions and has a problem with remembering when people visit. The nurse implements a memory notebook. This notebook will benefit the patient by:

A. Having the answers to frequently asked questions written down
B. Continually reinforcing the plan of care by serving as an aid memory when read
C. Having family, friends, and health care providers leave notes to aid in the patient's memory of events
D. All of the above

43. A patient sustains a mild traumatic brain injury in a football game. Which of the following is the most accurate description of a mild brain injury?

A. Presence of unconsciousness, or seizure activity following the brain injury
B. Completely back to normal within 24 hours of the injury
C. Infants present with irritability, lethargy, or vomiting following brain injury
D. Headache, dizziness, irritability, fatigue, or poor concentration are reported after brain injury

44. This intracranial injury is one of the most common types of brain injuries, it is one of the leading causes of death in people with traumatic brain injury, and is one of the most devastating. These patients come to the emergency room unconscious and in vegetative states. What is this injury called?

A. Diffuse axonal injury
B. Acquired brain injury

    C. Hypoxic brain injury
    D. Encephalopathy

45. Which of the following mechanisms of injury does not represent the risk of a diffuse axonal injury?

    A. Shaken baby syndrome
    B. Sports-related injuries
    C. Penetrating wound to brain
    D. Automobile collisions

46. A patient is brought to the emergency department after being found with a decreased level of consciousness on the beach and is noted to have a scalp laceration. On arrival, the patient is very agitated and uncooperative. After 30 minutes, the patient becomes completely obtunded. What would be the best explanation for these changes in mentation?

    A. The agitation is from hypoglycemia that has progressed into diabetic ketoacidosis making the patient obtunded.
    B. The agitation is because of hypoxia that has progressed to hypercapnia resulting in the patient being obtunded.
    C. The agitation is most likely because of being intoxicated and has progressed to the patient being obtunded as a result of being impaired.
    D. The agitation is the result of hypotension that has progressed to hypoxia resulting in the patient being obtunded.

47. The pediatric population is anatomically more prone to cranial injuries because of all of the following except:

    A. The head is heavier and larger
    B. White matter is not well myelinated
    C. The neck is shorter
    D. The occiput is prominent until the 10th year

Maxillofacial Trauma

MECHANISM OF INJURY

◼ *What is the mechanism of injury that can result in nasoorbitalethmoidal (NOE) injury?*

◼ **A direct blow to the nasal region**

Following injury to the nasal region, the medial orbital wall can be damaged, causing injury to the ethmoid region. The ethmoid bone is paper thin and is connected to the cribriform plate. Fracture of the ethmoid bone may be associated with a cribriform fracture and an orbital roof fracture.

> ▶ **HINT:** A loss of smell is commonly associated with an NOE injury as a result of direct injury to cranial nerve (CN) I (olfactory).

◼ *What is the mechanism of injury for a "blowout" fracture?*

◼ **Direct blow to the orbital globe**

Orbital blowout fractures occur when a blunt force is applied directly to the orbital globe. A blowout fracture can cause entrapment, most commonly of the inferior or medial rectus muscle. An isolated orbital blowout fracture is the fracture of the orbital walls without associated fractures of the orbital rims.

> ▶ **HINT:** Global entrapment following a blowout fracture causes restriction of eye movement.

◼ *A penetrating trauma to the roof of the mouth can result in injury to which structure?*

◼ **Brain**

Penetrating trauma to the roof of the mouth can result in the object entering the brain and causing significant brain trauma. The angle of the penetrating object to the oral cavity or the face can determine whether the brain is involved in the trauma. Lacerations to the floor of the mouth can extend to the pharynx, tonsil, submaxillary triangle, or hyoid bone.

◼ *What is a common cause of facial trauma in a front-impact motor vehicle collision?*

◼ **Airbag**

A common mechanism of injury for maxillofacial trauma includes high-velocity impact, including a motor vehicle collision with airbag deployment.

■ *Violence or assault is most commonly associated with injuries to which region of the face?*

■ **Midface**

Violence or assault is most commonly associated with injuries to the nose, maxillary, zygoma, and frontal bones, which are components of the midface.

▶ **HINT:** Women are more likely to experience facial fractures than men following a similar impact to the face.

■ *Which injury is commonly associated with blunt facial trauma and what should it be assessed for?*

■ **Cervical spine injury**

Applying blunt force to the face may cause hyperextension of the neck, causing a cervical injury. The care provided by prehospital and emergency room health care providers should include cervical stabilization until injury has been ruled out.

▶ **HINT:** A blow to the back of the head can cause the neck to hyperflex with the face impacting an object, causing a cervical injury with facial fractures.

■ *What is the most prominent clinical sign of an optic nerve laceration?*

■ **Immediate blindness**

Common mechanisms of injury that result in blindness include penetrating trauma to the eye and sudden acceleration or deceleration movement of the head. Other symptoms of eye injuries include diplopia, or blurred vision. Traumatic injuries to the eye can result in delayed or immediate blindness in the involved eye (Box 2.1).

▶ **HINT:** Diplopia can result from orbital fractures with extracoular entrapment from "blowout" fracture.

Box 2.1 Trauma-Induced Blindness

Immediate or Early-Onset Blindness	Delayed or Late-Onset Blindness
Vitreous hemorrhage (posterior portion)	Retinal detachment
Prolapse globe contents	Hemorrhage
Intraocular foreign body	Glaucoma
Optic nerve laceration	
Occipital lobe hemorrhage	

TRAUMATIC INJURIES

■ *What is an associated injury that is considered life-threatening?*

■ **Airway obstruction**

Associated injuries with facial trauma include cervical spinal injuries, airway obstruction, and brain injury. Airway obstruction is a potentially life-threatening associated injury. Facial trauma is not considered a priority of care unless it involves an airway obstruction.

▶ **HINT:** Injuries that affect the airway and breathing are the most common answers for questions regarding life-threatening injuries.

■ *What is a significant complication that can occur with scalp lacerations?*

■ **Bleeding**

Scalp and facial lacerations can result in extensive blood loss as a result of dense vasculature and therefore may become life-threatening from hemorrhage. Facial injuries can cause injury to the temporal artery, leading to an arterial bleed.

■ *What type of LeFort fracture results in isolated movement of the maxilla?*

■ **LeFort I fracture**

The level of facial mobility following a trauma defines the type of LeFort fracture present. Isolated maxilla movement is a LeFort I fracture and is commonly called a "free floating" maxilla. LeFort I fracture is caused by a horizontal fracture through the maxillary body, causing a detachment of the entire maxilla at the level of the nasal floor.

This fracture results from a horizontal or downward force applied to the anterior face.

> ▶ **HINT:** To assess for a LeFort I fracture, the maxilla is held with the thumb and forefinger, and an attempt is made to move the maxilla gently as not to cause further separation and injury.

■ *What is the injury that is classified as a LeFort II fracture?*

■ **Separation of the midface**

A LeFort II fracture is a separation of the midface in a pyramidal shape (similar to the appearance of an oxygen facemask). The fracture pattern is a result of a horizontal impact to the upper midface. A LeFort II fracture is a LeFort I fracture plus an extension of the fracture through the orbital rim, medial orbital wall, ethmoid sinuses, and nose. It is associated with a sinus roof or cribriform fracture and cerebrospinal fluid leak.

> ▶ **HINT:** A LeFort II fracture line is similar to the shape and size of an oxygen facemask.

■ *What is the injury that is classified as a LeFort III fracture?*

■ **Total craniofacial separation**

A LeFort III fracture is a total craniofacial separation. This is commonly called a *craniofacial disjuncture.* The impact of a LeFort III fracture is a downward oblique impact that separates the facial skeleton from the skullbase. The floor, roof, and lateral and medial walls of the orbit can be injured in a LeFort III fracture.

> ▶ **HINT:** Gently rocking the maxilla produces movement of the entire midface, independent of the skull.

■ *What is a severe eye injury that can occur following a sudden acceleration or deceleration movement of the head?*

■ **Optic nerve avulsion**

A sudden deceleration or acceleration force to the head or eye region can result in the avulsion or laceration of the optic nerve. The symptoms include a sudden-onset blindness immediately following the injury. An example of a deceleration injury is a motor vehicle collision in which the victim's moving head impacts a windshield.

> ▶ **HINT:** Traumatic brain injuries to the occipital region can result in visual losses, typically in the same visual fields bilaterally, but do not cause a total unilateral blindness.

■ *What is the term for an accumulation of blood in the anterior chamber of the eye?*

■ **Hyphema**

A hyphema is an accumulation of blood that disperses in layers within the anterior chamber of the eye. The amount of visual impairment is related to the amount of occlusion from the hemorrhage. A severe or complete loss of vision is caused by the obscuring of the entire anterior chamber of the eye with blood. Associated symptoms may include a deep aching eye pain and increased intraocular pressures.

> ▶ **HINT:** The mechanism of injury for hyphema is a direct blow to the globe of the eye.

■ *What type of eye injury causes a decrease in intraocular pressure following a facial trauma?*

■ **Perforated globe**

Traumatic injury to the eye can cause globe rupture, which results in a lowering of intraocular pressure. A normal intraocular pressure is about 15 mmHg. A low pressure is less than 10 mmHg and indicates a globe rupture. A high intraocular pressure may be caused by retrobulbar hemorrhage.

> ▶ **HINT:** A direct blow to the globe can result in a hyphema, or accumulation of blood within the anterior chamber of the globe.

ASSESSMENT/DIAGNOSIS

■ *A facial fracture that results in loss of sensation may involve damage to which CN?*

■ **CN V (trigeminal)**

CN assessment following facial trauma is important when assessing for complications (Box 2.2). CN V (trigeminal) is responsible for sensation across the forehead, cheek, and jaw. An injury to the peripheral portion of the CN can cause loss of sensation.

> ▶ **HINT:** CN assessment is important following facial trauma. CNs II to VII are the most commonly injured CNs following a facial trauma.

Box 2.2 Commonly Injured Cranial Nerves

Cranial Nerves	Assessment
CN II	Visual acuity
CN III, IV, VI	Extraocular eye movement
CN V	Sensory; determined by light touch or pinprick to forehead, cheek, and jaw
CN VII	Symmetry of facial expressions

CN, cranial nerve.

■ **What is the trauma nurse looking for while palpating the face and skull during the assessment?**

■ **Bony depression**

Assessment following trauma involving the head and neck is for underlying skull deformities or depression under the area of the scalp, or facial laceration that would indicate bony fractures. Laceration of the scalp may be explored with a finger or blunt instrument to determine the depth of the laceration.

> ▶ **HINT:** Displacement of the inner table (thinner wall) of the frontal sinus can result in dural involvement.

■ **A trauma patient presenting with epistaxis and nasal discoloration is most likely to have sustained what type of injury?**

■ **Nasal fracture**

Edema, epistaxis, deformity, nasal obstruction, pain, and discoloration are signs of a nasal fracture. The recognition of a nasal fracture leads the trauma nurse to assess for complications of nasal fractures, including obstruction of nasal passages with clots.

> ▶ **HINT:** Following facial trauma, overt nasal deformity may not be immediately noticeable because of facial edema.

■ **When looking at the patient's profile, the nose appears to have an abnormal "pug" appearance. What is the most likely injury?**

■ **NOE injury**

Injury of the NOE region results in the patient's profile having the appearance of a depression or a "pug" nose. The frontal view of injury to the NOE region appears to be widened and flattened with the illusion of the eyes being farther apart (called *telecanthus*). This is a result of the disruption of the medial canthal ligaments.

> ▶ **HINT:** Telecanthus is present when the intercanthal distance is greater than 30 to 35 mm; a definitive diagnosis is determined by a distance greater than 45 mm.

■ **What is the primary finding of a blowout orbital fracture with entrapment?**

■ **Restricted eye movement**

Following an orbital blowout fracture, the bony pieces impinge on the extraocular muscles, causing restricted eye movement. This is frequently called *entrapment*. Following orbital trauma, the trauma nurse should evaluate vision, eye movement, pupil size and reaction, lid appearance, cornea, and conjunctiva.

> ▶ **HINT:** Orbital blowout fractures may have the presence of enophthalmos (globe recedes posteriorly).

■ **A patient with pain on opening the mouth with limited jaw movement may have what type of facial injury?**

■ **Mandibular fracture**

Mandibular fractures result in a limited ability to open the mouth and produce significant pain on opening the mouth or clenching the jaws. A malocclusion or deviation of the jaw indicates either mandibular or maxillary injury. Another sign of mandibular or mental nerve injury is numbness over a portion of the mandibular body. During the assessment of a mandibular fracture, the temporomandibular joint is palpated bilaterally as the patient opens and closes their mouth.

> ▶ HINT: In mandibular fractures, airway obstruction can occur because the tongue is secured to the muscle attached to the mandible and a fracture can cause loss of tongue control.

■ *What should the trauma nurse assess on a patient with lower facial trauma?*
■ **Inside of the mouth**

Following lower facial trauma, the inside of the mouth should be assessed for breaks in the skin, ecchymosis, clots, exposed bone, or bone fragments. Severe injuries of the mandible are characterized by fragmentation of bone and teeth, and disruption of adjacent soft tissue. Hematomas present in the mouth, soft tissue injuries in the oral cavity, or blood accumulating in the hypopharynx can cause upper airway obstruction.

> ▶ HINT: As a result of facial injuries, large amounts of blood can be swallowed, so signs of bleeding may not be apparent until the patient vomits blood.

■ *Following a traumatic injury to the face, the patient presents with stridor. What would be the trauma nurse's concern about the patient?*
■ **Partial airway obstruction**

Stridor, drooling, and cyanosis are some potential signs of arterial airway obstruction. Following a traumatic injury to the face, airway obstruction may be caused by swelling, hematoma, bleeding, or laryngeal obstruction. Injury to the vagus or hypoglossal nerve with facial trauma can cause vocal cord or hemi-tongue paralysis, contributing to airway obstruction following facial trauma.

> ▶ HINT: Blood or vomit aspiration following facial trauma can cause laryngo-spasm, which contributes to upper airway obstruction.

■ *In the trauma intensive care unit (ICU), patient develops a "beachball" appearance of the face. What is the most likely LeFort classification of the facial fracture?*
■ **LeFort III**

The LeFort III fracture involves a total craniofacial separation and commonly develops massive swelling , which results in a "beachball" face. Upper airway obstruction can occur and intubation may be required early, or an emergency cricothyroidotomy may be necessary if a complicated obstruction occurs.

■ *When the patient's nose and chin are against the x-ray plate, what is the radiographic view called?*
■ **Water's view**

A Water's view x-ray is taken with the nose and chin against the x-ray plate. It is used to identify injuries to maxillofacial bones; maxillary sinus; nasal bones; frontal processes of maxilla, zygoma, and zygomatic arch; and coronoid process of the mandible, orbit, ethmoid, and frontal sinuses. Caldwell's view involves placing the forehead and nose against the x-ray plate; it provides a different angle used to evaluate structures similar to those seen in Water's view. A lateral facial x-ray is used to identify nasal bones; frontal sinus; and multiple, small maxillofacial floors.

> ▶ **HINT:** CT scans commonly have replaced plain films and are considered the "gold standard" to evaluate facial trauma.

- **What is used to identify presence of corneal abrasions?**
- **Fluorescein staining**

Identification of surface eye injuries, such as corneal abrasion, is determined with fluorescein staining and examination with Wood's light or a slit-lamp. The area of abrasion will appear as green under fluorescent illumination (Box 2.3).

> ▶ **HINT:** The recommendation for staining is with fluorescein strips to prevent contamination and eye infections with drops.

Box 2.3 Signs of Serious Eye Injury

Sudden decrease vision or blurred vision
Photophobia
Diplopia
Abnormal papillary reaction
Proptosis
Eye pain
Eye redness or ecchymosis
Hyphema

> ▶ **HINT:** Diplopia can be unilateral or bilateral depending on the mechanism of injury.

MEDICAL/SURGICAL INTERVENTIONS

- **What is the initial management of intraoral arterial bleeding from penetrating trauma?**
- **Secure airway and pack the throat**

In penetrating injuries, bleeding in the intraoral or pharyngeal tissue may be caused by injury to the carotid artery, internal jugular vein, and/or their branches. With intraoral injuries, secure the airway and pack the throat to control pharyngeal bleeding. Continued blood loss may require an emergent angiography. Deep tongue lacerations may cause injury to the lingual artery and require suturing of the arterial laceration.

> ▶ **HINT:** Blood from the oral cavity can be aspirated or swallowed.

■ *What is the preferred method for obtaining an airway in a trauma patient with significant injuries?*

■ **Endotracheal intubation**

Mask ventilation of a facial trauma may be difficult and advanced airways may be indicated. Securing an airway following facial trauma is best performed with endotracheal intubation, if possible.

> ▶ **HINT:** In patients with maxillofacial trauma and airway obstruction, emergency cricothyroidotomy can be performed to temporarily obtain an airway.

■ *Following an ocular injury, what is used to reduce eye movement to facilitate healing?*

■ **Eye patch**

An eye patch or shield is used to reduce movement of the affected eye. This is used with retinal injuries to allow healing. Eye patches and shields may also be used to protect the affected eye from light if photophobic. Any impaled objects in the eye should be stabilized and the unaffected eye patched.

> ▶ **HINT:** A suspected or open-globe injury should not be covered with a patch because of the resulting pressure on the globe.

NURSING INTERVENTIONS

■ *A patient presents to the emergency room bleeding profusely from a scalp laceration. What would be an appropriate nursing intervention to control the blood loss?*

■ **Maintain direct pressure**

To limit blood loss, trauma nurses can attempt to control blood loss from facial or scalp wounds with direct pressure or pressure dressings.

> ▶ **HINT:** A stapler or stitches may be required on the scalp or facial laceration for quick control of blood loss until formal repair may be done.

■ *What is the cosmetic risk of inadequate cleansing of facial wounds?*

■ **Scarring**

Cleansing of the debris from facial abrasions is important to prevent the embedding of the debris called *tattooing*. Contamination of foreign debris can cause deep tissue infections, which destroy the tissue and affect the tissue's ability to reconstruct. When cleaning, only debride dead tissue because compromised tissue may still survive in this highly vascular area. Large foreign bodies imbedded in the scalp and face need to be removed to prevent cellulitis and abscesses.

> ▶ **HINT:** Do not shave eyebrows. They can serve as landmarks for approximation of wound edges in the upper face and may not grow back.

■ *What is an appropriate nursing intervention to control epistaxis following a nasal fracture?*

■ **Direct pinch pressure**

The trauma nurse can attempt to control epistaxis with direct pinch pressure on the nose for about 10 to 30 minutes without release, which is usually sufficient. If this fails to control the bleeding, nasal packing can be used. Posterior epistaxis requires posterior packing or balloon tamponade. Nonsurgical management of nasal fracture may include butterfly stitches placed across the dorsum of the nose or a moldable thermoplast nasal splint applied within 1 week.

> ▶ **HINT:** The trauma nurse assessing the function of the nose can occlude one side and have the patient sniff through the other nostril. Compare both sides for the ability to pass air.

■ *Which complication of facial injuries would require immediate surgical intervention?*

■ **Airway obstruction**

Airway obstruction is a life-threatening complication of facial fractures and requires securing a surgical airway.

■ *What is the primary intervention for managing ocular chemical injuries?*

■ **Irrigation**

Copious, continuous irrigation with a crystalloid solution, such as normal saline, should begin immediately following exposure to chemical solutions to the eye.

> ▶ **HINT:** Neutralization with causative agents is not recommended with ocular chemical injuries.

■ *What is the recommended position to place the patient in following an ocular injury resulting in an increase intraocular pressure?*

■ **Elevate the head of bed (HOB)**

A patient with elevated intraocular pressure should be placed with the HOB elevated to assist in lowering the pressure. If unable to elevate the HOB, place the patient in a reverse Trendelenburg position.

> ▶ **HINT:** Instruct the patient to avoid the Valsalva maneuver, coughing, or bending forward following ocular trauma and increased intraocular pressures.

■ *When would it be contraindicated to instill eye drops following an ocular trauma?*

■ **Global rupture**

Instillation of eye drops may be used to manage pain, infection, or inflammation but is contraindicated in open globe injuries. Corneal injuries are managed with normal saline drops or artificial tears to keep the cornea moist and prevent further injury.

> ▶ **HINT:** The eye may be covered with a sterile, moist saline eye-patch to prevent corneal drying and injury.

COMPLICATIONS

■ *A patient with facial fractures presents to the emergency room with nasal drainage. What is the potential complication in this patient?*

■ **Cerebrospinal fluid (CSF) leak**

Facial fractures can result in basal skull fractures and dural tears, causing a CSF leak. Signs of dural involvement in facial fractures include pneumocephalus and CSF. CSF may leak from the nose, ears, or from the facial lacerations.

> ▶ **HINT:** Pneumocephalus is diagnosed with a noncontrast CT scan and is demonstrated by air in the cranium (not just in the sinuses).

■ *What is the most commonly associated injury with a LeFort I fracture?*

■ **Loose or broken teeth**

Loose or broken teeth are complications of maxillary fractures. Following a LeFort I fracture, the upper jaw and mouth are inspected for loose, broken, or missing teeth; open sockets; palate defects; and broken or missing dentures.

> ▶ **HINT:** A sign of a LeFort I fracture includes malocclusion of teeth.

■ *What is a long-term complication of a LeFort II fracture?*

■ **Loss of smell**

Damage to the olfactory nerve may cause temporary and permanent loss of smell.

> ▶ **HINT:** One of the signs of loss of smell is the inability to taste food.

■ *What is a potential complication of an injury damaging the medial canthus of the eyes?*

■ **Disruption of the lacrimal duct**

Injury near the medial canthus raises the suspicion of a potential lacrimal duct injury. Disruption of the lacrimal duct leads to epiphora or tear overflow, which is a result of outflow obstruction. Repair of lacrimal duct injury includes cannulation of the lacrimal duct with a silastic tube that remains in place for 3 to 6 months. This is called *dacryocystorhinostomy*.

> ▶ **HINT:** Excessive tearing and the appearance of a "pug" nose indicate injury to the medial canthus and lacrimal ducts.

■ *A laceration across the cheek presents with clear fluid drainage. What is the most likely injury or complication of the laceration?*

■ **Parotid duct injury**

Parotid duct (also called *Stenson's duct*) injuries may occur with wounds to the cheek or submental region. A cheek laceration can cause injury to the parotid ducts, resulting in clear fluid draining from the laceration. The parotid duct arises deep within the parotid gland and emerges from the superior third of the gland and then courses below the zygomatic arch into the buccal space entering the oral cavity. Treatment of a parotid duct injury is to temporarily cannulate with a silastic tube or repair with primary reanastomosis, ductal ligation, or placement of an interposition graft. Disruption of a parotid duct without repair may result in a parotid fistula or sialocele (salivary cutaneous fistula) (Box 2.4).

▶ **HINT:** CN VII (facial nerve) travels through the parotid gland and can be injured in lacerations and penetrating injuries.

Box 2.4 Complications of Traumatic Facial Injury

Traumatic Injury	Complications
Nasal fracture	Epistaxis, occluded nasal passages, hematoma nasal septum, CSF leak, abscesses
Zygomatic fracture	Malunion, endopthalmos, diplopia
Mandibular fracture	Airway obstruction, fragmentation of bone and teeth,
Oral cavity injury	Airway obstruction, traumatic brain injury, abscess, hematoma, CN dysfunctions

CN, cranial nerve; CSF, cerebrospinal fluid.

■ *Which causes greater damage to the eye: an alkali or an acid chemical burn?*

■ **Alkali**

Chemical injuries to the eye can be caused by either exposure to an alkali or acid substance. An alkali substance disrupts the cell membrane causing rapid penetration of the substance and extensive, severe tissue injury. Acidic substances do not penetrate the tissue and cause less injury and tissue damage, but can still cause corneal damage.

▶ **HINT:** Signs of chemical injury to the eye include corneal opacification, pain, and eyelid swelling.

■ *Following a corneal abrasion, the patient returns to the emergency department with the complaint of an increasing gray spot in the affected eye. What is the most likely complication?*

■ **Corneal infection**

A corneal infection is a potential complication following a corneal abrasion or injury. Corneal abrasions are frequently treated with antibiotics to lower the risk of infection. Symptoms of a corneal infection are increased pain in the affected eye and an enlargement of the grey area on the cornea. Infection can cause a permanent decrease in visual acuity, and incomplete healing can result in recurring attacks of eye pain, tearing, and photophobia.

▶ **HINT:** If a foreign body is left and not removed, it becomes a nidus of infection.

Questions

1. On receiving a trauma patient with facial trauma the airway should be closely inspected and assessed by checking for all of the following except:

   A. Vocalization
   B. Presence of loose teeth or foreign objects
   C. Chin-lift maneuver
   D. Presence of blood or secretions

2. When assessing a patient with facial injuries from a trauma, the trauma nurse should assess for symmetry and for the presence of edema or swelling. Which of the following is *not* a sign of a possible facial fracture?

   A. Discoloration or bruising on face
   B. Loss of ability to open jaw
   C. Loss of corneal reflexes
   D. Loss of facial tissue

3. Ms. Ruiz comes into the emergency room with a facial laceration from a piece of glass. The laceration is deep and clear fluid is leaking out of the site. What is the most likely type of injury sustained?

   A. Posterior table fracture with dural injury
   B. Pneumocephalus
   C. Maxillary fracture
   D. Mandible fracture

4. Scalp and facial lacerations can result in significant blood loss because of dense vasculature. All of the following are ways to address this injury except:

   A. Pressure dressing
   B. Holding direct pressure
   C. Stapler
   D. Skin adhesives

5. What medication would not be appropriate to use when cleansing a deep facial laceration?

   A. Normal saline
   B. Antibiotic solution
   C. Hydrogen peroxide
   D. Lidocaine

6. A patient sustains a large wound to the forehead and left eyebrow. The nurse is cleansing the wound and prepping to suture the site. The nurse delegates retrieval of needed supplies to the paramedic. The nurse requests normal saline, lidocaine, gauze, a suture set, sutures, and a razor. Which of these is an inappropriate request?

A. Lidocaine
B. Suture set
C. Normal Saline
D. Razor

7. The nurse receives a patient with a maxillofacial injury. Which of the following is *not* a recommended nursing intervention for the care of this patient?

   A. Place the patient in High-Fowler's position
   B. Place an orogastric tube
   C. Apply warm compress to the face
   D. Control external bleeding with direct pressure

8. A patient comes in with a nasal injury. Edema is clearly noted and the patient is experiencing significant epistaxis. The nurse has been applying direct pressure by pinching the nose for the past 25 minutes without control of bleeding. Which of the following interventions is *not* appropriate in this situation?

   A. Cauterization
   B. Balloon tamponade
   C. Ribbon gauze impregnated with petroleum jelly packing
   D. Surgical reduction of the nose

9. A hematoma of the septum can cause severe deformity and complications. Which of the following is *not* actually caused by the hematoma in the septum?

   A. Severe deformity of septum
   B. Abscess in nasal passage
   C. Central nervous system (CNS) infection
   D. Cerebrospinal fluid (CSF) leak

10. Cranial nerve (CN) I is located in the nasoorbitalethmoidal (NOE) region and it should be assessed with all of the following acquired injuries except a(n):

    A. Cribriform fracture
    B. Orbital roof fracture
    C. Maxillary fracture
    D. Frontal lobe injury

11. A 32-year-old man was hit in the left eye by a baseball during practice. He initially sustained an orbital hematoma. The patient now returns to the emergency room with complaints of decreased vision in the left eye and a loss of color vision. Which of the following mechanisms of injury best describes this patient's traumatic optic nerve injury?

    A. Indirect injury to the optic nerve
    B. Direct injury to the optic nerve
    C. Blunt force directly to the optic nerve
    D. Penetrating injury to the optic nerve

12. Mr. Henry comes to the emergency room with an impaled stick in the eye, which occurred while hiking. The impaled stick was removed by the patient before arrival. The patient is noted to have a hyphema and restricted extraocular movements. Which of the following injuries should the trauma nurse suspect based on the clinical findings?

    A. Direct brain injury
    B. Internal carotid injury
    C. Cerebrospinal fluid (CSF) leak
    D. Orbital fracture

13. When a patient suffers an ocular trauma, it is important for the nurse to obtain a thorough history. Which of the following questions would *not* be an important inquiry for this type of patient?

    A. Does the patient have blepharospasm?
    B. Does the patient have dysphonia?
    C. Has the patient ever had eye surgery?
    D. Does the patient wear glasses or contact lenses?

14. A patient comes in with periorbital ecchymosis from a baseball hitting the orbit. The nurse is assessing the patient's vision, eye movement, pupil size and reaction, and conjunctiva. What is missing from the nurse's assessment in this injury?

    A. Applying direct pressure to assess for globe stability
    B. Inverting eyelid and looking for lacerations
    C. Performing a halo test
    D. Presence of enophthalmos

15. A patient with a zygomatic fracture can present with all of the following except:

    A. Pain with opening of the mouth
    B. Frontal view as the appearance of a flattened cheekbone
    C. Rounded medial palpebral fissure
    D. Palpable step-off deformity

16. In this particular facial fracture, airway assessment is vital because the tongue can lose control and occlude the airway. What is this type of fracture?

    A. Mandibular fracture
    B. Zygomatic fracture
    C. Oral cavity injury
    D. Nasoorbitalethmoidal (NOE) injury

17. Mr. Carrington attempted suicide by shooting himself in the mouth with a pistol. Bullet wounds penetrating the pharyngeal area carry a risk of damaging the carotid artery. What should be the order of events to take care of this patient?

    A. Pack the throat to control bleeding, intubate the patient, and send for angiography
    B. Send for angiography, intubate the patient, and pack the throat to control bleeding
    C. Intubate the patient, pack the throat to control bleeding, and send for angiography
    D. Intubate the patient, send for angiography, and pack the throat to control bleeding

18. Complications of a patient who sustains an oral cavity injury can be extensive. Which of the following is *not* considered a complication that can occur following oral cavity trauma?

    A. Massive hemorrhage
    B. Aneurysm formation
    C. Cerebrospinal fluid (CSF) leak
    D. Injury to cranial nerve (CN) III

19. A soft tissue injury to the lateral side of the face was suffered after a patient got hit in the face with a hockey puck. Clear fluid is leaking from the wound. Why is this symptom occurring?

    A. Injury to the parotid gland or the parotid duct
    B. Injury to the sublingual gland
    C. Injury to the submandibular gland
    D. Injury to the submandibular and Stensen duct

20. The face is anatomically divided into three areas. Which of the three areas include the zygoma, maxilla, and the nasal bones?

    A. Upper third
    B. Middle third
    C. Lower third
    D. None of the above

21. A 16-year-old patient got hit in the mouth with a softball. The patient is experiencing epistaxis, swelling, and missing teeth. How would the nurse assess the patient for a possible LeFort type I fracture?

    A. Rock the maxilla back and forth and watch for movement of the midface.
    B. Face separation from the cranium is noted on rocking the maxilla.
    C. Rock the maxilla to assess whether the maxilla is independent from the remainder of the face.
    D. Place two fingers in the lower jaw and assess whether it moves freely.

22. The LeFort II fracture is a LeFort I fracture with the addition of which of the following facial fractures?

    A. Mandible
    B. Zygomaticomaxillary complex
    C. Ethmoid sinus
    D. Lateral orbital wall

23. Which of the following is more commonly associated with a LeFort III fracture than a LeFort II fracture?

    A. Loss of consciousness
    B. Cerebrospinal fluid (CSF) leaks
    C. Risk of airway obstruction
    D. Orbital fractures

24. Which of the following x-ray procedures position the patient's nose and chin against the x-ray plate to identify injuries to maxillofacial bones?

    A. Caldwell's view
    B. Water's view
    C. Lateral view
    D. Mandible view

25. All of the following are examples of complications resulting from facial trauma except:

    A. Aspiration pneumonia
    B. Loss of vision
    C. Loss of hearing
    D. Hemorrhage

26. A trauma patient suffered a facial injury with damage to cranial nerve (CN) VII (facial) nerve. The trauma nurse is providing education to the patient regarding expectations following reanastomosis of the nerve. Which of the following would be incorrect information?

    A. It may take up to 2 years to recover function
    B. Routine use of artificial tears is recommended
    C. Eyelids may be taped shut after surgery
    D. Facial, sensory, and motor losses postoperatively are permanent

27. Which of the following is the most likely method for treating a parotid duct injury?

    A. Tube cannulation for 3 to 6 months
    B. Removal of the duct
    C. Bypass procedure
    D. Self-limiting, does not require intervention

28. Mr. Gold was injured in a collision with another person while playing football. He is drooling, lethargic, and noted to have stridor. His face appears elongated. Which of the following is the priority for this patient's obvious facial trauma?

    A. Obtaining a CT scan for a suspected brain injury
    B. Obtaining an airway
    C. Assessing for a cerebrospinal fluid (CSF) leak
    D. Assessing for a subconjunctival hemorrhage

29. Which of the following is *not* true regarding surgical interventions for facial fractures?

    A. The primary treatment is wiring
    B. The primary treatment is open reduction with internal fixation
    C. Surgical procedures may be delayed for up to 1 week
    D. Titanium is the choice of metal for craniofacial plates

30. Which of the following is a common mechanism for ocular injuries?

    A. Motor vehicle collision (MVC)
    B. Thermal injuries
    C. Machinery
    D. Firearms

31. This patient has experienced a mild traumatic brain injury. Following the injury, the patient is complaining of ocular pain, tearing, redness, blurred vision, and a headache. Which of the following is most likely the cause for the presenting symptoms?

A. Subconjunctival hemorrhage
B. Corneal abrasion
C. Choroidal hemorrhage
D. Retinal necrosis

32. Which of the following is an ocular injury that may occur as a result of blunt force trauma to the head and is associated with traumatic brain injury?

A. Choroidal hemorrhage
B. Commotio retinae
C. Retinal necrosis
D. Corneal abrasions

33. The trauma nurse is caring for a patient in the burn unit following a burn to the face from a grease fire. The patient's eyelids are burned. Which of the following complications would *not* be experienced because of this injury?

A. Exposure of the cornea and ocular surface
B. Corneal abrasions
C. Contraction of the eyelids
D. Hymphema

34. Orbital floor fracture acquired from low-impact trauma that occurs without an orbital rim fracture is commonly called?

A. Pure orbital floor fracture
B. Impure orbital flood fracture
C. Blow out fracture
D. LeFort I fracture

35. A patient has an orbital blowout fracture. This injury has caused entrapment of the ocular muscles and extraocular eye movements are restrained. The nurse explains the procedure that is going to be performed to determine the presence and severity of the entrapment. Which of the following is the correct process for this injury?

A. Oral antibiotics and nasal decongestants
B. Needle decompression of the ocular muscle
C. Reconstruction of the orbital floor and medial wall with mesh, synthetic orbital plates, or bone grafting.
D. Forceps used to grab the rectus muscle and rotate the globe in all directions

36. A patient presents with an obvious orbital injury. Radiographic studies confirm an orbital injury. The patient is light-headed, awake, nauseous, and has vomited once. The patient's heart rate is 52 beats per minute (bpm) and blood pressure is 128/94 mmHg.

The nurse knows that there is an immediate need for an evaluation for possible surgical intervention because the patient:

A. Most likely has entrapment of extraocular muscles
B. Has signs of oculocardiac reflex
C. Most likely has an intracranial hemorrhage
D. Has symptoms of retrobulbar hemorrhage

37. Mr. Jacobs comes to the nurse postoperatively after orbital floor reconstruction surgery from a traumatic orbital fracture. The nurse knows that the postoperative care of the patient is important because of the increased risk of retrobulbar hemorrhage. All of the following would be medications that may be administered to prevent this complication except:

A. Stool softeners
B. Antiemetics
C. Beta blockers
D. Anticoagulants

38. A patient presents to the emergency room with corneal abrasion. The nurse is explaining to the orienting new nurse the treatment of this type of injury. Which of the following is a correct statement regarding the treatment for a corneal abrasion injury?

A. Apply a light semi-pressure dressing to the eye
B. Tape the dressing from the forehead to the ear
C. Administer oral antibiotics for 14 days
D. Apply a firm-pressure dressing to the eye

39. A patient presented in the emergency room because of increased eye pain. The patient reports that fragments of sawdust entered his eye last week. On examination, there is an enlarged gray area on the corneal surface. What is this reflective of?

A. Conjunctivitis
B. Corneal infection
C. Conjunctival infection
D. Corneal abrasion

40. Ocular injury is diagnosed based on a thorough nursing assessment, including an external inspection of the eye, pupillary assessment, and all of the following except:

A. Photo documentation
B. Extraocular eye movement
C. Careful slit-lamp examination
D. Vision acuity measurement

41. A foreign object is suspected in the patient's eye. Which of the following diagnostic studies ordered should be questioned by the trauma nurse?

A. Ultrasound
B. CT
C. X-ray
D. MRI

42. Mr. Shee comes into the emergency room after a boxing injury to the eye. External examination, visual acuity, and pupillary assessment are performed on admission. His tonometry reading is 23 mmHg. Which of the following treatments would be inappropriate for Mr. Shee?

    A. Diamox Sequels
    B. Timolol
    C. Fluvoxamine
    D. Glycerin

43. Ocular injury caused by chemical or thermal burns requires copious irrigation, topical steroids, and antibiotics. Which would be the correct way to irrigate an eye with this type of injury?

    A. Irrigate 1 L of fluid with Morgan lens and test pH; if pH is not neutral, sweep fornices with cotton swab to remove crystallized particles
    B. Irrigate with 500 mL of fluid with Morgan lens, test pH, if pH is not neutral, sweep fornices with cotton swab to remove crystallized particles
    C. Irrigate 1 L of fluid with Lewis lens and test pH; if pH is neutral, sweep fornices with cotton swab to remove crystallized particles
    D. Irrigate 500 mL of fluid with Lewis lens and test pH; if pH is neutral, sweep fornices with cotton swab to remove crystallized particles

44. Which of the following types of chemical burn to the eye has the ability to penetrate deeper tissue and causes damage to the intraocular structures, leading to glaucoma and cataracts?

    A. Acid
    B. Base
    C. Neutral
    D. Corrosive

45. When a nurse receives a patient with an orbital trauma, the eye needs to be shielded for protection until an ophthalmologist can come to evaluate the patient. What is used to shield the eye?

    A. Fox shield
    B. Tungsten shield
    C. Suction shield
    D. Uvex shield

Neck Trauma

MECHANISM OF INJURY

■ *What portion of the neck is the most exposed to a traumatic injury?*

■ **Anterior neck**

The neck is well protected posteriorly with the spine and inferiorly with the chest. The most common areas of neck injuries are the anterior and lateral regions. The larynx and trachea are situated anteriorly, and are the most exposed to injury.

> ▶ **HINT:** The neck is divided into three zones or regions that are used to assist with the assessment of neck injuries (Box 3.1).

Box 3.1 Zones of the Neck

Zone 1	Base of the neck, divided by the thoracic inlet inferiorly and cricoid cartilage superiorly
Zone 2	Midportion of neck and region from cricoid cartilage to the angle of the mandible
Zone 3	Superior aspect of neck, bounded by the angle of the mandible and the base of the skull

■ *What is it called when a person experiences neck pain following sudden flexion–extension of the neck?*

■ **Whiplash**

Whiplash occurs when there is a sudden flexion followed by extension of the neck. This commonly occurs with the mechanism of front-end collision and results in neck pain. The pain originates from the stretching of the ligaments and muscles in the neck region.

> ▶ **HINT:** Bony involvement or more significant injuries have been ruled out before the diagnosis of whiplash.

TRAUMATIC INJURIES

■ *Which is the most anterior structure in the neck that is most commonly injured in neck trauma?*

■ **Trachea**

The trachea and larynx are located most anteriorly, and thus are more commonly involved in injury. The neck is a condensed area with multiple structures that may be involved in the injury. Trauma to the neck can cause airway (trachea), gastrointestinal (esophagus), neurological (spinal cord, phrenic nerve, brachial plexus, and cranial nerves), vascular (carotid artery and jugular vein), glandular (thyroid and parotid), and musculoskeletal injuries.

▶ **HINT:** Understanding the location of each structure can assist the trauma nurse in identifying the issues.

■ *Which of the zones of injury in the neck region present with the most obvious injuries?*
■ **Zone 2**

Zone 2 is the region in which the injuries are more likely to be apparent and less likely to present with occult injuries. The structures in zone 2 are more likely to be symptomatic on admission than the other two zones in the neck region.

▶ **HINT:** Most carotid injuries are associated with zone 2 injuries (Box 3.2).

Box 3.2 Structures at Risk Based on Location of Injury

Zone 1	Great vessels Trachea Esophagus Lung apices Cervical spine Spinal cord Cervical nerve roots
Zone 2	Carotid and vertebral arteries Jugular veins Pharynx Larynx Trachea Esophagus Cervical spine Spinal cord
Zone 3	Salivary gland Parotid gland Esophagus Trachea Vertebral bodies Carotid arteries Jugular vein Cranial nerves

■ *Which of the zones of the neck have the highest morbidity and mortality with injury?*
■ **Zone 1**

Zone 1 injuries are associated with the highest morbidity and mortality and, in general, have the poorest outcomes. Blunt trauma to the neck region causing a vascular injury is also associated with high morbidity and mortality.

▶ **HINT:** Penetrating injuries most commonly affect zone 2 because of accessibility.

ASSESSMENT/DIAGNOSIS

■ *A patient develops hoarseness and hemoptysis following a blunt neck trauma. What is the most likely injury?*

■ **Laryngeal or tracheal injury**

The signs of neck injury are dependent on the region involved in the trauma. Laryngeal and tracheal injuries can present as hoarseness and hemoptysis (Box 3.3).

> ▶ **HINT:** A penetrating injury to the trachea commonly results in a hissing or sucking sound, with froth or bubbling at the site of injury.

Box 3.3 Signs and Symptoms of Neck Injuries

Laryngeal and tracheal injury	Hoarseness Hemoptysis Stridor Drooling Dyspnea
Esophageal and pharyngeal injury	Dysphagia Bloody saliva Bloody nasogastric aspirate
Carotid injury	Decreased level of consciousness Hemiparesis Deviated gaze Facial droop Thrill or bruit
Jugular vein injury	Hematoma Hypotension
Cranial nerve injury	Facial (CN VII) facial drooping Glossopharyngeal (CN IX) dysphagia Vagus nerve (CN X) hoarseness Spinal accessory nerve (CN XI) weak shoulder shrug Hypoglossal nerve (CN XII) deviation of tongue

CN, cranial nerve.

■ *What is the recommended diagnostic study for neck injuries?*

■ **CT scan**

When bone or soft tissue injuries are suspected, CT scans are useful in diagnosing the injuries. Clinically subtle signs of larynx injuries are best recognized with a CT scan. CT angiograms (CTA) can detect vascular injuries in the neck region quickly, although a conventional angiogram produces the most definitive result. Conventional angiograms can be used preoperatively to determine surgical needs, including whether injury is intrathoracic.

> ▶ **HINT:** CTA in hemodynamically stable patients significantly decreases the rate of negative exploration without an increase in missed injuries.

MEDICAL/SURGICAL INTERVENTIONS

■ *What is the priority of care in a neck injury?*

■ **Airway**

Airway and hemorrhage are the two most immediate risks following a neck injury. Obtaining an airway is a priority of care for a patient who has sustained a neck injury. Direct injury to the trachea, either penetrating or blunt, can cause a loss of airway. Swelling in the neck region can compress the trachea, also resulting in the loss of airway. In rare cases, emergency cricothyroidotomy may be required to immediately secure an airway. Excessive vigorous attempts at intubation may worsen the patient's status by causing further injury. Awareness of potential laryngeal injury is important before intubation even when securing an airway in an emergency.

> ▶ **HINT:** Patients with rapidly developing hematomas in the neck should have the airway secured.

■ *Persistence in difficulty of breathing despite intubation and ventilation may indicate what type of injury?*

■ **Pneumothorax**

Signs of respiratory distress even after intubation and ventilation suggest the presence of a pneumothorax. Tracheal injury can result in a pneumothorax or tension pneumothorax. The management includes needle decompression and chest tube placement.

> ▶ **HINT:** If there is a persistent pneumothorax, suspect a tracheal injury.

■ *Which zone of injury in the neck region might require an emergency sternotomy for repair?*

■ **Zone 1**

Injuries located in zone 1 of the neck may require a median sternotomy for repair of intrathoracic injuries. This incision may extend to the sternocleidomastoid or subclavicular regions as well. Endovascular interventions with stent placements have been used in some vascular injuries within this zone.

> ▶ **HINT:** Subluxation or dislocation of the mandible may be required in zone 3 injuries.

NURSING INTERVENTIONS

■ *What is the best way to control hemorrhage in the neck region?*

■ **Direct pressure**

Bleeding from the neck is best controlled by direct pressure. Impaled objects should be left in place until surgical repair is available. It is not recommended to blindly clamp a transected vessel because of the potential damage that can occur to surrounding structures. When the injury is to the pharynx, direct pressure may not adequately control the hemorrhage and may require cricothyroidotomy and packing.

▶ **HINT:** Intravenous (IV) access should be avoided in the affected side because of the potential disruption of ipsilateral venous circulation.

COMPLICATIONS

■ *What is the potential risk if a neck wound is probed or locally explored outside of the operating room?*

■ **Hemorrhage**

It is not recommended to locally explore or probe a traumatic wound to the neck in the emergency room or outside of the operating room. This can result in dislodgement of clots, hemorrhage, and air embolus (Box 3.4).

▶ **HINT:** Placing a patient in mild Trendelenburg position may decrease the risk of air embolization with an open wound to the neck.

Box 3.4 Complications

Hemorrhage/hypovolemic shock
Expanding hematoma
Airway obstruction
Open trachea
Paralysis
Hemoptysis
Hematemesis and aspiration
Air embolus
Arteriovenous fistula
Tracheoinnominate fistula
Esophagocutaneous fistula
Pneumothorax or tension pneumothorax
Infections or sepsis

▶ **HINT:** Oral secretions are a major source of infection in neck wounds.

Questions

1. An 84-year-old woman fell down a flight of stairs; she is currently in a cervical collar and is complaining of neck pain reported as 8 out of a 10-point scale. She remains awake, alert, and oriented. Her vital signs are blood pressure 94/62 mmHg, respiratory rate of 16 and regular, heart rate of 59 beats per minute (bpm), oxygen saturation is 98%, and oral temperature is 98°F. On assessment she is unable to move her lower extremities. The nurse is now suspecting neurogenic shock and the first intervention should be:

   A. Start an IV bolus of normal saline
   B. Start Levophed intravenous drip to keep systolic blood pressure (SBP) greater than 100 mmHg
   C. Place the patient on a nonrebreather mask and prepare for possible intubation
   D. Start a Cardizem drip to keep heart rate greater than 60 bpm

2. A city bus was involved in a collision and four patients present to the emergency department with neck fractures. There is one patient with a C4 injury still on a backboard, another with a T9 fracture and abdominal breathing, one with a C8 fracture, and the last suffered a C6 injury with edema. The nurse should expect which patient(s) to require intubation.

   A. The C4 and C6 injury
   B. The patient with the T9 fracture
   C. The C6 and C8 injury patients
   D. The C4, C8, and T9 patients

3. Mr. Martinez presents to the emergency room after a motor vehicle collision. He is currently maintained with cervical spine precautions. He is awake, alert, oriented, and does not have any tenderness on palpation of the spine. Which would be the most appropriate diagnostic intervention?

   A. Clear cervical spine with physical examination.
   B. Obtain a full set of lateral, odontoid, and flexion–extension x-rays
   C. Obtain a CT scan of the neck
   D. Obtain an MRI of the neck

Part II

Clinical Practice: Trunk

Part II

Clinical Procedures

Thoracic Trauma

MECHANISM OF INJURY

■ *The thoracic cavity extends from the first rib to which structure?*

■ **Diaphragm**

The thoracic cavity extends from the first rib to the diaphragm. The diaphragm level can vary anywhere from the fourth intercostal space (ICS) on exhalation to the lower costal margin (10th rib) on maximal inhalation.

> ▶ **HINT:** A penetrating trauma at the nipple level can result in either chest or abdominal trauma depending on whether the patient took a deep breath in or let a breath out.

■ *A patient presents with a sternal fracture. What is the significance of the injury that the trauma nurse should be aware of?*

■ **Force of impact**

Fracture of the sternum requires a great force of impact so is associated with significant intrathoracic injuries, such as myocardial contusion and aortic dissection. The trauma nurse should be aware of the correlation between the sternal fracture and significant intrathoracic injuries, which may be life threatening.

> ▶ **HINT:** Fractures of ribs 1 to 3, femur, and scapula all require a significant force of impact.

■ *Which kind of mechanism causes an open pneumothorax: blunt or penetrating?*

■ **Penetrating**

An open pneumothorax is caused by penetrating trauma to the chest. It is also called a *sucking chest wound* and is caused by a large defect in the chest wall, causing equilibration of pressures between intrathoracic and atmospheric pressure. An open pneumothorax can also accumulate air in the pleural space during inspiration, leading to profound hypoventilation and hypoxia.

> ▶ **HINT:** If the penetrating wound to the chest is greater than two thirds the diameter of the trachea, air will flow in and out of the wound (least resistance to airflow).

■ *Which side (right or left) of the diaphragm is more likely to be injured following chest trauma?*

■ **Left**

The majority of diaphragm injuries from blunt trauma occur on the left side. The most common blunt injury is large posterior lateral tears on left diaphragm. The right diaphragm may be more protected by the liver and requires a greater force of impact to injure, thus resulting in higher mortality. Lateral impact is the most common mechanism of injury to result in a diaphragm injury on the ipsilateral side.

> ▶ **HINT:** Penetrating injuries to the diaphragm cause small tears and may have a delayed presentation of weeks to years later as the injury enlarges and gradual herniation of stomach or bowel occurs.

■ *What is the most common mechanism of injury that results in a pulmonary contusion?*

■ **Compression–decompression**

The mechanism of injury is commonly a compression–decompression impact on the thoracic cavity. This causes the lungs to be compressed between the anterior chest wall and the thoracic spine, increasing the pressure within the lungs. Contusions are a result of the increased pressure.

> ▶ **HINT:** Pulmonary contusions are commonly associated with chest wall injuries, including rib fractures.

■ *A trauma patient is identified as having a sternal fracture. What cardiac injury is the most common after a significant blunt force impact to the chest?*

■ **Cardiac contusion**

Sternal fractures are commonly associated with cardiac contusions (cardiac injury) and pulmonary contusions (pulmonary injuries; Box 4.1).

> ▶ **HINT:** Any injury that occurs as a result of a significant force of impact to the chest can be associated with myocardial contusion.

Box 4.1 Associated Injuries With Cardiac Contusions

Chest wall bruises
Multiple rib fractures
Flail chest
Sternum fracture
Pulmonary contusion
Pericardial tamponade
Coronary artery laceration
Cardiac valve rupture

■ *What is a common thoracic injury that occurs because of a sudden deceleration mechanism of injury?*

■ **Thoracic aortic transection/aneurysm**

The most common mechanism of injury for a thoracic aortic transection or aneurysm is a sudden deceleration mechanism of injury. The ligamentum arteriosum secures the aorta near the aortic arch, called the *level of the isthmus*. During a sudden deceleration, the aorta moves except at the point of the ligament, causing a transection and, potentially, an aneurysm to form at that level.

> ▶ **HINT:** The deceleration can be horizontal (such as in a motor vehicle injury) or vertical (such as in a fall).

TRAUMATIC INJURIES

■ *What is one of the most common injuries that occurs with a blunt trauma to the chest?*

■ **Rib fracture**

Rib fractures are probably the most common injury in blunt chest trauma. The fractures of ribs 1 through 3 are associated with significant intrathoracic injuries because of the force of impact required to fracture these ribs.

> ▶ **HINT:** Associated injuries with fracture of ribs 1 to 3 may include aortic aneurysms, tracheobronchial, and vascular injuries.

■ *What is an associated injury with the fractures of ribs 10 to 12 on the right side?*

■ **Liver injury**

A fractured rib can be displaced, causing injury to the underlying structures. On the right, ribs 10 to 12 cover the liver and on the left cover the spleen. Fracturing of ribs 10 to 12 can cause injury to liver or spleen, depending on the side involved. Impacting ribs 4 to 12 can cause them to have a "bowing" effect, resulting in a midshaft fracture.

> ▶ **HINT:** Shoulder harness seat belts can cause fractures of ribs 10 to 12. The driver is at a greater risk for right-sided rib fractures and liver injury, whereas the passenger is at a greater risk for spleen injuries.

■ *A patient presents in the emergency department with paradoxical chest wall movement following a motor vehicle collision (MVC). What would be the most likely injury the patient has sustained?*

■ **Flail chest**

A flail chest involves three or more fractures at two or more places resulting in a freely moving segment of chest wall. Paradoxical movement of the chest wall is a hallmark sign in a flail chest (Box 4.2).

> ▶ **HINT:** Sternal fractures may also cause a flail chest and paradoxical chest wall movement.

Box 4.2 Signs of Flail Chest

Dyspnea
Bruising anterior chest wall
Crepitus
Positioning to splint chest wall
Paradoxical chest wall movement

> ▶ **HINT:** Muscle spasms will splint the ribs, making a flail not always readily recognizable. Muscle relaxants will emphasize the presence of flail chest.

■ *An injury to the internal mammary artery can result in what type of injury?*

■ **Hemothorax**

Hemothorax is caused by lung parenchymal lacerations, injuries to intercostal vessels, and injuries to the internal mammary artery. Both blunt and penetrating injuries to the chest can result in hemothorax.

> ▶ **HINT:** Hemothorax is a potential source of significant blood loss.

■ *What is the most common site of injury in the trachea and bronchial area?*

■ **Bifurcation of mainstem bronchus**

Following blunt mechanism to the chest, the most common site of bronchial injury is at the bifurcation of the mainstem bronchus about an inch from the carina. If the injury does occur below the carina, the chest radiograph will show mediastinal air.

> ▶ **HINT:** Injury above the level of the carina can result in a delayed presentation such as unresolved pneumothrorax.

■ *What pulmonary injury is commonly associated with a flail chest?*

■ **Pulmonary contusion**

A blunt force significant enough to cause rib fractures and a flail chest can also cause the capillary vessels within the lungs to rupture, allowing blood to enter the interstitium and alveoli. Inflammation and edema develop in the lungs within a couple of hours after the injury. Lacerations to the lung tissue can also occur.

> ▶ **HINT:** Pulmonary contusions may be small and localized with minimal symptoms, or large, involving one or both lungs with life-threatening symptoms.

■ *Which cardiac chamber is most likely to be injured in a blunt mechanism of injury to the chest?*

■ **Right ventricle**

The right ventricle lies closest to the anterior chest wall and, because of its location, is more commonly injured following a blunt chest trauma. The atria are less commonly injured because they are smaller than the ventricles.

> ▶ **HINT:** The complication of thrombus formation in the cardiac chambers is most common in the right ventricle because of the involvement of the right ventricle in blunt chest injuries.

ASSESSMENT/DIAGNOSIS

■ *What diagnostic examination should be considered in patients with fractures of the first rib?*

■ **Arteriogram**

A diagnostic chest x-ray may have difficulty visualizing the first rib and may miss a fracture in this area. Arteriogram should be considered following fracture of ribs 1 through 3 because the force of impact and the vascular structures underlying those ribs can result in significant arterial injuries, including damage to the subclavian artery or vein.

> ► **HINT:** Clavicle fracture is not usually serious but a jagged edge of the clavicle bone may also injure the subclavian artery or vein.

■ *What is the most definitive diagnosis for a bronchial injury?*

■ **Bronchoscopy**

An injury above the level of the carina may not demonstrate mediastinal air on chest radiograph. The most definitive diagnosis is with a bronchoscopy.

> ► **HINT:** Bronchial injuries are commonly diagnosed by the presence of symptoms.

■ *What is an obvious sign of a diaphragm injury with bowel herniation?*

■ **Bowel sounds in chest**

On assessment, bowel sounds heard in the chest, especially on the left side, indicate a significant diaphragm injury and bowel herniation into the thoracic chest. This is commonly associated with increased work of breathing and diminished breath sounds.

> ► **HINT:** Diaphragmatic injuries are associated with hemothorax. Chest tubes should be placed cautiously to avoid injury to the herniated bowel.

■ *What radiographic examination is most specific to diaphragm injury?*

■ **MRI**

The most prominent feature found on a chest radiograph is elevation of hemidiaphragm and potentially a bowel pattern in the chest.

■ *What is the finding on a chest x-ray that indicates the presence of a pulmonary contusion?*

■ **Infiltrates may be unilateral or bilateral and have the appearance of acute respiratory distress syndrome (ARDS). This is caused by fluid in both the pulmonary parenchyma and alveoli.**

> ► **HINT:** Severe pulmonary contusions can progress into ARDS.

■ *What is the most specific diagnostic study used to identify a thoracic aortic aneurysm?*

■ **Arteriogram**

A chest x-ray is a screening tool used on trauma patients and can identify a widened mediastinum (Box 4.3), but is not specific to a thoracic aortic aneurysm. An arteriogram is recommended to visualize the aorta. An invasive aortagram is the most specific study for an aortic injury but a CT arteriogram is less invasive and is used as a screening tool.

> ▶ **HINT:** The most common site for a traumatic aortic injury is the level of the isthmus.

Box 4.3   Findings on Chest X-Ray for Thoracic Aortic Injury

Widened mediastinum
Loss of aortic knob
Presence of left apical cap

■ *A patient is admitted for 24-hour monitoring following an MVC with a result of a bent steering wheel. What injury may be suspected in this patient?*

■ **Cardiac contusion**

Cardiac arrhythmias, including life-threatening ventricular arrhythmias, may occur following cardiac contusion and require cardiac monitoring for at least 24 hours.

> ▶ **HINT:** Other workup of a patient with suspected cardiac contusion includes 12-lead EKG, cardiac enzymes, and an echocardiogram.

■ *What diagnostic technique is commonly used to evaluate the chest for the presence of pericardial blood?*

■ **Focused assessment sonography for trauma (FAST) technique**

FAST is an ultrasound technique used to evaluate both abdominal and thoracic cavities. It is used to detect the presence of blood or fluid (effusion) in the pericardial space.

> ▶ **HINT:** FAST has the advantage of being able to be performed rapidly in the emergency department for hemodynamically unstable trauma patients.

MEDICAL/SURGICAL INTERVENTIONS

■ *Following the placement of a chest tube in a trauma patient, the nurse notes 1,500 mL of bloody output immediately on placement. What would the nurse expect the physician to do to manage this injury?*

■ **Thoracotomy**

A hemothorax with greater than 1,000 to 1,500 mLs of blood on the initial insertion of a chest tube or greater than 200 mL/hr for 4 hours indicates the need for a thoracotomy. Accumulation of blood in the pleural space with a hemothorax can compromise ventilatory effort by compressing the lung tissue, resulting in hypoxemia as well as hemorrhagic shock as a result of excessive loss of blood.

> ▶ **HINT:** Early surgical management for a large hemothorax is recommended to prevent complications of ongoing blood loss, empyema, and late fibrothorax.

■ *What is the priority of care in patients with diaphragmatic injuries and herniated bowel?*

■ **Airway and breathing**

The herniation of bowel into the chest cavity increases the thoracic pressures and interferes with ventilation. The cornerstone of treatment of diaphragmatic injuries is intubation and ventilation to protect the airway.

> ▶ **HINT:** Placement of a nasogastric tube can assist with decompression of the bowel and limit herniation.

■ *What type of mechanical ventilation may be considered in trauma patients with severe unilateral pulmonary contusion and severe hypoxemia?*

■ **Independent lung ventilation (ILV)**

ILV is considered in patients with significant unilateral pulmonary contusion and severe hypoxemia that cannot be corrected. Positive end-expiratory pressure (PEEP) is recommended in managing patients with pulmonary contusions, but in patients with unilateral lung involvement, the unaffected lung can become overdistended and the affected lung underventilated. This is called *maldistribution of ventilation*.

> ▶ **HINT:** Pressure control modes of ventilation and high-frequency oscillatory ventilation (HFOV) may be used in patients with bilateral pulmonary contusions who have failed with conventional ventilation.

■ *Following a paracentesis, the blood aspirated is placed in a container and agitated. It does not form clots. This indicates the blood was aspirated from which space?*

■ **Pericardial space**

Blood aspirated from the pericardial space is defibrinated, so the blood does not clot. If the needle would have punctured the ventricle and aspirated blood is from the ventricular chamber, then the blood will clot.

> ▶ **HINT:** Blood from the pleural space is defibrinated and does not clot.

■ *A patient with cardiac contusion becomes hypotensive. What pharmacological intervention may be used to improve the patient's hemodynamic status?*

■ **Dobutamine (Dobutrex)**

Dobutamine is a positive inotropic agent that increases myocardial contractility. Patients with cardiac contusion frequently experience decreases in myocardial contractility and ejection fractions. Improving contractility will improve blood pressure and hemodynamics.

> ▶ **HINT:** Administering vasoconstrictive agents to increase blood pressures in patients with cardiac contusions may actually worsen their hemodynamics because of the increase in resistance (afterload) on the heart.

■ *A patient with a thoracic aortic injury presents to the intensive care unit with a blood pressure of 194/98 mmHg and a heart rate of 106 beats per minute. The trauma nurse would expect that the physician would order which class of medication to lower the patient's blood pressure?*

■ **Beta-blocker**

A beta-blocker will block adrenergic activity and lower the blood pressure. This will lower the risk of further injury to the aorta and aortic rupture. Beta-blockers decrease the heart rate, also limiting injury to the aorta. Alpha-blockers, such as nipride, will lower the blood pressure but cause a reflex tachycardia that may worsen the aortic injury.

> ▶ **HINT:** Esmolol is a beta-blocker that is short acting and titratable. It is commonly used to manage the blood pressure in patients with traumatic aortic aneurysms.

■ *In a suspected tension pneumothorax, what intervention can be performed before a chest tube can be placed?*

■ **Needle thoracentesis**

If the patient is suspected of having a tension pneumothorax and is hemodynamically unstable, a needle thoracentesis can be performed to rapidly reverse the life-threatening symptoms. The 14-gauge (G) needle is placed in the second ICS, midclavicular on the affected side.

> ▶ **HINT:** The definitive treatment of tension pneumothorax is the placement of a chest tube to decompress the pneumothorax.

■ *What is a concern of intubating a patient with tracheobronchial injury?*

■ **Further injury**

The blind placement of an endotracheal tube on a patient with a tracheobronchial injury can cause further injury. A flexible bronchoscope can be useful in guiding the placement of the endotracheal tube, limiting the risk of further injury.

> ▶ **HINT:** Positive pressure mechanical ventilation can worsen the pnuemothorax by forcing air into the pleural space.

NURSING INTERVENTIONS

■ *What is the primary goal for managing a patient with rib fractures?*

■ **Pain management**

Management of rib fractures includes pain management, usually with oral analgesics, including opioids, nerve blocks, epidural, or intrapleural analgesia if pain is severe.

> ▶ **HINT:** In patients with flail chest, administration of analgesia will decrease pain and may relax the intercostal muscles, making paradoxical chest wall movement of flail more obvious.

■ *During assessment of a trauma patient in the emergency room, the nurse notes diminished breath sounds on the left side with dullness to percussion. What is the most likely cause?*

■ **Hemothorax**

If diminished breath sounds on the affected side are found, it indicates a collapsed lung and is commonly found with a pneumothorax. The presence of dullness on percussion indicates the presence of fluid or blood such as a hemothorax. A pneumothorax will have hyperresonance with percussion over the affected side.

> ▶ **HINT:** Clinical presentation of hemothorax includes dullness to percussion, decreased breath sounds on affected side, and flat neck veins resulting from blood loss.

■ *What type of dressing is recommended to manage an open-sucking chest wound before definitive treatment?*

■ **Three-sided dressing**

A three-sided dressing works as a flutter valve. It allows air to leave but not to reenter the pleural space. An occlusive dressing could result in a tension pneumothorax.

> ▶ **HINT:** A flutter valve may also be used to manage the open pneumothorax.

■ *Following a blunt chest injury, a patient in the trauma intensive care unit demonstrates subcutaneous air, cough, hemoptysis, and persistent subcutaneous emphysema. What is the most likely injury?*

■ **Bronchial injury**

Symptoms of a bronchial injury may be delayed by several days after injury. Bronchial injury commonly recognized by the symptoms, especially an unresolving pneumothorax (Box 4.4).

> ▶ **HINT:** Tracheobronchial injuries are more likely to be caused by a penetrating trauma and should cause a high suspicion.

Box 4.4   Symptoms of Tracheobronchial Injuries

Noisy breathing
Dyspnea
Airway obstruction
Hemoptysis
Cough
Hoarseness
Subcutaneous emphysema: neck, face, or suprasternal
Progressive mediastinal air
Persistent pneumothorax
Tension pneumothorax

■ *A patient in the emergency room presents with a penetrating trauma of the left chest. If the patient continues to be unresponsive to fluids and remains hemodynamically unstable, then the trauma nurse should suspect which injury?*

■ **Pericardial tamponade**

Penetrating trauma is the most common mechanism of injury for pericardial tamponades. A pericardial tamponade commonly presents with hemodynamic instability despite adequate fluid resuscitation. The development of tamponade produces a reduction of filling of ventricles during diastole and a decrease in output.

> ▶ **HINT:** Cardiac tamponade is caused by bleeding into the pericardial sac caused by a ruptured coronary artery, lacerated pericardium, or an injury to the myocardium in trauma patients.

■ *What is considered the Beck's triad associated with cardiac tamponade?*

■ **Increased jugular venous distension, hypotension, and muffled heart sounds**

The increased jugular venous distension is caused by impedance to filling the ventricle during diastole, hypotension is caused by decrease in cardiac output, and muffled heart sounds occur because of the accumulation of blood in the pericardial sac. If the patient has other associated injuries with significant blood loss, the jugular venous distension will be absent (Box 4.5).

> ▶ **HINT:** Diminished amplitude of the QRS complex may also be associated with pericardial tamponade because of the fluid collection around the heart.

Box 4.5 Symptoms of Pericardial Tamponade

Increased jugular venous distension
Hypotension
Muffled or distant heart sounds
Pulsus paradoxus
Pulsus alternans
Cyanosis
Dyspnea
Pulseless electrical activity (PEA)
Tachycardia
Pericardial friction rub

> ▶ **HINT:** Pulsus paradoxus is the decrease in systolic blood pressure during inspiration, whereas pulsus alternans is an alternating weak and strong pulse.

■ *A trauma patient is admitted to the trauma intensive care unit following a blunt trauma to the chest. The patient was intubated in the emergency room and is on a mechanical ventilator. One day posttrauma, the nurse notes an increase in peak inspiratory pressures (PIP). What would be the most likely cause?*

■ **Pulmonary contusion**

The combination of atelectasis, blood and fluid, and interstitial edema produces a decrease in pulmonary compliance and an increase in peak inspiratory pressures. The findings of pulmonary contusions frequently occur within 24 to 48 hours after injury and are commonly associated with a blunt chest injury. The triad of physiological changes associated with pulmonary contusion is hypoxemia, intrapulmonary shunting, and reduced pulmonary compliance (Box 4.6).

> ▶ **HINT:** ARDS may also present with an increase in PIP but will commonly occur 48 to 72 hours after a traumatic injury.

Box 4.6 Symptoms of Pulmonary Contusion

Shortness of breath
Diffuse crackles
Tachypnea
Hypocarbia
Blood-tinged or bloody sputum
Wheezes
Increased work of breathing
Increased peak airway pressures
Infiltrates on chest x-ray
Tachycardia
Hypoxemia

- ■ *Following fluid resuscitation and patient stabilization, what is the most appropriate fluid management to prevent worsening of pulmonary contusions?*
- ■ **Limit fluid intake**

Trauma patients should not have excessive restrictions of fluid replacement while the patient is unstable and requiring fluid to manage hemodynamics. After the trauma patient is stabilized hemodynamically, then restriction of fluids may limit pulmonary contusions and associated complications.

> ▶ **HINT:** Restricting fluids initially in a hemodynamically unstable patient following a trauma can significantly decrease tissue perfusion and worsen outcomes.

- ■ *A driver of a motor vehicle involved in a front-end collision suddenly develops short runs of ventricular tachycardia. What would be the most likely cause of the arrhythmias?*
- ■ **Cardiac contusion**

Complications of myocardial contusions include arrhythmias. These arrhythmias can range from supraventricular tachycardia and rapid ventricular response atrial fibrillation to lethal ventricular arrhythmias. Atrioventriclular (AV) blocks may also be associated with cardiac contusions (Box 4.7).

> ▶ **HINTS:** The most common arrhythmia with myocardial contusion is sinus tachycardia. Cardiac contusion can cause signs of decreased perfusion to tissues because of the decrease in ejection fraction and cardiac output.

Box 4.7   Signs of Cardiac Contusion

Tachycardia
Decreased urine output
Hypotension
Chest pain
Increased jugular venous distention
Arrhythmias
ST segment changes (elevation)
T-wave changes

■ *A patient with multiple rib fractures on the right is noticed to have rapid shallow breathing and limited movement. What is the most appropriate intervention by the trauma nurse?*

■ **Provide pain management**

Patients with multiple rib fractures experience significant pain and breathing deeply increases the painful response. Managing the patient's pain can allow the patient to breath deeper and more effectively with less splinting. Splinting places the patient at an increased risk for atelectasis and pneumonia.

> ▶ **HINT:** The use of multimodal pain management is recommended to manage pain to allow deeper breathing without the respiratory depression of opioids.

COMPLICATIONS

■ *What is the life-threatening complication of a pneumothorax?*

■ **Tension pneumothorax**

In a tension pneumothorax, the air builds in the pleural space, becomes trapped, and the increased pressure causes the mediastinum to shift. The shifting of the mediastinal structures causes the compression of the aorta and inferior vena cava. This results in a life-threatening hemodynamic instability. Needle decompression, with 14- to 18-gauge angiocath at the second to third ICS midclavicular, is the emergency treatment until a chest tube can be placed.

> ▶ **HINT:** The trauma nurse should palpate the trachea for deviation. The trachea will be deviated away from the side of the tension pneumothorax.

■ *What is a long-term pulmonary complication of pulmonary contusions?*

■ **Pulmonary fibrosis**

Contused lungs from trauma commonly demonstrate fibrosis on chest x-ray within 1 to 6 years after injury. The vital capacity and air volumes are also significantly decreased because of the fibrosis. Patients with pulmonary contusions are more likely to develop ARDS.

> ▶ **HINT:** The fibrosis can also be found in ARDS, which has very similar physiological effects following the injury or insult.

■ *An echocardiogram may be used to evaluate a patient with a myocardial contusion several days after injury. What late complication of a cardiac contusion can be identified with an echocardiogram?*

■ **Intracardiac thrombus**

The decrease in contractility and ejection fraction, which occurs with contusion of the myocardium, can lead to blood stasus in the cardiac chambers and thrombus formation. The use of echocardiogram can identify the thrombus in the cardiac chambers. The identification of depression of myocardial contractility and cardiogenic shock can be identified early with echocardiogram and are complications of cardiac contusion.

> ▶ **HINT:** Transesophageal echocardiogram is more sensitive than a transthoracic approach in identifying intracardiac thrombus.

■ *A trauma patient experiences pulseless electrical activity (PEA) during fluid resuscitation. What traumatic injury is most likely to have occurred?*

■ **Pericardial tamponade**

One of the causes of PEA is pericardial tamponade. This is caused by the pericardial restriction of the heart, which limits filling of the cardiac chambers and the ability for mechanical contractility. Electrical activity is not affected so the patient has a discernable rhythm on the monitor, but no mechanical activity.

> ▶ **HINT:** Pericardial tamponade is considered to be a constrictive cardiomyopathy.

■ *Which blunt cardiac injury has one of the highest mortalities?*

■ **Cardiac rupture**

Blunt forces to the chest increase the intrathoracic pressure resulting in the rupture of a cardiac chamber. This carries a high mortality. Transection of the ascending aorta is fatal in most cases.

> ▶ **HINT:** Emergency thoracotomy on a patient with blunt trauma cardiac arrest is rarely successful.

Questions

1. The nurse receives a patient following a motor vehicle collision. The driver was unrestrained and the airbag did not deploy. The patient has a respiratory rate of 42 breaths per minute, obvious paradoxical movement of the chest wall, and presents in severe respiratory distress requiring intubation. The nurse is suspecting what type of injury?

   A. Three or more fractures in two or more places
   B. Fracture of the sternum
   C. Rib fractures involving ribs 4 to 6
   D. Clavicle fracture

2. A patient was stabbed in the right lateral chest. The patient presents in the emergency department moaning in pain and breathing 40 breaths per minute. The nurse finds the patient has hyperresonance on the right side. After radiographic studies are completed, it is confirmed that a pneumothorax is present on the right. The nurse assists in setting up for chest-tube insertion. After the chest tube is placed, the nurse notes that there is continuous bubbling in the water-seal chamber. Which of the following is the best method for the nurse to use to address this problem?

   A. Place the chest tube below the level of the chest to facilitate drainage
   B. Pinch the chest tube at the insertion site and determine whether the bubbling stops
   C. Replace the chest drainage unit immediately
   D. Obtain a chest x-ray immediately

3. Rib and sternal fractures are commonly associated with other severe injuries. Which of the following correctly matches the location of the injury to the associated complications?

   A. Left lower rib fractures and hepatic lacerations
   B. Right lower rib fractures and splenic rupture
   C. Sternal fracture with cardiac contusion
   D. Left lower rib fracture with great vessel injuries

4. A patient presents to the emergency department with dysphonia and dyspnea after aspirating a fish bone. The physician suspects that the patient has a tracheal rupture and begins to prepare for intubation. What is the most definitive way to confirm the diagnosis of a tracheal rupture?

   A. Bronchoscopy
   B. Chest x-ray
   C. CT of the chest
   D. Ultrasound

5. A patient comes into the emergency room after involvement in a motor vehicle collision. The car was traveling at a high speed of about 90 miles per hour and ran into a telephone pole. The patient was unrestrained and there were no airbags in the vehicle. The patient is unresponsive on arrival with a blood pressure of 80/40 mmHg, absent pedal pulses, and bounding radial pulses. There is severe chest wall ecchymosis and a loud systolic murmur. What is this patient's expected injury?

A. Descending aortic injury
B. Pericardial tamponade
C. Blunt cardiac injury
D. Ascending aortic injury

6. A patient comes in after a T-bone motor vehicle collision during which the patient was struck on the right lateral side. The patient has a blood pressure of 91/60 mmHg, a heart rate of 119 beats per minute, with cool, clammy skin. CT of the abdomen revealed a liver laceration with evidence of active bleeding and the CT of the chest revealed widened mediastinum. What is the priority of care in this situation?

A. Control the abdominal hemorrhage
B. Prepare for the operating room for repair of the aortic transection
C. Prepare for a pericardial window to be performed
D. Blood pressure control

7. Which of the following patients presenting with an aortic injury would require immediate surgery to repair the aorta?

A. Patients who need to be transferred to other facilities for treatment
B. Associated severe brain injury
C. Stable injury less than 5 cm
D. Expanding aortic transection

8. Mr. Carson comes into the emergency room with a machete lodged in his chest. He is hypotensive and is displaying pulsus paradoxus. The nurse is actively transfusing the patient with blood products and intravenous fluids are being administered. Mr. Carson now becomes unconscious and cyanotic. Which intervention would be most appropriate in this situation?

A. Pericardiocentesis
B. Expedited transfer to the operating room
C. Open thoracotomy
D. Obtain an emergency arteriogram of the aorta

9. A patient with a pulmonary contusion has a decrease in pulmonary compliance and an increase in airway pressures. This is related to all of the following except:

A. Interstitial edema
B. Hypercarbia
C. Atelectasis
D. Presence of blood and fluid

10. A patient who suffered a femur fracture is 2 days postoperative and begins to report chest pain on inspiration. The nurse assesses the patient and discovers an oxygen saturation of 92% on 2 L via nasal cannula, a respiratory rate of 27 breaths per minute, and a heart rate of 112 beats per minute. All of the following imaging studies may be used to diagnose a pulmonary embolism (PE) except for which one?

A. Computed tomography angiogram (CTA) of chest
B. Pulmonary angiogram
C. Chest x-ray (CXR)
D. Ventilation perfusion scan

11. Ventilation techniques used in the treatment of patients with pulmonary contusions include all of the following except:

A. Increasing positive end-expiratory pressure (PEEP)
B. Maintaining low plateau pressures
C. Decreasing respiratory rates
D. Utilize pressure control ventilation

12. Myocardial cell necrosis, infiltration of leukocytes, absorption of hemorrhage, and healing by scar formation make myocardial contusions very similar to what other disease process?

A. Myocardial infarctions
B. Hemorrhagic contusions
C. Pulmonary contusions
D. Liver lacerations

13. What is the physiological difference between a myocardial contusion and a myocardial infarction?

A. There is no necrotic zone in myocardial contusions.
B. There is no ischemic zone in myocardial contusions.
C. There is no healthy cardiac tissue in myocardial infarctions.
D. There is no necrotic zone in myocardial infarctions or myocardial contusions.

14. A patient comes in with a cardiac contusion and multiple rib fractures following a motor vehicle collision. The trauma nurse performs a 12-lead EKG and draws blood for cardiac enzyme studies. What other diagnostic procedures would be appropriate for this patient?

A. Echocardiography
B. Radionuclide angiography
C. Transesophageal echocardiogram (TEE)
D. All of the above

15. A trauma patient comes into the emergency room with a traumatic aortic transection, and is lethargic and difficult to arouse. The spouse is at the bedside and the physician explains that immediate surgery is necessary. The spouse is contemplating whether or not to sign the consent form for the procedure. The nurse should disclose:

A. This surgery is necessary and will decrease the mortality rate for the patient.
B. The surgery will not make much of a difference at this point, the mortality rate is high with or without surgical intervention.
C. The surgery is not really an emergency and can wait until the patient wakes up.
D. The surgery is necessary and will decrease the mortality rate for the patient from 90% to 40%.

16. The nurse is caring for a patient who sustained a fall from a second-story home. The patient's voice begins to get hoarse and the nurse notices some swelling over the base of the neck. Which of the following assessments is indicated to assess for aortic injuries?

    A. Pupillary reactions
    B. Pulses in upper and lower extremities
    C. Bowel sounds
    D. Skin color changes

17. All of the following are screening or diagnostic tests for diagnosing patients with traumatic aortic aneurysms except:

    A. Computerized tomography angiography (CTA)
    B. Aortography
    C. Sonography
    D. x-ray

18. A patient admitted with a traumatic aortic aneurysm is most likely to have which one of the following performed during the surgical repair of the aorta to prevent complications?

    A. Autotransfusion from the chest tube
    B. Clamped aorta without distal canalization
    C. Partial left heart bypass
    D. Aortic bypass with autologous graft

19. During cross-clamping to surgically manage a traumatic aortic aneurysm, hypotension can occur below the clamp, whereas hypertension can occur above the clamp. What are the possible complications caused by the cross-clamping?

    A. Right lung pneumonia
    B. Myocardial infarction
    C. Graft infection
    D. Atelectasis

Abdominal Trauma

MECHANISM OF INJURY

■ *The spleen is most commonly injured in which type of trauma: blunt or penetrating?*

■ **Blunt**

Common organs injured by blunt mechanism are the solid organs such as spleen, liver, and pancreas. Entrapment of the abdominal wall against the vertebral column and compression of the abdomen increases the pressure within the abdominal cavity, and causes solid organs to rupture. Hollow organs are more susceptible to collapse during the increased pressure.

> ▶ **HINT:** Other mechanisms of injury in blunt trauma to the abdomen include changing of organ position and puncture of organs with bony fractures.

■ *During sudden deceleration in a blunt trauma, movement of abdominal organs most commonly causes tearing of which abdominal organ?*

■ **Duodenum**

During energy transfer, shearing forces may cause tearing at the attachment points of ligaments. The duodenum is secured by the ligament of Treitz; therefore a sudden deceleration results in the tearing of the duodenum at the level of the ligament.

> ▶ **HINT:** This is a similar mechanism to the tearing of the aorta during a sudden deceleration mechanism because of the arch secured by the ligamentum of arteriosum.

■ *Seat belts can increase injury to which body system?*

■ **Abdomen**

Seat belts can change the patterns of blunt trauma by increasing abdominal injuries. They decrease the severity of injury and lower the number of traumatic brain injuries but can increase the abdominal trauma. Lap belts lie across the lower abdomen and can increase abdominal organ injuries. Handlebars on bicycles and motorcycles can impact the abdomen during a crash and result in a higher incidence of abdominal trauma.

> ▶ **HINT:** A bent steering wheel in a motor vehicle collision (MVC) is associated with more significant abdominal injuries to the driver.

■ *Following an MVC, the driver of the vehicle with a shoulder harness on during the collision is more likely to injure which abdominal organ?*

■ **Liver**

The harness seat belt is secured across the left shoulder to the right hip, with the belt lying across the area of the liver. On impact, the liver is compressed, resulting in an injury.

> ▶ **HINT:** A passenger with a shoulder harness is more likely to damage the spleen.

■ *Which mechanism, gunshot or stab wound, is more likely to result in an abdominal organ injury requiring surgical management?*

■ **Gunshot wound**

Gunshot wounds are associated with a 96% to 98% chance of a significant intra-abdominal injury requiring surgery and have a higher mortality rate than stab wounds. Stab wounds are associated with a 30% to 40% chance of surgical injury and have a lower mortality than gunshot wounds. Gunshot wounds are associated with a greater kinetic energy and destruction of tissue than stab wounds, which may not enter the peritoneum.

> ▶ **HINT:** Gunshot wounds to the abdomen are more likely to have an exploratory laparotomy with minimal diagnostic workup before the surgery.

TRAUMATIC INJURIES

■ *Where is the pancreas located in the abdominal cavity: the intraperitoneal or retroperitoneal space?*

■ **Retroperitoneal**

The abdominal cavity is divided into the peritoneal and retroperitoneal spaces. The peritoneal cavity contains the stomach, small intestine, liver, gallbladder, transverse colon, sigmoid colon, upper one third of rectum, part of the bladder, and uterus. The retroperitoneal space contains part of the duodenum, ascending colon, descending colon, kidneys, part of the bladder, pancreas, and major vessels.

> ▶ **HINT:** Retroperitoneal organ injuries can be more difficult to diagnose than intraperitoneal injuries.

■ *The abdomen can be divided into three regions. What is the region that extends from the xiphoid process to the pubic bone between the anterior axillary lines called?*

■ **Anterior abdomen**

In injuries to the abdomen, the abdomen can be divided into three regions: anterior, thoracoabdominal, and flank and back. The anterior abdomen extends from the xiphoid process to the pubic bone between the anterior axillary lines. The flank and back region is posterior to the anterior axillary lines, and the thoracoabdominal area extends from the nipple line to the costal margin.

> ▶ **HINT:** The division of the abdomen into regions can assist in determining potential organ injuries in penetrating stab wounds.

■ *Penetrating trauma to the back, flank, or buttocks can result in injury to which body system?*

■ **Abdominal trauma**

The flank and back are regions of the abdomen, and penetrating injuries in these regions can result in trauma to the abdomen. Penetrating injuries to the diaphragm are harder to recognize than blunt injuries, and may require laparoscopy or surgical exploration.

> ▶ **HINT:** A missed occult injury to the diaphragm may have a delayed presentation of shortness of breath because of herniated stomach or bowel into the thoracic cavity.

■ *Which diaphragm, right or left, is more likely to be injured in a blunt abdominal trauma?*

■ **Left**

Rupture of the left diaphragm is more common than the right because the liver protects the diaphragm on the right. Following a diaphragm injury, the stomach or small bowel may herniate into the thoracic cavity. The trauma nurse may be able to auscultate bowel sounds in the chest cavity if this occurs.

> ▶ **HINT:** The presence of asymmetrical chest wall movement may indicate an injury to the diaphragm, liver, or spleen.

■ *A nasogastric (NG) tube is placed following penetrating abdominal trauma and bloody aspirate is obtained. What organ is most likely injured?*

■ **Stomach**

Stomach injuries are commonly caused by penetrating trauma. The most common sign of a stomach injury is blood in the NG aspirate.

> ▶ **HINT:** Signs of stomach injury following trauma include rapid onset of epigastric pain, tenderness and signs of peritonitis because of the release of gastric contents, and free air on abdominal x-ray.

■ *Which abdominal organ is most likely to be injured in both blunt and penetrating trauma?*

■ **Liver**

The most frequently injured organ is the liver because of its size and location. It is a solid organ and hence is more commonly injured in blunt abdominal trauma. The driver's liver is also frequently injured in a motor vehicle collision due to the location of the shoulder harness. It is also commonly damaged with penetrating injuries because of its size.

> ▶ **HINT:** The high mortality caused by liver injury is the result of hemorrhage (early) or peritonitis and sepsis (late).

■ *Which portion of the esophagus is most commonly injured following penetrating trauma?*

■ **Cervical region**

The esophagus is not commonly injured. The most common mechanism of injury is penetrating trauma and occurs more frequently in the cervical region of the esophagus. The abdominal portion is rarely injured.

> ▶ **HINT:** Injury results in fluid accumulation in the lungs and respiratory distress.

■ *A hematoma of the spleen is blood accumulation in which part of the spleen?*

■ **Capsular portion of the spleen**

A hematoma in the spleen is an accumulation of blood in the capsular portion of the spleen. If the capsule ruptures, it is then called a *laceration*.

▶ **HINT:** A splenic hematoma can be monitored for a bleeding complication and managed with observation instead of surgical management.

ASSESSMENT/DIAGNOSIS

■ *Which abdominal organ injury may present with a delayed presentation?*

■ **Duodenum**

Secretions in the stomach are acidic but are alkaline in the duodenum. Perforation of the stomach results in rapid, acute signs of peritonitis, whereas the spillage of alkaline fluid into the abdominal cavity is not an immediate irritant of the peritoneum. Duodenal ruptures may have referred pain to back, chest, shoulder, and testicles (retroperitoneal injury).

▶ **HINT:** Presentation may be delayed and presents with septic peritonitis (Box 5.1).

Box 5.1 Delayed Presentation

Fever
Elevated white blood cell count
Jaundice
High intestinal blockage
Third-spacing
Elevated bilirubin and amylase
Hypovolemia

■ *Free air in the abdomen may indicate the presence of rupture to which type of abdominal organs?*

■ **Hollow organs**

Hollow organs are air filled and when ruptured will demonstrate "free air" in the abdomen. Solid organ rupture will not present with free air on radiographic x-rays.

▶ **HINT:** Free air found on radiographic studies indicates the need for immediate surgery for a significant organ injury.

■ *Which diagnostic radiographic study is best able to identify the severity of organ injury?*

■ **CT scan**

Advantages of CT scan include the ability to grade the severity of injury, as well as to be able to view the retroperitoneal cavity and the intra-abdominal injuries. The ability to grade injuries allows for some patients to be observed following injury rather than undergo surgical management. The disadvantage is that there is a need to transport unstable patients to perform the CT scan.

▶ **HINT:** An abdominal CT scan can identify the organ involved and the severity of organ injury; thereby, lowering the incidence of negative laparotomies.

■ *What is bruising in the flank area because of bleeding in the retroperitoneal cavity called?*

■ **Grey-Turner sign**

Grey-Turner's sign is ecchymosis (or bruising) in the flank area resulting from bleeding in the retroperitoneal space. Cullen's sign is ecchymosis around the umbilicus and indicates bleeding in the peritoneal cavity. The trauma nurse should inspect the patient's abdomen for bruising, abrasions, and lacerations, which may indicate intra-abdominal organ injury.

▶ **HINT:** Grey-Turner's and Cullen's signs may not appear for several hours or days following the trauma.

■ *While assessing the patient, the trauma nurse finds a "board-like" abdomen. What does this finding indicate?*

■ **Peritonitis**

A "board-like" abdomen is the result of involuntary spasm of abdominal muscles resulting from peritonitis. Muscle guarding is an increased voluntary contraction of the abdominal muscles in an effort to prevent pain.

▶ **HINT:** Rebound tenderness is pain or abdominal activity following sudden withdrawal of stimulus such as fingers.

■ *An upright chest x-ray (CXR) is obtained following a trauma. The findings include free air, which indicate injury to what type of organ?*

■ **Hollow organ rupture**

An upright CXR and left lateral decubitus are used to identify free air (ruptured hollow organ), indicating the presence of a hollow organ injury. This is an indication for an exploratory laparotomy.

▶ **HINT:** Supine abdominal radiographs can identify retroperitoneal free air, gross organ injury, and presence of blood or foreign objects in the abdominal cavity.

■ *What is the advantage of a CT scan compared to a diagnostic peritoneal lavage (DPL)?*

■ **It reveals retroperitoneal injuries.**

The advantage of a CT scan compared to DPL is the scan's ability to view the retroperitoneal cavity as well as intra-abdominal injuries. The other advantage is the CT scan's ability to identify the organ involved and grade the severity of injury. Disadvantages of CT scan include the expense and difficulty in scanning an unstable patient. CT scan is the diagnostic modality of choice in monitoring nonoperative solid visceral injuries.

▶ **HINT:** CT scan may miss injuries to the mesentery and small bowel, thus limiting the diagnostic effectiveness of CT scan for these injuries.

■ *Which is the noninvasive and repeatable test that can be used to evaluate hemoperitoneum at the bedside following a blunt trauma?*

■ **Abdominal ultrasound**

Ultrasonography of the abdomen is preferred more than abdominal CT scan in hemodynamically unstable trauma patients. It is a noninvasive, quick, inexpensive, and repeatable test that can be used to evaluate hemoperitoneum. Most trained technicians should be able to identify free fluid greater than 200 mL with an abdominal sonography.

> ▶ **HINT:** Ultrasonography is less reliable than CT scans for grading the severity of abdominal organ injuries and excluding hollow visceral injuries.

■ *What is the ultrasonography technique used to rapidly evaluate the abdomen following a blunt trauma?*

■ **Focused abdominal sonography technique (FAST)**

FAST is a technique used to rapidly evaluate the abdomen for traumatic injuries. One of the advantages of using FAST in the emergency department is that the patient does not have to be transported to imaging to obtain a CT scan. Exploratory laparotomy is indicated in hemodynamically unstable patients with a positive FAST, indicating evidence of hemoperitoneum. It can estimate the amount of blood in the abdomen and identify candidates for observation, thus preventing unnecessary laparotomies.

> ▶ **HINT:** A penetrating stab wound to the abdomen evaluated with the FAST technique can have false negatives.

■ *Which abdominal organ is more difficult to evaluate for injury with a diagnostic laparoscopy?*

■ **Bowel**

A laparoscope can observe the diaphragm, liver, spleen, anterior stomach, uterus, ovaries, cecum, and sigmoid colon. It is more difficult for a complete examination of the bowel, flexures of colon, and retroperitoneum, and may miss injuries in these areas. Some corrections of injuries can be performed during diagnostic laparoscopy such as ligating bleeders or closing lacerations.

> ▶ **HINT:** Diagnostic laparoscopy may be indicated with penetrating injuries when there is a high likelihood that the injury is tangential to the abdomen.

■ *A supraumbilical approach for a DPL is more accurate than below the umbilicus in a patient with what type of associated injury?*

■ **Pelvic fracture**

DPL is a procedure used to diagnose occult intra-abdominal bleeding in abdominal trauma. A below-the-umbilicus DPL performed on a patient with a pelvic fracture can result in a false positive and an unnecessary exploratory laparotomy. The technique of performing the DPL above the umbilicus lowers this risk. Disadvantages of DPL include the inability to diagnose retroperitoneal injuries, inability to determine type or extent of injury, and potential of a missed ruptured hollow viscera if performed early after the injury.

> ▶ **HINT:** Relative contraindications for DPL include advanced pregnancy, pelvic injuries, previous multiple abdominal surgeries, morbid obesity, advanced cirrhosis, and coagulopathy.

■ *If an emergency DPL is performed in a patient with suspected abdominal trauma, what red blood cell (RBC) level would indicate a positive lavage?*

■ **Greater than 100,000 mm³**

An RBC count greater than 100,000 mm³ is considered positive with a DPL and is an indication for exploratory laparotomy (especially if the patient is hemodynamically unstable). Other signs of positive DPL frequently include white blood cell (WBC) levels greater than 500 mm³, or elevated amylase, alkaline phosphate, or bilirubin in the lavage fluid.

> ▶ **HINT:** If a DPL is performed, an elevated WBC has no diagnostic value in the early postinjury period (less than 4 hours).

■ *What would be the best intervention in a hemodynamically stable patient with a grade II liver laceration?*

■ **Observation**

A hemodynamically stable grade II liver laceration can be observed without an exploratory laparotomy in most situations without other significant abdominal organ injuries. Observation of patients with abdominal organ injuries should include hemodynamic monitoring, serial frequent physical assessment, and serial labs (especially hemoglobin [Hgb] and hematocrit [Hct]).

> ▶ **HINT:** Unnecessary laparotomy can increase complications, length of stay, and mortality following stab wounds and blunt abdominal trauma.

MEDICAL/SURGICAL INTERVENTIONS

■ *What would be the most appropriate intervention for a patient with blunt abdominal trauma presenting with obvious signs of peritonitis?*

■ **Exploratory laparotomy**

Obvious signs of peritonitis are an indication for an exploratory laparotomy following a blunt abdominal trauma. Other indications for exploratory laparotomies indicate unexplained shock, impalement, evisceration of bowel or omentum, significant bleeding from NG tube, ongoing hemodynamic instability, or free air on x-ray.

> ▶ **HINT:** Signs of peritonitis should be recognized following an abdominal injury and include abdominal tenderness, board-like abdomen, elevated WBC count, fever, and other signs of sepsis.

■ *What is the first priority in an exploratory laparotomy following an abdominal trauma with hemodynamic instability?*

■ **Locate and control hemorrhage**

The first priority in exploratory laparotomy following abdominal trauma is to locate and control hemorrhage. The second priority is to locate colonic injury to control fecal contamination, then identify injuries to abdominal organs and structures, followed by repair to the damaged tissues and organs. The third and fourth priority identifies injuries to abdominal organs and structures, and repair of damage to tissues and organs.

> ▶ **HINT:** The combination of bowel and liver injury significantly increases risk of posttraumatic infections.

■ *A penetrating trauma to the stomach results in devitalized tissue. What is the best surgical intervention for this patient?*

■ **Debridement of devitalized tissue**

Treatment of stomach injury includes debridement of devitalized tissue and closure with sutures or a partial gastrectomy if the injury is extensive.

> ▶ **HINT:** Following stomach repair, an NG tube may be present for 3 to 5 days with specific instructions not to reposition the NG tube. Repositioning an NG tube after gastric repair can cause damage to the anastomosis or sutures.

■ *What is the primary surgical management of small bowel injuries?*

■ **Debridement and resection**

The key to successful surgical repair of the small bowel is debridement. All devitalized tissue and marginally injured bowel should be resected. Most small bowel injuries can be closed after simple debridement, resection, and suturing.

> ▶ **HINT:** All but 50 cm of the entire small bowel can be resected without compromise (total length is 260 cm).

■ *During the exploratory laparotomy, the liver is noted to be profusely bleeding. What is the most commonly used technique to control bleeding called?*

■ **Damage control**

If intra-abdominal hemorrhage is severe, the trauma surgeon may pack the liver bed, use fibrin glue (sealant made from concentrated fibrinogen and thrombin), and/or selective hepatic artery or portal vein ligation temporary closure, and planned reoperation to control coagulopathic bleeding. This is frequently referred to as *damage control surgery*.

> ▶ **HINT:** After the damage control surgery, the trauma nurse assesses for uncontrolled hemorrhage, monitors coagulation studies, and administer agents to reverse the coagulopathy.

■ *What is a common practice for treating a grade I liver laceration following a blunt abdominal trauma?*

■ **Observation**

Simple injuries (grade I to II) may be observed. A nonoperative course is taken for these minor hepatic injuries with no evidence of bleeding. If surgically managed, surgery usually includes suture or application of topical agents to control bleeding or electrocautery.

> ▶ **HINT:** This involves observation in the intensive care unit (ICU) with frequent vital signs, complete blood count (CBC) and prothrombin time (PT)/partial thromboplastin time (PTT) monitoring.

■ *What is a commonly used fecal diversion following a colon injury?*

■ **Double-barrel traverse colostomy**

Double-barrel transverse colostomy involves the complete division of the bowel and each part is brought to the surface. One opening puts out stool and one puts out just mucus.

Loop colostomies are easily constructed and taken down, but may not completely divert fecal material from the distal segment of the colon. A colostomy is made either at the site of the colon injury or proximal to the site to protect distal repair.

> ▶ **HINT:** In a right colon injury, colostomies are avoided because of the difficulty of the procedure. Right colon injuries are typically treated with primary repair or hemicolectomy.

■ *A grade V rupture of the spleen typically requires what type of intervention?*

■ **Splenectomy**

A splenectomy is the recommended procedure for a grade IV to V splenic injury. These injuries involve vascular injuries that produce major devascularization or completely shatter the spleen.

> ▶ **HINT:** Surgical repair of the spleen is called a *splenorrhaphy.*

■ *What is a nonoperative treatment of a splenic or liver injury used to control bleeding?*

■ **Embolization**

Embolization of splenic and hepatic arteries in patients with contrast extravasation and ongoing blood loss can be used to control the hemorrhage. This is a nonoperative management of abdominal bleeding from the liver or spleen.

> ▶ **HINT:** Grades IV and V liver or splenic injuries may require surgery because of the increased severity of injury.

NURSING INTERVENTIONS

■ *Percussion over the right upper quadrant (RUQ) following an acute liver injury produces what type of sound?*

■ **Dullness**

Signs of traumatic liver injuries include tenderness over right lower ribs or RUQ, dullness to percussion, signs of peritoneal irritation, and increased abdominal girth.

■ *Following a stomach injury and partial gastrectomy, the patient has a NG tube. What is a common order regarding the care of the NG tube?*

■ **Do not reposition**

The NG tube is placed intraoperatively. Repositioning the NG tube can cause injury to the anastomosis or sutures.

> ▶ **HINT:** Following stomach repair postop an NG tube may be present for 3 to 5 days.

■ *A Kehr's sign indicates the presence of which abdominal organ injury?*

■ **Spleen**

Symptoms of traumatic splenic injury include profound bleeding, positive Kehr's sign, Saegesser's sign, and Ballance's sign (Box 5.2).

Box 5.2 Signs of Splenic Injury

Saegesser's sign	Pain in the neck area because of irritation of the phrenic nerve
Kehr's sign	Pain radiates to the left scapula
Ballance's sign	Dullness over left flank

> ▶ **HINT:** Pain associated with spleen injuries includes generalized abdominal pain with localized pain in the left upper quadrant (LUQ).

- *A patient presents in the trauma ICU with abdominal pain that worsens with movement and rebound tenderness. What is the most likely cause of the pain?*
- **Peritonitis**

The symptoms of peritonitis include diffuse abdominal pain, rebound tenderness to board-like abdomen, which worsens with movement. Peritonitis frequently results from hollow organ rupture or spillage of bowel contents into the peritoneal cavity.

> ▶ **HINT:** The Markel test is used to assess for peritonitis. Strike the patient's heel with a fist. If this elicits abdominal pain, it is a possible indication of peritonitis.

- *Which abdominal organ injury may lack peritoneal signs?*
- **Duodenum**

Duodenal injuries frequently lack signs of peritonitis soon after trauma. This is because of the neutral to alkaline pH in the duodenum. The injury may produce abdominal pain and vomiting. After several days, the patient may develop leukocytosis and fever along with abdominal pain, indicating the presence of septic peritonitis.

> ▶ **HINT:** A board-like abdomen indicates presence of peritonitis.

COMPLICATIONS

- *Soon after blunt abdominal trauma and an exploratory laparotomy, the patient develops respiratory distress and bilateral fluffy infiltrates. What is the most likely complication?*
- **Abdominal compartment syndrome (ACS)**

Intra-abdominal pressure (IAP) is a compartment pressure that can be monitored and measured. It is defined as a steady-state pressure concealed within the abdominal cavity. When the pressure increases in the abdominal cavity to the extent of causing organ dysfunction or failure, it is now known as ACS. ACS causes decreased tidal volume and increased ventilatory pressures leading to respiratory distress and bilateral fluffy infiltrates (Box 5.3).

> ▶ **HINT:** Closing an abdominal cavity after surgery can result in ACS with multiple complications, including acute respiratory distress, acute renal failure, dehiscence and evisceration of bowel, sepsis, and multiple organ failure (MOF).

Box 5.3 Three Factors of ACS

Factors	Indications
Abdominal organ volume	Grossly swollen bowel (occupies several times the original space)
	Excessive crystalloid resuscitation
Presence of space-occupying substances (blood, ascites, tumor, free air)	Bleeding, leakage of abdominal contents, bowel edema
	Blood or blood clots
Abdominal wall compliance	Acute respiratory failure, abdominal surgery, major trauma/burns, prone positioning, central obesity

ACS, abdominal compartment syndrome.

- ■ *What pressures can be monitored to assess for the presence of ACS?*
- ■ **Bladder pressures**

ACS monitoring is performed by the measurement of bladder pressure, which can be obtained through a Foley catheter. A normal IAP is approximately 5 to 7 mmHg, whereas the normal range in critically ill patients is from 5 to 15 mmHg of pressure. It is not uncommon to find a pressure of 15 to 20 mmHg in abdominal trauma patients or those with sepsis. ACS is defined as an IAP greater than 20 mmHg with organ involvement (Box 5.4).

▶ HINT: IAP in morbidly obese patients often ranges from 9 to 14 mmHg.

Box 5.4 Grading IAP

Grade	IAP
I	12 to 15 mmHg
II	16 to 20 mmHg
III	21 to 25 mmHg
IV	Greater than 25 mmHg

IAP, intra-abdominal pressure.

- ■ *What is the potential neurological complication of ACS?*
- ■ **Increased ICP**

There is a direct relationship between elevated IAP and ICP. The increased pressure is referred to the thoracic cavity from the abdominal region, increasing the thoracic pressure. This decreases the jugular venous drainage and increases the pressure within the cranium. This is very important in trauma patients with traumatic brain injuries.

▶ HINT: Refractory intracranial hypertension has been treated successfully using abdominal decompression or neuromuscular blocking agents (relaxes abdominal muscles thus lowering pressures).

- ■ *What is the surgical management of ACS?*
- ■ **Decompression**

An excessively high IAP or progressive or refractory ACS typically requires a decompressive laparotomy. Many trauma surgeons leave the abdomen open following major laparotomies to prevent ACS.

▶ **HINT:** Surgical decompression of the abdomen frequently causes hypotension because the sudden perfusion of the mesenteric vascular bed.

■ *Following a decompressive abdominal surgery, what type of wound coverage is recommended?*
■ **Negative pressure dressing**

Negative pressure systems control the abdominal contents, manage third-space fluids, and facilitate wound closure. Vacuum-assisted fascial closure (VAFC) systems provide constant tension on the abdominal wound edges, facilitating the ability to successfully perform a late fascial closure.

▶ **HINT:** The goal of temporary closure is to create a tension-free closure of abdomen without elevating IAP.

■ *What is a potential late complication of abdominal trauma involving the small intestines?*
■ **Intestinal adhesions or obstruction**

Internal scarring following abdominal surgery can result in intra-abdominal adhesions leading to obstruction (Box 5.5).

Box 5.5 Late Complications of Abdominal Trauma

Peptic ulcers
Intestinal obstruction (adhesions or strictures)
Hernia (midline or ostomy sites)
Fistulas
Chronic abscesses
Cholelithiasis and cholecystitis

▶ **HINT:** Duodenal fistulas cause acidosis secondary to loss of bicarbonate from pancreatic juices.

■ *What is the major potential complication following a splenectomy that requires preventive management?*
■ **Pneumococcal infections**

A concern is an overwhelming postsplenectomy sepsis (OPSS), which can occur because of the loss of some immune responses. A large percentage of the OPSS occurs within 1 year postsplenectomy but can occur several years later too. Pneumococcal infections are associated with high mortality following a splenectomy.

▶ **HINT:** Before discharge, the vaccination Pneumovac needs to be given to a patient following a splenectomy.

■ *What metabolic abnormality occurs with a draining fistula following stomach injury?*

■ **Metabolic alkalosis**

Fistulas that form after gastric injury repair cause metabolic alkalosis because of the loss of hydrogen chloride (HCL) and potassium (K^+). The loss of gastric acids increases the pH.

> ▶ **HINT:** Duodenal fistulas can cause metabolic acidosis secondary to loss of bicarbonate from pancreatic juices. Jejunal fistula produces low volumes of neutral pH fluid with little change in acid or base balance.

■ *Which combination of abdominal organ injury has been found to increase mortality?*

■ **Liver and colon**

The combined intra-abdominal injuries of liver and colon have the highest mortality risk because of increased septic peritonitis. Intra-abdominal abscess formation occurs because of foreign-body fragments, necrotic tissue, blood, or bile remaining at site of injury. The combination of spillage of stool and blood clots leads to abdominal infections.

> ▶ **HINT:** Postoperative fluid collections or abscesses can be drained by CT-guided placement of a catheter.

■ *Which electrolyte abnormality commonly occurs following pancreatic injury?*

■ **Hypocalcemia**

Calcium is sequestered into the pancreas following an injury. Hypocalcemia presents with tetany, prolonged QT interval, and muscle cramping. Close monitoring of ionized calcium and treatment with calcium are important in the care of pancreatic trauma patients.

> ▶ **HINT:** The life-threatening complication of hypocalcemia is torsades de pointes.

Questions

1. Referring to the anatomy of the abdomen, what contains the stomach, small intestine, liver, gallbladder, transverse colon, sigmoid colon, upper third of rectum, part of the bladder, and the uterus?

   A. Peritoneal cavity
   B. Retroperitoneal space
   C. Splenic flexure
   D. Pleural space

2. All of the following are possible mechanisms of injury to organs in blunt abdominal trauma except:

   A. Entrapment between vertebral column and impacting forces
   B. A sudden decrease in uniform pressure
   C. Changes in organ position
   D. Puncture from bone fractures

3. During the assessment of an abdominal trauma patient, the nurse inspects the abdomen, auscultates it, and then performs percussion of the abdomen during secondary survey. The nurse palpates hyperresonance. This finding is most indicative of which of the following?

   A. Presence of air
   B. Presence of blood
   C. Fluid accumulation
   D. Possible solid mass

4. A patient comes to the emergency department following a motorcycle collision. The patient was wearing a helmet and thrown from the bike about 10 ft. The patient just returned from receiving a CT scan of the head, neck, back, and abdomen. The results revealed a 2-cm liver laceration. The patient asks the nurse whether surgery is needed. What is the best response?

   A. "The liver laceration is 2 cm, it is categorized as a grade III, and most likely needs a surgical intervention."
   B. "The liver laceration is 2 cm, it is categorized as a grade I, and surgery is usually not warranted."
   C. "The liver laceration is 2 cm, it is categorized as a grade IV, and immediate surgery is needed."
   D. "The liver laceration is 2 cm, it is categorized as a grade II, and usually does not require surgery."

5. The nurse is assessing a patient with a blunt abdominal trauma injury. The patient has hypoactive bowel sounds, abdominal pain, and dullness on percussion of the abdomen. Blood pressure is 121/82 mmHg, heart rate is 99 beats per minute (bpm), respiratory rate is 20 breaths per minute with an oxygen saturation of 98% on 4 L via nasal cannula. What diagnostic study as known to the nurse is the best choice with this clinical presentation?

A. CT of the abdomen
B. CT with intravenous contrast of the abdomen
C. Diagnostic peritoneal lavage (DPL)
D. CT with oral contrast of the abdomen

6. The trauma nurse is teaching a nurse about proper nursing interventions for a patient with an abdominal injury. The nurse questions the new nurse about the rationale for inserting a gastric tube and aspirating the gastric contents. All of the following would be acceptable answers except:

A. Inserting a gastric tube decompresses the stomach
B. Inserting a gastric tube increases vagal stimulation
C. Inserting a gastric tube prevents aspiration
D. Inserting a gastric tube minimizes leakage contamination of the abdominal cavity

7. The patient is currently in the intensive care unit (ICU) after being admitted yesterday with an abdominal injury. The original CT scan revealed intestinal bleeding. There is a repeat CT scan ordered for this morning. The patient was questioning why the test is being ordered so soon after the original scan. Which of the following rationales is not accurate?

A. A repeat CT scan evaluates ongoing bleeding.
B. A repeat CT scan evaluates for a pseudoaneurysm.
C. A repeat CT scan evaluates abdominal distention.
D. A repeat CT scan evaluates stabilization of the injury.

8. A patient has suffered an abdominal gunshot wound. The abdomen is open and there is evisceration of abdominal contents. The nurse has secured an airway and cannulated two veins to infuse crystalloid solutions. How should the nurse address the abdominal wounds?

A. Attempt to place abdominal contents back into the cavity
B. Place a sterile dressing over the site and the intestines
C. Irrigate the site and leave open
D. Place a sterile dressing over the site and cover the intestines with vaseline gauze

9. Ms. Cross sustained a liver laceration during a rollover motor vehicle collision (MVC). When evaluating her, the nurse should place extra emphasis when assessing:

A. Distal and proximal pulses
B. Localized pain to palpation and bony crepitus sites
C. Auscultation of lung sounds and percussion for signs of pneumothorax or hemothorax
D. Abdominal distention, pain with palpation, and dullness to percussion

10. All are true regarding penetrating injuries to the abdomen except:

A. Gunshot wounds are associated with a 96% to 98% chance of significant intra-abdominal injury.
B. Solid organs are more likely to be injured.
C. Stab wounds are associated with a 30% to 40% chance of injury to the abdomen.
D. Tangential injuries occur when objects enter the abdomen, but not into the abdominal cavity.

11. Mr. Bartow was riding a bicycle, hit the curb, and fell onto the handlebars. The nurse performing his assessment did not observe areas of abdominal bruising or distension, and the abdomen is soft on palpation with bowel sounds present in all four quadrants. Which of the following missing assessments would indicate a possible abdominal injury?

    A. Waiting 30 minutes and reassessing for bowel sound changes
    B. Auscultation of possible abdominal bruit
    C. Assessing abdominal pain on a scale of 1 to 10
    D. Lack of rectal tone

12. A patient comes to the emergency room after being pinned between two vehicles in a parking lot. The patient is reporting abdominal pain and has a blood pressure of 101/59 mmHg, pulse is 114 beats per minute (bpm), respiratory rate is 33 breaths per minute, and an oxygenation saturation of 96% on a nonrebreather mask. All of the following are likely signs of acute abdominal trauma except:

    A. Abdominal distention
    B. Tachycardia
    C. Absent bowel sounds
    D. Board-like abdomen

13. Diagnostic examinations for an abdominal trauma patient include all of the following except:

    A. CT of the spine
    B. CT of the abdomen
    C. Chest x-ray
    D. Abdominal x-ray

14. A morbidly obese patient comes to the emergency room with a gunshot wound to the abdomen. The patient is complaining of severe abdominal pain. The nurse is reviewing the plan of care with the physician, what order should the nurse question?

    A. Focused assessment sonography for trauma (FAST) examination
    B. Peritoneal lavage
    C. Diagnostic laparoscopy
    D. CT scan of the abdomen

15. The focused assessment sonography for trauma (FAST) is a rapid, bedside examination that is most helpful when examining patients with hemodynamic instability. This is utilized to examine patients with all of the following except:

    A. Brain injury
    B. Pericardial tamponade
    C. Free fluid in the pelvis
    D. Intraperitoneal hemorrhage

16. In what area of the body is the focused assessment sonography for trauma (FAST) not utilized?

    A. Chest
    B. Pelvis
    C. Neck
    D. Flanks

17. A patient presented to the hospital with a blunt injury to the abdomen. The patient was treated and admitted to the unit for close observation. Two days later, the patient spikes a fever of 102°F, has an elevated bilirubin level, board-like abdomen, and is jaundiced. The nurse is highly suspicious of:

    A. Liver failure
    B. Gallstones
    C. Sepsis
    D. Peritonitis

18. The American Association for the Surgery of Trauma (AAST) has developed a grading system for splenic injuries in order to guide proper treatment and interventions. What grade splenic injury would involve a laceration of vessels producing devascularization to more than 25% of the spleen?

    A. Grade I
    B. Grade II
    C. Grade III
    D. Grade IV
    E. Grade V

19. The spleen is the most commonly injured visceral organ in blunt abdominal trauma in both adults and children. Nonoperative management is the current standard of practice for patients who are hemodynamically stable with low-grade splenic injuries. All of the following are interventions with this type of stable splenic injury except:

    A. Bed rest
    B. Limited oral intake
    C. Serial hemoglobin (Hgb) and hematocrit (Hct) levels
    D. Repeat CT scan within 24 hours

20. The nurse is precepting a new intensive care unit (ICU) nurse in the trauma unit. The patient they are caring for is diagnosed with abdominal compartment syndrome (ACS) and the orientee is preparing to perform bladder pressure readings. Which of the following statements by the orientee would require correction by the preceptor?

    A. "An indwelling bladder catheter needs to be inserted using sterile technique."
    B. "The transducer needs to be leveled to the symphysis pubis."
    C. "Installation of 200 mL of dextrose into the bladder should be performed before pressure reading is obtained."
    D. "The physician needs to be notified for pressure readings greater than 20 mm Hg."

21. The physician comes into the patient's room and tells him that he has a minor pancreatic injury from his motor vehicle accident today. After the physician leaves, the patient asks the nurse, "What happens now? Do I need surgery? How is this going to be fixed?" The best response would be:

    A. "We most likely have to take you to the operating room to remove the pancreas."
    B. "We most likely have to take you to the operating room to aggressively debride the pancreas."
    C. "We have to make sure you are up to date on your vaccinations."
    D. "We might have to place a temporary drain in the area of the pancreas."

22. A patient sustained a liver laceration 10 days before that had been repaired and also underwent a splenectomy. The nurse has stabilized the patient and now is preparing the patient for transfer to the trauma telemetry unit. While reviewing the labs, the nurse notes that the complete blood count (CBC) results are:

    Red blood cell (RBC): 5.1
    White blood cell (WBC): 10
    Hemoglobin (Hgb): 9.4
    Hematocrit (Hct): 37
    Platelet: 519

    On which of the following medications should the patient be placed before transfer?

    A. Lovenox
    B. Neulasta
    C. Aspirin
    D. Folic acid

23. Ms. Swartz is now being discharged and the nurse prepares the patient's discharge instructions. It is most important to instruct Ms. Swartz to seek medical attention if she experiences:

    A. Fever and chills
    B. Nausea and vomiting
    C. Purplish red spots on the skin
    D. All of the above

24. A 14-year-old male patient was riding his bicycle and performing tricks when he fell over the handlebars. He is complaining of midepigastric abdominal pain. The nurse knows that a pancreatic injury should be identified early because delayed treatment in these injuries increases morbidity and mortality. All of the following are indicative of a pancreatic injury except:

    A. Midepigastric abdominal pain
    B. Leukocytosis
    C. Elevated serum lactate level
    D. Elevated serum amylase level

25. An elevated serum amylase may be useful in diagnosing pancreatic injury, but amylase can also be elevated in other injuries, including all of the following except:

    A. Splenic trauma
    B. Hepatic trauma
    C. Facial trauma
    D. Duodenal trauma

26. The American Association for the Surgery of Trauma (AAST) developed a classification system for grading pancreatic trauma injuries. Which of the following grades would indicate a major laceration to the pancreas without ductal injury or tissue loss would be graded as?

    A. Grade I
    B. Grade II
    C. Grade III
    D. Grade IV
    E. Grade V

27. A small 8-year-old girl came into the emergency room after being involved in a motor vehicle collision (MVC). She was restrained with a lap belt in the rear passenger seat of the vehicle. She has ecchymosis on her lower abdomen, and has decreased motor and sensory function to her bilateral lower extremities. What is the suspected injury sustained?

    A. Seat belt compression
    B. Seat belt syndrome
    C. Pelvic fracture
    D. Cervical fracture

28. A 5-year-old boy was hit in the right lateral chest with a baseball bat. The radiographic results reveal no rib fractures but the patient is crying and saying that his chest hurts. The nurse should still be assessing the patient for a possible:

    A. Cardiac injury
    B. Liver injury
    C. Renal injury
    D. Lung contusion

29. The nurse is assessing a crying pediatric patient complaining of "belly" pain who has marked abdominal distention. The trauma nurse should expect which test to be performed?

    A. CT of the abdomen
    B. Focused assessment sonography for trauma
    C. Peritoneal lavage
    D. X-ray of kidneys, ureter, and bladder

6

Genitourinary Trauma

MECHANISM OF TRAUMA

■ *What is the most common mechanism of injury for urethral injury?*

■ **Straddle injury**

Blunt mechanism usually results in posterior urethral injury. An example is a straddle injury, which occurs when the bulbous urethra is compressed against the symphysis pubis. Common causes are motor cycle collision, horseback-riding injuries, and bicycle injuries. Penetrating mechanism is secondary to gunshot wounds, stab wounds, self-instrumentation, and perineal impalement after falls.

> ▶ **HINT:** Urethral damage is less common in women because the urethra is short, mobile, and protected by the symphysis pubis. There is a greater chance of injury in males because the urethra is longer and fixed by a ligament.

■ *Are ureteral injuries more commonly a result of blunt or penetrating trauma?*

■ **Penetrating**

The most common cause for ureteral injury is penetrating trauma. A blunt mechanism of injury is rare mechanism of injury. A severe deceleration mechanism may cause an avulsion of the ureter from the ureteropelvic junction.

> ▶ **HINT:** Colon and bowel injuries commonly occur concomitant with ureter injuries.

■ *What is the most common blunt mechanism of injury that causes bladder rupture?*

■ **Motor vehicle collision (MVC)**

MVC is the most common cause of a ruptured bladder and is associated with full bladders. Compression of a full bladder by the lap belt during a sudden deceleration impact causes the dome of the bladder to rupture into the intraperitoneal space.

> ▶ **HINT:** History of prior bladder surgery, irradiation, or malignancy may weaken the bladder and make the bladder prone to rupture.

■ *What injury may be associated with posterior urethral injuries?*

■ **Pelvic fracture**

Posterior urethral injuries may accompany pelvic fractures. Presence of a known pelvic fracture and blood at the meatus would be a significant red flag for the presence of urethral injury.

▶ **HINT:** Remember, blood present at the meatus indicates that the trauma nurse should not attempt to insert an indwelling bladder catheter.

■ *What type of genitourinary injury can occur with intercourse?*
■ **Penile fracture**

Penile fracture can occur with forceful bending of the erect penis during intercourse. Amputations of the penis or testicle can occur because of self-mutilation, assaults, and industrial trauma.

▶ **HINT:** Blunt trauma to the scrotum can result in rupture of the testicles.

TRAUMATIC INJURIES

■ *What traumatic injury is most commonly associated with extraperitoneal bladder rupture (EBR)?*
■ **Pelvic fracture**

The majority of EBR ruptures occur with pelvic fractures. A cystography is recommended in patients with pelvic fractures because of high association of bladder injuries.

▶ **HINT:** Acetabular fractures are not commonly associated with bladder injuries.

■ *Which kidney is most commonly injured in a trauma?*
■ **Right kidney**

The right kidney is the most frequently injured because of its lower position and less protection from the posterior rib cage. Increased injuries to the kidneys occur with a deceleration mechanism, back and flank injuries, or rib fractures.

▶ **HINT:** Kidneys are well protected from trauma by the vertebral column, are surrounded by perirenal fat pads, capped by the adrenal glands, and protected anteriorly by abdominal viscer.

■ *What is the most commonly injured structure within the renal system?*
■ **Kidney**

The kidney is the most commonly injured organ within the renal system. Blunt mechanisms of injury account for the majority of these injuries.

▶ **HINT:** Kidney damage can cause significant blood loss and a life-threatening injury. Avulsion of the renal artery and complete loss of blood flow to the kidney is called a *pedicle injury*.

■ *Following a straddle injury, if the Buck's fascia remains intact, the ecchymosis is confined to which structure?*
■ **Penis**

The urethra is divided into the anterior and posterior compartments. The anterior urethra is composed of the bulbar and penile urethra. The narrowest portion of the urethra is the meatus.

If Buck's fascia is intact, the ecchymosis of urethral disruption is confined to the penis or perineum. The posterior urethra is composed of prostatic and membranous urethra, and neurovascular erectile mechanism, which runs posterolateral and adjacent to the posterior urethra.

> ▶ **HINT:** Symptoms of urethral injury depend on whether the anterior or posterior urethra is injured in the trauma.

ASSESSMENT/DIAGNOSIS

■ *What is a common finding that would require urological imaging to be performed?*

■ **Hematuria**

Gross hematuria requires a series of urological imaging to diagnose an injury to the urological system. Microscopic hematuria in the presence of hemodynamic instability should also be an indication for an evaluation. Gross hematuria is a cardinal sign of kidney and bladder injuries.

> ▶ **HINT:** Hematuria is not always present in all urological injuries but is an indication for a urological radiographic series.

■ *What is the gold standard diagnostic study used to identify renal injury?*

■ **CT scan**

A CT scan is the gold standard for evaluating the renal system following blunt trauma. A CT scan can be used to identify injury to the kidneys and grade the severity of the injury (Box 6.1). A CT arteriogram may also be used to identify vascular injuries to the renal artery or renal vein. An MRI is equivalent to a CT in identifying and grading the severity of the renal injury. An MRI is more capable of differentiating an intrarenal hematoma from a perirenal hematoma.

> ▶ **HINT:** Ultrasound has not been found to be accurate in identifying injuries of the renal system.

Box 6.1 Renal Injury Scale

Grade I	Contusion	Microscopic or gross hematuria with normal urologic studies
Grade I	Hematoma	Subcapsular, nonexpanding without parenchymal laceration
Grade II	Hematoma	Nonexpanding perirenal hematoma confined to renal retroperitoneum
Grade II	Laceration	Less than 1 cm parenchymal depth of renal cortex without extravasation
Grade III	Laceration	Great than 1 cm parenchymal depth of renal cortex without collecting system rupture or urinary extravasation
Grade IV	Laceration	Parenchymal laceration extending through the renal cortex, medulla, and collecting system
Grade IV	Vascular	Main renal artery or vein injury with contained hemorrhage
Grade V	Laceration	Complete shattered kidney
Grade V	Vascular	Avulsion of renal hilum that devascularizes the kidney

■ *What diagnostic study is most frequently used to evaluate ureteral injuries?*
■ **Intravenous pyelogram (IVP)**

IVP is a diagnostic study used to view the kidneys, ureters, and bladder. Contrast dye is administered intravenously and consecutive x-rays are obtained to evaluate renal function; identify extravasation of dye from the kidneys, ureters, or bladder; and determine devitalized segments of the kidney or abnormal ureteral deviation. An IVP has a high false negative rate in penetrating injuries and is not reliable for diagnosis in that population.

> ▶ **HINT:** No single diagnostic test can be used to evaluate the renal system and an IVP may be combined with cystogram and CT scan.

■ *What diagnostic study should be performed before cystogram if the patient presents with blood at the meatus?*
■ **Retrograde urethrogram**

A retrograde urethrogram is used to evaluate the urethra and diagnose urethral rupture by presence of extravasation of dye (Box 6.2). It may be performed before a cystogram to assure the urethra is intact without injury before inserting a catheter into the bladder to perform the cystography.

> ▶ **HINT:** Although blood at the meatus and a high-riding prostate are commonly associated with urethral injury, the absence of such findings does not rule out the presence of urethral injury.

Box 6.2 Indications for Retrograde Urethrogram

Straddle injury
Significant deceleration mechanism
Blood at meatus
High-riding prostate
Perineal butterfly hematoma
Scrotal or perineal crepitus
Inability to pass indwelling catheter

■ *What is the diagnostic study that is best used to identify a bladder rupture?*
■ **Cystogram**

CT of the abdomen is inadequate to identify a bladder rupture. A cystogram is the most accurate diagnostic study and can be used to differentiate intraperitoneal from an extraperitoneal bladder rupture. The normal bladder is shaped like a teardrop. It may appear distorted by the presence of a pelvic hematoma. Cystography is the most sensitive for a submucosal tear of the bladder wall.

> ▶ **HINT:** CT cystography is another option to evaluate the integrity of the bladder and is about equal to a conventional cystography.

■ *What is the diagnostic study of choice to identify urethral injuries?*
■ **Retrograde urethrogram**

A retrograde urethrogram is used to identify the presence of both anterior and posterior urethral injury. The presence of extravasation of dye indicates an injury.

> ▶ HINT: It is also important to use the retrograde urethrogram to determine whether the injury is partial or complete.

MEDICAL/SURGICAL INTERVENTIONS

■ *What is an indication for surgical management of kidney injury?*

■ **Pedicle injury**

A pedicle injury is the avulsion of the renal artery from the aorta, resulting in complete loss of blood flow to the kidney. The kidney is mobile in the retroperitoneum, and the main renal artery connected to the aorta undergoes excessive stretch, causing arterial injury. The injury may be an avulsion or rupture of the intimal layer, forming a thrombus causing arterial occlusion and renal ischemia.

> ▶ HINT: Indications for surgical management also include ongoing hemorrhage, penetrating mechanism, and a pulsatile or expanding hematoma.

■ *What is the nonoperative management of hematuria in a stable patient?*

■ **Bed rest**

Bed rest may be ordered for 24 to 72 hours, or until hematuria is cleared, in patients presenting with gross hematuria but are hemodynamically stable.

> ▶ HINT: Nonoperative management of renal trauma may include angiography and embolization to control bleeding.

■ *What is the purpose of a stent being placed in the ureter following surgical repair?*

■ **Maintain patency**

A stent is placed in ureters to maintain alignment, assure patency during healing, ensure tension-free anastomosis, and prevent urinary extravasation. Surgical management of ureteral injuries typically involves debridement and anastomosis of the ureters with the goal of water-tight closures. If large segments of the ureters are damaged, a transureteroureterostomy can be performed in which one ureter is anastomosed to the other.

> ▶ HINT: Extravasation of urine can cause the development of a uroma.

■ *What is the most common nonoperative management of an EBR?*

■ **Suprapubic catheter**

A suprapubic catheter is placed to drain urine and allow the bladder to heal. The catheter is usually left in place for 7 to 10 days and then the bladder is reevaluated by cystogram for continued extravasation. If extravasation persists, the catheter may remain in place for another 7 to 10 days. The majority of bladder ruptures can be managed with catheter placement and drainage alone. Intraperitoneal bladder ruptures (IBR) may require surgical repair, intraperitoneal irrigation, and catheter placement.

> ▶ **HINT:** An indication for surgical management EBR includes avulsion of the bladder, neck, or concomitant injury to vagina or rectum.

■ *A complete injury of the anterior or posterior urethra typically requires what type of management?*

■ **Placement of suprapubic catheter**

Complete disruption of the anterior or posterior urethra is an indication for a suprapubic catheter to be placed for urinary diversion. The patient may undergo an observational period while the associated pelvic fracture and hematoma stabilize. Definitive management may include surgical repair or reconstructive procedure.

> ▶ **HINT:** An incomplete injury may be management with a urethral-placed catheter by a urologist.

NURSING INTERVENTIONS

■ *What clinical finding would be a contraindication for the placement of an indwelling bladder catheter?*

■ **Blood at the meatus**

If blood is present at the meatus, under no circumstances should a Foley be placed. Other contraindications to insertion of a bladder catheter include scrotal hematoma, perineal hematoma, or high-riding prostate.

> ▶ **HINT:** If resistance is met with insertion of a bladder catheter, stop the insertion. If the bladder catheter is inserted without a urine return, do not inflate the balloon.

■ *A patient presenting with hematuria and flank pain following an MVC may have experienced injury to which urological structure?*

■ **Kidneys**

A common presentation of kidney trauma is hematuria and flank pain. Hematuria is an important sign for injury to several of the urological structures but, in combination with flank pain, it is more likely an injury to the kidneys.

> ▶ **HINT:** Ureter injuries will not have hematuria in 20% to 45% of the cases.

■ *The presence of vaginal bleeding following a straddle injury in a female may indicate what type of injury?*

■ **Urethral injury**

Although women are less likely to experience urethral injuries, the presence of vaginal bleeding, external genitalia, or significant incontinence in the presence of pelvic fractures should be a high suspicion of a urethral injury.

> ▶ **HINT:** Men are more likely to experience urethral injuries because they have longer urethras.

■ *What type of bladder injury may present with an inability to void and acute abdominal signs?*

■ **Intraperitoneal Bladder Rupture (IBR)**

A complete rupture of the dome of the bladder results in extravasation of urine into the peritoneal cavity. The common presenting signs include an inability to void and acute abdominal signs such as abdominal pain or tenderness, fever, and peritoneal irritation. IBR are also associated with shock symptoms of hypotension and tachycardia (Box 6.3).

▶ **HINT:** Extraperitoneal bladder rupture (EBR) usually occurs at the lateral end or base of the bladder and is associated with pelvic fractures.

Box 6.3 Symptoms of Intraperitoneal and Extraperitoneal Bladder Rupture

Intraperitoneal Bladder Rupture	Extraperitoneal Bladder Rupture
Suprapubic tenderness	Pain with urination
Peritoneal irritation	Suprapubic tenderness
Ileus	Reddened suprapubic area
Inability to void	Necrosis of tissue suprapubic area
Hypotension	
Fever	
Abdominal pain	
Abdominal tenderness	

■ *What is the triad of symptoms found in urethral injuries?*

■ **Blood at meatus, inability to void, and distended palpable bladder**

The classic triad of symptoms includes blood at meatus, inability to void, and distended palpable bladder (Box 6.4).

▶ **HINT:** The diagnostic test to evaluate for presence of urethral injury is a retrograde urethrogram.

Box 6.4 Symptoms of Anterior and Posterior Urethral Injuries

Anterior Urethral Injury	Posterior Urethral Injuries
Perineal pain	Inability to void
Blood at meatus	Blood at meatus
Penile and perineal edema	Distended bladder
Distended bladder	Butterfly perineal bruising
Inability to void (occasionally be able to void)	High-riding prostate with rectal exam
Scrotum swelling	
Ecchymosis of scrotum	
Necrosis of scrotal tissue (late sign)	

COMPLICATIONS

■ *What is a complication of a delayed presentation of a ureter injury?*

■ **Peritonitis**

Delayed presentation appears as peritonitis. These symptoms include onset of fever, development of an ileus, abdominal mass, and hematuria, as well as an increase in serum creatinine levels (Box 6.5).

> ▶ **HINT:** Delayed presentation injuries may be managed initially with endoscopic or interventional procedures followed by delayed surgical management.

Box 6.5 Complications of Ureteral Injuries

Infection
Ureteral strictures
Urinary ascites
Uroma
Fistula formation with bowel

■ *What is the most common complication of urethral injury managed with a suprapubic catheter alone?*

■ **Stricture formation**

The placement of a suprapubic catheter alone without a urethral-placed bladder catheter has a high incidence of stricture formation in the urethra. This is typically managed with urethroplasty (Box 6.6).

Box 6.6 Complications of Urethral Injuries

Impotency
Strictures
Incontinence
Obstruction

Questions

1. A patient arrives to the emergency room following a motor vehicle collision (MVC). The patient was restrained and the airbag deployed. What injuries should the nurse suspect when a lap belt is utilized?

   A. Injuries to the colon and the bladder
   B. Injuries to the bladder and the small intestine
   C. Injuries to the stomach and the colon
   D. Injuries to the small intestine and the stomach

2. A patient who sustained bilateral leg fractures after falling off of a ladder is now experiencing nausea and has not had a bowel movement since before admission. The nurse suspects a possible bowel obstruction. What is the most important concern with a diagnosis of bowel obstruction?

   A. Nutrition
   B. Bowel ischemia
   C. Placing a nasogastric tube to low-wall suction
   D. Administering a soapsuds enema

3. A patient has sustained a straddle injury after horseback-riding accident. The patient is complaining of suprapubic pain and has the inability to urinate. The nurse suspects a bladder injury and knows that treatment modalities differ according to the type of bladder injury. Which of the following diagnostic procedures would be most appropriate to diagnose a bladder injury?

   A. Pelvic x-ray
   B. CT cystography
   C. Bladder ultrasound
   D. Kidney ureter bladder (KUB) x-ray

4. A patient came into the emergency department after a bicycle injury. The patient hit a curb, flew off the bike, and landed on his back. The patient complains of lower back pain and abdominal tenderness. Considering the method of injury, what would be the most probable injury sustained?

   A. Kidney rupture
   B. Acute tubular necrosis
   C. Hemorrhagic injury to the kidney
   D. Vascular damage to the renal artery

5. A patient was sitting on a glass table that broke, causing a penetrating injury to the pelvis. The basic metabolic panel results came back with blood urea nitrogen (BUN) = 26, creatinine level = 2.1 mg/dL, glucose = 99 mg/dL. A pyelogram is obtained and results are pending. In the meantime, the patient becomes febrile, develops hematuria and a firm abdomen. The nurse suspects:

   A. Peritonitis
   B. Ureteral injury
   C. Kidney injury
   D. Sepsis

6. A 32-year-old male patient had a bicycle accident, landed on the crossbar, and sustained a straddle injury. He is experiencing an inability to void, blood at the meatus, and butterfly bruising to the scrotal area. These symptoms are expected with what type of injury?

   A. Medial urethral injury
   B. Anterior urethral injury
   C. Posterior urethral injury
   D. Injury at Buck's fascia

7. Treatment for a urethral tear includes all of the following except:

   A. Intravenous antibiotics
   B. Urethral catheter
   C. Suprapubic catheter
   D. Alpha-adrenergic blockers

Obstetrical Trauma

MECHANISM OF INJURY

■ *What is the most common mechanism of injury for obstetrical trauma?*

■ **Motor vehicle collision (MVC)**

A frequent mechanism for trauma in pregnant women is an MVC. As a driver of the vehicle, during impact, the steering wheel can cause damage to the gravid abdomen. Third trimester holds the greatest risk because of the enlarged abdomen and closeness to the dash and steering wheel.

> ▶ HINT: Other mechanisms of injury in pregnant trauma patients include falls, domestic violence, and gunshot wounds.

■ *The gait disturbances of a pregnant woman can lead to what type of traumatic injury?*

■ **Falls**

Falls may be common because of gait disturbances and altered balance. The relaxation of the pelvic girdle ligaments causes changes in balance. Although an increase in fatigue and risk of presyncopal and syncopal episodes in pregnant women also contribute to falls.

> ▶ HINT: The enlarged uterus contributes to the imbalance and as the pregnancy progresses through the trimesters, fall risks increase.

■ *What is a significant risk of fetal death in house fires with pregnant women?*

■ **Carbon monoxide poisoning**

Burns and smoke inhalation during pregnancy can cause carbon monoxide poisoning, which can be fatal to the fetus. Carbon monoxide poisoning is most commonly associated with house fires. Battering and spousal abuse during pregnancy is another mechanism of injury and the pregnancy may be the precipitating factor in some of the domestic violence cases.

> ▶ HINT: Fetal survival is directly related to gestational age.

TRAUMATIC INJURIES

■ *What is a common genitourinary traumatic injury during the third trimester of pregnancy?*

■ **Bladder rupture**

The bladder is more elevated and compressed by the uterus in pregnant women, therefore it is more likely to rupture with blunt force trauma. There is also an increase in glomerular filtration and urinary frequency (Box 7.1).

Box 7.1   Genitourinary Considerations

Increased glomerular filtration rate
Glycosuria
Hypocalcemia
Hypophosphatemia
Hypomagnesemia
Decreased serum creatinine levels

> ▶ **HINT:** Calcium, phosphate, and magnesium levels may decrease during pregnancy and require monitoring following a trauma.

ASSESSMENT/DIAGNOSIS

■ *What information would be important when obtaining a history of a pregnant trauma patient?*

■ **Gestational age of the fetus**

When obtaining a medical history in a pregnant woman following a trauma, the following information should be included: gestational age, status of pregnancy, parity, maternal Rh factor, and delivery history. The trauma nurse should determine whether the patient has had a previous cesarean section (C-section), which may direct the delivery, if necessary.

> ▶ **HINT:** The trauma nurse should also question the pregnant trauma patient regarding history of any previous abortions or premature deliveries.

■ *What is a common respiratory physiological change that results in hypocarbia?*

■ **Chronic hyperventilation**

Pregnant women commonly have $PaCO_2$ levels of 25 to 30 mmHg because of chronic hyperventilation. Normal respiratory changes with pregnancy include a chronic state of hyperventilation, increased tidal volumes by as much as 40%, and increases in vital capacity by 100 mL to 200 mL (Box 7.2).

Box 7.2   Normal Respiratory Changes in Pregnancy

Tachypnea
Hypocarbia
Increased tidal volume
Increased vital capacity
Elevated diaphragm
Elevated PaO_2
Decreased functional residual capacity

▶ **HINT:** Normal physiological changes, which occur during pregnancy, can affect the assessment, interventions, and outcomes during a trauma.

■ *What changes occur with the circulating blood volume in pregnant women?*

■ **It increases**

Normal cardiovascular change with pregnancy includes hypervolemia. The blood volumes increase by the 10th week, with an increase of as much as 50% by the 34th week of pregnancy. Acute blood loss can lead to a decrease in perfusion to the uterus and fetus (Box 7.3).

▶ **HINT:** The normal hypervolemic state during pregnancy can mask a 30% gradual blood loss or 10% to 15% acute blood loss.

Box 7.3 Cardiovascular Changes in Pregnant Women

Hypervolemia
Tachycardia
Left-axis deviation
T-wave flattening or T-wave inversion
Elevated ST segments
Q-waves
S3 gallop

▶ **HINT:** Heart rate can increase by 15 to 20 beats per minute (bpm) by the second trimester of pregnancy; therefore, if the heart rate in a pregnant trauma patient reaches 70 bpm, this is considered to be bradycardia.

■ *What is the assessment technique used to evaluate the fetus in a trauma patient?*

■ **Fetal heart tones (FHTs)**

Following a trauma, the pregnant woman should have FHT assessed to identify fetal distress. FHTs are audible with Doppler by weeks 10 to 12. A normal FHT is 120 to 160 bpm, and rates more than 160 bpm or less than 120 bpm are signs of distress. FHT is the fifth vital sign in pregnancy. Continuous cardiotocographic monitoring is recommended following a trauma or the presence of meconium.

▶ **HINT:** Fetal tachycardia progressing to bradycardia suggests fetal anoxia.

■ *What is the purpose of palpating the abdomen of the pregnant trauma patient when assessing the fetus?*

■ **To assess fundal height**

The uterus is palpable between weeks 12 and 14, and is located at the top of the umbilicus between weeks 18 and 22. A palpated fundal height is used to determine gestational age in weeks of the fetus. Fundal height is measured by determining the distance from the symphis pubis to the top of the uterus.

▶ **HINT:** Fundal height that is higher than the expected gestational age may indicate an abruptio placenta or uterine rupture.

MEDICAL/SURGICAL INTERVENTIONS

■ *Following a fatal MVC, when should a C-section be performed?*
■ **During cardiopulmonary resuscitation (CPR)**

Perimortem C-section is determined by the gestational age and duration of maternal arrest. A viable fetus is above 23 to 28 weeks gestational age and it should be performed within 4 to 5 minutes of the cardiac arrest. The C-section should be performed while CPR is in progress.

NURSING INTERVENTIONS

■ *In what position should the trauma nurse place the pregnant trauma patient while lying on the stretcher?*
■ **Tilted to the side**

If a pregnant woman in the third trimester is lying supine, the enlarged uterus compresses the vena cava and aorta, impeding venous return and cardiac output. The pregnant trauma patient should be rolled to her side.

> ▶ **HINT:** Placing a pregnant patient supine can result in hypotension.

■ *When obtaining x-rays on a pregnant trauma patient, what should the nurse do?*
■ **Place a lead apron over patient's abdomen**

When obtaining radiographic studies on a pregnant trauma patient, shield the uterus with a lead apron. This decreases the radiation exposure of the fetus.

> ▶ **HINT:** The use of MRI is preferred to CT when evaluating a pregnant trauma patient because of the exposure of radiation with CT scans.

■ *In what position would the trauma nurse place the pregnant patient with a prolapsed cord?*
■ **Trendelenburg's position with knee–chest position**

If a cord prolapse is present following a trauma, relieve cord compression by placing the patient in Trendelenburg's position with knee–chest position, if the mother's injuries allow.

> ▶ **HINT:** Insert a gloved hand into the vagina and cradle the cord in the palm of the hand with the fingertips elevating the fetus with a prolapsed cord.

COMPLICATIONS

■ *Because of the relaxation of the gastroesophageal sphincter during advanced pregnancy, what is a potential complication of pregnant woman?*
■ **Aspiration**

Pregnant women experience relaxation of the gastroesophageal sphincter, delayed gastric emptying, and ileus, which can all contribute to vomiting and aspiration. Abdominal palpation assessing for tenderness is not reliable in the pregnant patient as abdominal guarding, tenderness, and rigidity are normal findings.

> ▶ **HINT:** Assume that the pregnant patient has a full stomach and is at risk for vomiting and aspiration.

■ *Immobilization of a pregnant trauma patient places the patient at a high risk for what complication?*

■ **Thromboembolic event**

Fibrinogen and factors VI, VIII, and IX increase during pregnancy, whereas circulating plasminogen levels decrease. This increases the risk of thromboembolism with immobilization. Coagulation studies do not typically change during pregnancy.

> ▶ **HINT:** Anemia can occur during pregnancy because erythrocyte production may not be maintained during pregnancy.

■ *A pregnant trauma patient is complaining of a headache and is noted to be hypertensive. What is the most likely complication of the pregnancy?*

■ **Preeclampsia**

Obstetric complications, such as eclampsia or preeclampsia, may present as changes in vision, headache, hypertension, edema, proteinuria, and seizure activity. Preeclampsia involves gestational hypertension, which is defined as a systolic blood pressure greater than 140 mmHg or diastolic blood pressure greater than 90 mmHg. The difference between preeclampsia and eclampsia is the presence of seizures in the latter (Box 7.4).

> ▶ **HINT:** The most severe form of eclampsia is called the *HELLP syndrome*: hemolysis, elevated liver enzymes, low platelets.

Box 7.4 Symptoms of Preeclampsia

Hypertension
Headache
Edema of hands, face, and sacrum
Visual changes
Nausea
Abdominal pain
Proteinuria
Albuminuria
Elevated creatinine and BUN
Decrease urine output

BUN, blood urea nitrogen.

> ▶ **HINT:** A complication of preeclampsia is acute kidney injury.

■ *The mother reports no fetal movement after a traumatic injury. What would that indicate?*

■ **Fetal demise**

No fetal movement following a trauma indicates fetal demise. FHT and ultrasound can be used to determine presence of fetal heart activity.

> ▶ **HINT:** Premature labor may indicate fetal injury or demise.

■ *Differentiation of amniotic fluid and urine can be determined by testing the fluid for what?*

■ **pH**

Following a trauma and suspected premature rupture of membranes (PROM), differentiation of amniotic fluid from urine may be determined by checking the pH of the fluid. Amniotic fluid has a pH of 7.0 to 7.5, whereas urine is more acidic and has a pH of 4.8 to 6.0. The physician may check for ferning under a microscope.

> ▶ **HINT:** Evidence of fluid pooling in the vagina, or leaking from the cervical os when the patient coughs, or when fundal pressure is applied, will help determine PROM.

■ *A pregnant trauma patient is admitted for PROM. Two days later, the patient exhibits an elevated white blood cell (WBC) count and fever. What is the most likely cause?*

■ **Amniotitis**

Amniotitis is an infection of the amniotic membranes following PROM. Signs of amniotitis include elevated WBC, maternal tachycardia, tender uterus, temperatures higher than 101°F or 38°C, and fetal tachycardia.

> ▶ **HINT:** Elevated WBC and fever indicate infection; the hint in the question is the reference to PROM.

■ *What would be a sign of premature labor following a trauma?*

■ **Bloody show with ruptured membranes**

The trauma nurse needs to recognize signs of labor that include a bloody show, ruptured membrane, and increased frequency of contractions. Following a trauma, the fetus is assessed for viability and injuries before the premature labor is stopped. If the fetus is found to be uninjured, labor can be inhibited with medications such as tocolytics (ritodrine hydrochloride, magnesium sulfate).

> ▶ **HINT:** When timing frequency of contractions during labor, they are timed from beginning of one to the beginning of the next.

■ *What is a predominant sign of an abruptio placentae in a pregnant trauma patient?*

■ **Vaginal bleeding**

Abruptio placenta occurs when the placenta separates or pulls away from the uterine wall, causing disruption of maternal–fetal circulation. An abruptio placentae can occur more than 48 hours after the initial trauma. Signs of abruptio placentae include vaginal bleeding, premature labor pains, abdominal pains, abdominal and uterine tenderness, expanding fundal height, maternal shock, fetal distress, and uterine rigidity.

> ▶ **HINT:** Early recognition of an abruptio placentae and treatment will increase the chance of survival for the fetus.

■ *What laboratory finding is the most specific to disseminated intravascular coagulation (DIC)?*

■ **Elevated D-dimer**

DIC is a potential complication with pregnant trauma patients. It presents with abnormal bleeding, bruising, petechiae, and organ dysfunction. The laboratory findings include an elevated prothrombin time/partial thromboplastin time (PT/PTT), decreased fibrinogen, decreased platelets, and increased D-dimer. There are many coagulopathies that will elevate the coagulation times and decrease the platelets, but DIC is the only coagulopathy that will elevate the D-dimer. The D-dimer measures the by-product of a clot.

> ▶ **HINT:** DIC is the only coagulopathy that causes the body to clot first and bleed second.

■ *An antigen–antibody reaction can occur if the mother is Rh negative or positive?*

■ **Negative**

Antigen–antibody reaction can occur if the mother is Rh negative. When the fetus is Rh positive and the mother is Rh negative, the mother is at risk for an antigen–antibody reaction from the mixing of fetal–maternal blood, causing a thrombolytic reaction. Kleihauer–Betke assay blood test can detect fetal blood cells in maternal circulation.

> ▶ **HINT:** Rh (D) immunoglobulin (RhoGAM) needs to be given within 72 hours of trauma if the mother is Rh negative.

Questions

1. Which of the following is the physiological reason a pregnant woman is commonly involved in falls?

   A. They have more syncopal episodes
   B. The pelvis girdle ligaments relax and develop a wide stance gait
   C. They experience bradycardic episodes
   D. They experience transient ischemic attacks (TIA)

2. What mechanism of injury typically has the lowest mortality rate in the pregnant patient subjected to trauma?

   A. Gunshot wound
   B. Stab wound
   C. Motor vehicle collision
   D. Fall

3. A 28-week pregnant patient comes in after being involved in a severe motor vehicle collision (MVC). The patient has shallow breathing, blood pressure of 89/48 mmHg, a heart rate of 52 beats per minute (bpm), and is currently being intubated. The patient loses a palpable pulse and cardiopulmonary resuscitative (CPR) efforts are being initiated. All of the following need to be done while resuscitation efforts are being performed with the exception of:

   A. Rapid estimation of gestational age assessment of fetal heart activity
   B. Vaginal or uterine examination and an assessment of vaginal bleeding
   C. Emergency C-section within 5 minutes of cardiac arrest
   D. Emergent call for the neonatal resuscitation team

4. When a pregnant patient presents with a blood pressure of 90/72 mmHg, what should be the first nursing intervention to address the situation?

   A. Repeat the blood pressure measurement
   B. Place the patient in reverse Trendelenburg position
   C. Assess the patient for symptomatic hypotension
   D. Place the patient on her left lateral side at 30 degrees

5. When a pregnant patient comes into the hospital for treatment, it is important to know how to measure fundal height in order to obtain an approximate gestational age. Approximately how many weeks gestation would be the fetal age if palpated at the level of the umbilicus?

   A. 20-weeks gestation
   B. 32-weeks gestation
   C. 12-weeks gestation
   D. 36-weeks gestation

6. A 32-week pregnant patient comes to the emergency room with a stab wound to the abdomen. The patient is requiring multiple blood transfusions and is blood type O negative. What distinct laboratory test is indicated to deliver proper treatment for this patient?

   A. Kleihauer–Betke test
   B. Beta human chorionic gonadotropin (HCG) level
   C. Prothrombin time (PT) and partial thromboplastin time (PTT) level
   D. Hemoglobin and hematocrit levels

7. A 28-week pregnant woman comes to the emergency department following a minor trauma. She begins to complain of a headache, blurred vision, and epistaxis. Which complication should the nurse be suspicious of?

   A. Preeclampsia
   B. Eclampsia
   C. Hypervolemia
   D. Status preclampsius

8. Pregnant women undergo a number of cardiovascular changes. A third-trimester-pregnant patient comes in complaining of mild chest pain. Her heart rate is 65 beats per minute (bpm) and regular, an S3 heart sound is auscultated, and inverted T waves and Q waves are present on the electrocardiogram. Which is considered abnormal in this patient's cardiac workup?

   A. S3 heart sound
   B. Heart rate of 65 bpm
   C. Inverted T waves
   D. Presence of Q waves

9. A woman who is 30 weeks pregnant was involved in a minor fender bender, but has decided to come to the hospital to get worked up. The nurse drew labs and collected a urine sample. The urine comes back with glycosuria. The complete blood count (CBC) results revealed a white blood cell (WBC) count of 24,000, hematocrit of 31.5%, and hemoglobin of 10.2 mg/dL. The basic metabolic panel came back with potassium of 4.0 mEq, calcium of 8.5 mg/dL, and magnesium of 1.5 mg/dL. Which of the following results is considered abnormal in the pregnant patient?

   A. Elevated WBC count
   B. Calcium 8.5 mg/dL
   C. Glycosuria
   D. Hematocrit 31.5 %

10. Ms. Rodriquez comes in to the emergency room after a motor vehicle collision (MVC). She was unrestrained and her airbag did deploy. She is 32 weeks pregnant and has sustained major injuries, especially to her left hip and head. While assessing her injuries, the heart monitor begins to alarm, Ms. Rodriquez is now in ventricular tachycardia. The nurse assesses for a pulse and she is pulseless, the nurse begins cardiopulmonary resuscitation (CPR), but because the patient is pregnant the nurse knows not to administer which of the following drugs during the code?

   A. Epinephrine
   B. Amiodarone
   C. Sodium bicarbonate
   D. All can be administered

11. A 22-year-old pregnant patient in her third trimester has arrived to the emergency department in respiratory distress. The patient was eating pistachios and got a shell lodged in her trachea. The shell was successfully retrieved and the patient is currently complaining of a sore throat and cough. An arterial blood gas (ABG) is collected and the results are: pH = 7.36, PaO_2 = 104 mmHg, SaO_2 = 95%, $PaCO_2$ = 30. Which of the following is the most correct interpretation of this ABG?

    A. Mild compensating respiratory acidosis
    B. Normal
    C. Compensated metabolic acidosis
    D. Respiratory alkalosis

12. All of the following are complications that pregnant patients can experience that cause an alteration in tissue perfusion except:

    A. Premature labor
    B. Increased metabolism
    C. Hypovolemia
    D. Interruption of venous flow

Part III

Clinical Practice: Extremity and Wound

Musculoskeletal Trauma

MECHANISM OF INJURY

■ *What type of spine fractures can occur when people jump from a significant height and land on their feet?*

■ **Compression fractures**

Compression fractures of the lumbar spine frequently occur when people fall or jump on their feet from significant heights. A common triad of fractures occurs with falls that include calcaneus, thoracolumbar, and bilateral wrist fractures. The triad is caused by the person landing on his or her feet (calcaneus fracture), the force causing compression fractures in the thoracolumbar spine, and the person falls forward on his or her wrists (bilateral wrist fractures).

> ▶ **HINT:** A direct impact on the top of the head can also cause compression fractures of the upper spine and is called *axial loading*.

■ *A motor vehicle/pedestrian collision causes a typical pattern of injury. What is this called?*

■ **Waddell's triad**

Motor vehicle/pedestrian injury commonly presents with a pattern of injury called *Waddell's triad*. The three injuries include bilateral femur fractures, blunt chest injury, and traumatic brain injury. This is classic with children who turn to face the approaching vehicle. The impact of the vehicle bumper occurs at the level of the femur (bilateral femur fractures), the child is thrown onto the hood of the vehicle (chest trauma), and then continues off the car, landing on the head (traumatic brain injury).

> ▶ **HINT:** Adult motor vehicle/pedestrian collisions may have a slightly different pattern of injury as adults will commonly turn to avoid being hit by the vehicle.

■ *Where is the most common point of impact on the dash in a front-seat passenger during head-on collision?*

■ **Bilateral knees**

A front-seat passenger in a motor vehicle collision (MVC) may sustain injury to bilateral knees from the impact of the dashboard, and hip fractures or posterior dislocations may be caused by the posterior directional force.

> ▶ **HINT:** If the passenger is not restrained with a shoulder harness, then the face is typically the point of impact on the dash.

■ *A history of frequent fractures or various stages of healing fractures may indicate what in pediatric patients?*

■ **Child abuse**

History of multiple fractures and emergency department (ED) visits, or various stages of healing fractures in children may be a sign of child abuse and should be further investigated. At ages 2 years and younger, ribs are very bendable and less likely to fracture, therefore rib fractures in children younger than 2 years indicate a significant force and should create a high suspicion of child abuse. Spiral fractures are a result of a "twisting" mechanism and are uncommon unintentional injuries in young children. A simple fall does not cause spiral fracture in children. A corner fracture or bucket handle fracture in a child is also especially predictive of child abuse as these occur with intentional injury.

▶ **HINT:** A corner fracture is a piece of bone avulsed from the fragile growth plate caused by a shearing mechanism, whereas a bucket fracture is similar but involves a larger piece of avulsed bone.

■ *What is a common fracture that occurs in an elderly person following a fall?*

■ **Femoral neck**

Fractures of the femoral neck are common in elderly patients. The elderly patient's bones with osteoporosis may actually fracture during ambulation causing the fall versus the fracture being the result of the fall itself.

▶ **HINT:** The comorbidities of osteoporosis and osteoarthritis in elderly patients increase their risk of fractures.

■ *What type of amputation involves a cut with well-defined edges?*

■ **Guillotine**

An amputation caused by a cut or guillotine type of mechanism has well-defined edges and is easier to reimplant. Crush injuries causing an amputation result in soft tissue damage and are less likely to be able to be reimplanted. A forceful stretching and tearing away of the tissue causing an amputation is called an *avulsion injury*.

▶ **HINT:** A clean guillotine amputation has the most success of reimplantation.

TRAUMATIC INJURIES

■ *What type of fracture results in a great amount of nerve and vascular injury?*

■ **Displaced fracture**

Bone disruption or displacement following an injury can result in injury to surrounding tissue, nerves, and blood supply. Trauma to the surrounding structures and bone can be caused by both blunt and penetrating injuries.

▶ **HINT:** Musculoskeletal trauma includes injuries to bone, joints, muscle, ligaments, nerves, and blood vessels.

■ *What type of injury may have occurred when there is a laceration over the site of the fracture?*

■ **Open fracture**

An open fracture occurs when the skin integrity over or near the fracture is open; this is typically a complete fracture (Box 8.1). The bone may or may not be protruding from the wound. An incomplete fracture occurs when the bone integrity is not completely disrupted.

> ▶ **HINT:** The trauma nurse should consider any lacerations or open wounds in the vicinity of the fracture as an open fracture.

Box 8.1 Grade of Open Fracture

Grade	Description
Grade I	Minimal soft tissue damage
Grade II	Wounds greater than 2 cm with a crush injury
Grade III	Associated with extensive tissue damage

> ▶ **HINT:** Grade III open fractures have a large amount of wound contamination and are associated frequently with nonviable tissue.

■ *What is the name of the fracture when the bone bends and the fracture is an incomplete fracture?*

■ **Greenstick fracture**

A greenstick fracture occurs when the bone bends and the fracture is incomplete. A comminuted fracture is the splintering of bone into multiple pieces following a blunt injury. A displacement is the lack of alignment of the ends of the bones, although an impaction injury occurs when the bones are wedged into each other.

> ▶ **HINT:** Greenstick fractures are more likely found in pediatric trauma patients than adults.

■ *What is the systemic response to a fat emboli called?*

■ **Fat embolism syndrome**

Fat embolism is the presence of fat particles within the microcirculation. Fat embolism syndrome is the systemic response and manifestation of fat embolism. Large numbers of patients with long-bone fractures have fat globules present in the blood, but only a few have symptoms of fat embolism.

> ▶ **HINT:** Symptoms of fat embolism syndrome are similar to a pulmonary embolism and can be indistinguishable from acute respiratory distress syndrome.

ASSESSMENT/DIAGNOSIS

■ *What would a low ankle–brachial index (ABI) indicate following a lower limb traumatic injury?*

■ **Decrease perfusion**

ABI measures the systolic blood pressure (SBP) in the ankles and is divided by the SBP in the brachial area. An ABI of 1 is normal, whereas an ABI of less than 0.9 indicates occlusive disease, and an ABI of less than 0.45 indicates significant decrease in blood flow.

■ *When assessing an extremity following a fracture, the nurse notes the patient has paresthesia. What type of injury is associated with the fracture?*

■ **Nerve injury**

Both motor and sensory abnormalities should be assessed following an extremity injury. The neurovascular examination of an extremity includes the five Ps: pain, pallor, pulseless, paresthesia, and paralysis. Of the five Ps, pain, paresthesia, and paralysis correlate to nerve injury, whereas pallor and pulselessness are used to assess arterial supply distal to the site of injury.

> ▶ **HINT:** A nerve that is lacerated or that has sustained significant injury may cause a loss of sensation to the affected extremity distal to the site of injury.

■ *An abnormal externally rotated leg may indicate what type of fracture?*

■ **Pelvic fracture**

Pelvic fractures can be a result of external rotation, lateral compression, abduction, and shearing forces. The trauma nurse should have a high suspicion for a pelvic fracture if the trauma patient has an abnormal rotation of a leg, especially an externally rotated leg.

> ▶ **HINT:** If a patient has sustained a pelvic fracture, the trauma nurse should assess for associated injuries such as blood at the meatus (renal trauma) and hemodynamic instability (hemorrhage).

■ *When performing an extremity assessment on a trauma patient, to what should the trauma nurse compare the affected extremity?*

■ **Unaffected extremity**

The trauma nurse should compare the affected extremity to the unaffected when performing assessment of the color, pulse, length of limb, sensory abnormalities, and function. When assessing the trauma patient, note whether the patient has full range of motion in all extremities unless contraindicated.

> ▶ **HINT:** Palpate pulses proximal and distal, and compare the pulses to the opposite side for strength and quality.

■ *What is the bedside assessment that can be performed to assess for the stability of a pelvis?*

■ **Press iliac crests together**

To assess for pelvic fractures and pelvic stability, the trauma nurse may press the iliac crests toward the midline noting any instability or increased pain. An unstable pelvic fracture exists when there is a fracture in more than one place of the pelvic ring, resulting in displacements on the ring.

> ▶ **HINT:** Never "rock" a pelvis if an injury is suspected. This may cause further damage to the internal structures.

■ *What is the initial diagnostic study for identifying fractures?*
■ **Radiographs**

Radiographs are used to identify fractures following extremity trauma. Recommended radiographs of an extremity should be of at least two views because a fracture may not be seen with just a single view. Common views obtained to identify a fracture are anterior–posterior and lateral views. An arteriogram should be obtained if there is a suspected injury to the vasculature with an extremity injury. A duplex Doppler ultrasonography may be used as an alternative to an angiogram and can be performed in the ED.

> ▶ **HINT:** Crepitus noted during palpation of an extremity indicates the possibility of an underlying fracture and a radiograph should be obtained.

■ *What monitoring should be used in patients with suspected pulmonary embolism?*
■ **Oxygen saturation**

The use of continuous oxygen-saturation monitoring is recommended to identify periods of transient hypoxia following a long-bone fracture because of fat embolism. Clinical symptoms of fat embolism include hypoxia, tachycardia, tachypnea, dyspnea, fever, and chest pain.

> ▶ **HINT:** Hypoxia because of a fat embolism is refractory to high levels of FiO_2 (fraction of inspired oxygen) and decreases lung compliance as a result of intrapulmonary shunting.

■ *What is the clinical symptom of a fat embolism that can be used to distinguish fat embolism from a pulmonary embolism?*
■ **Petechiae**

The appearance of petechiae on the upper trunk, axilla, chest, conjunctiva, and mucous membranes is a hallmark sign of a fat embolism and is present in about 50% of the cases. There is no specific test to diagnose fat embolism.

> ▶ **HINT:** This petechial rash usually resolves within 24 hours of the fat embolism syndrome.

■ *What is considered to be the hallmark of compartment syndrome?*
■ **Pain beyond pain medications**

Pain beyond pain medications is a hallmark sign of compartment syndrome, whereas pain on passive movement is an early sign of compartment syndrome. Pain on passive movement is assessed by moving the distal portion of the extremity and determining the presence of pain (i.e., calf injury can be assessed by the examiner moving the foot up and down).

▶ **HINT:** Compartment syndrome can produce pain beyond pain medications, paresthesia, and paralysis (or weakness of the involved extremity) early in the presentation.

■ *What finding on assessment of an extremity at risk for compartment syndrome would indicate irreversible tissue injury?*

■ **Loss of a pulse**

Pulses and capillary refill remain intact in the presence of compartment syndrome because it involves the collapse of arterioles and veins, not the major arteries. In compartment syndrome, once a pulse is lost, it is too late to salvage the extremity because of irreversible tissue damage.

▶ **HINT:** A presentation of compartment syndrome may include a decrease in the sensation of the affected extremity because of the damage of the nerves within the fascial compartment; this is an earlier sign than a loss of a pulse.

■ *What is considered a normal compartmental pressure in an extremity?*

■ **10 mmHg**

Extremity compartment pressures can be measured in patients suspected of experiencing compartment syndrome. A normal compartment pressure is 10 mmHg of pressure. A compartmental pressure greater than 30 mmHg requires a surgical open fasciotomy to relieve the pressure.

▶ **HINT:** The physical examination may be primarily used to recognize compartment syndrome.

■ *Compartment syndrome in the forearm and wrist can be assessed by asking the patient to perform what movement?*

■ **Flexion and extension of fingers**

The volar compartment contains flexors and pronator muscles of the forearm and wrist, median and ulnar nerve, ulnar and radial artery. Compartment syndrome occurring in the volar compartment presents with weakness in flexors of finger and thumb. The trauma nurse can assess the volar compartment by having the patient extend and flex a thumb and finger, or perform finger abduction or adduction movements.

▶ **HINT:** The patient maintains flexion of fingers and experiences pain on extension.

MEDICAL/SURGICAL INTERVENTIONS

■ *When would an extremity trauma become a higher priority of care in a multisystem trauma patient?*

■ **Potential loss of limb**

Injury to an extremity is not considered a high priority in managing a multiple trauma patient, unless it involves a potential loss of limb or hemodynamic instability. Vascular injuries are of a higher priority because of lack of perfusion to the extremity and potential loss of limb.

> ▶ **HINT:** A loss of pulse distal to the extremity injury indicates vascular involvement and may require surgical management to restore perfusion to the limb.

■ *When immobilizing a limb following a traumatic injury, how much of the extremity should be immobilized?*

■ **Joint above and below injury**

Proper immobilization includes immobilization of the joint above and below the injury. An extremity that has an obvious deformity, crepitus, edema, or vascular compromise should be immobilized. Immobilization devices should be checked frequently, monitored for swelling, with padded splints placed to prevent further injury. Air splints may be used to decrease edema.

> ▶ **HINT:** Any rigid material can be used as a splint and, in lower extremities, one limb can be splinted against the other. Splinting of a pelvic fracture may be performed with a folded sheet that is clamped or knotted in the front.

■ *The trauma nurse knows not to reposition which type of fracture to immobilize with splints?*

■ **Open fracture**

In an open fracture with protruding bone or a comminuted fracture, do not reposition the extremity to immobilize the fracture. Excessive manipulation of a fractured extremity can cause further injury to surrounding structures and increase bleeding into tissues.

> ▶ **HINT:** If the nurse suspects any neurovascular compromise from an external splint, the splint should be removed, adjusted, and reapplied.

■ *What is the primary goal of placement of external fixators on a pelvic fracture?*

■ **Limit blood loss**

An external fixator is frequently used to stabilize pelvic fractures and limit blood loss. External fixation is accomplished with percutaneous pins connected to a rigid frame. Therapeutic embolization in interventional radiology is also used to control hemorrhage associated with pelvic fractures.

> ▶ **HINT:** Damage-control procedures may be required to prevent hemorrhage and death.

■ *What type of medication is frequently ordered following vascular repair?*

■ **Antithrombotics**

Following surgical vascular repair in patients with extremity trauma, anticoagulation or antiplatelet therapy may be initiated to prevent formation of clots and graft occlusion. Vasopressors should be used cautiously because of the significant vasoconstriction in the peripheral circulation, causing loss of perfusion to the affected limb.

> ▶ **HINT:** Frequent neurovascular checks should be performed following vascular injury and surgical repair.

■ *What is the best intervention to decrease the incidence of fat emboli?*

■ **Fixation of fracture**

Long-bone fracture is associated with higher incidence of fat emboli. The best intervention to prevent fat embolism is to fixate the fracture. Early stabilization and fixation of the long-bone fracture has been shown to decrease the incidence of fat embolism. Immediate stabilization of long-bone fracture is not always possible in multisystem trauma patients but should be performed as soon as possible to prevent fat embolism.

> ▶ **HINT:** Manipulation of an extremity with a long-bone fracture can increase the risk of fat embolism.

■ *Following a traumatic amputation, what is the best initial method to use to prevent blood loss from the remaining stump?*

■ **Direct pressure**

The initial management of a traumatic amputation is to control the blood loss. This should be attempted first by applying direct pressure to the wound. If this does not control the blood loss, then apply a tourniquet as close to the stump as possible to minimize the amount of tissue ischemia caused by the tourniquet.

> ▶ **HINT:** Most amputated parts experience vasoconstriction, which limits the blood loss.

■ *What specific care of the amputated part increases the time from amputation to reimplantation?*

■ **Placing on ice**

Appropriate care of the amputated body part is to remove the dirt and debris from the part, then wrap it in gauze dressing moistened with saline. The amputated part should then be wrapped in a towel, enclosed in a sealed bag, and placed on ice. Cooling the extremity increases the time to reimplantation. Cooling the amputated part decreases the metabolic rate and inhibits bacterial growth.

> ▶ **HINT:** The amputated part should not be directly exposed to the ice or submerged in ice to prevent frostbite and further tissue damage.

■ *In the ED, what is the best cleansing solution to be used on the amputated part?*

■ **Aqueous penicillin**

Initial emergency care of the amputated part is to wash it with isotonic solution then wrap it in sterile gauze moistened with solution of aqueous penicillin (1,000,000 U in 50 mL Ringer's lactate). Do not use antiseptics, hydrogen peroxide, iodine, or other solutions on the amputated part.

> ▶ **HINT:** The use of betadine on the amputated part can cause the extremity to be unable to be reimplanted and should be avoided.

■ *What systemic complication of a trauma can limit the ability to reimplant and salvage an amputated extremity?*

■ **Hypotension**

The extent of the skeletal and soft tissue damage, and the duration of the limb ischemia are clinical variables used to predict whether the limb is salvageable. Severe hypotension worsens chances of being able to reimplant an extremity because of ischemic injuries.

> ▶ **HINT:** Success of reimplantation in elderly victims is not as good as in younger patients.

■ *A loss of bone in a lower extremity amputation limits reimplantation because of what complication?*

■ **Limb length discrepancy**

A large loss of bone in lower extremity amputations results in limb length discrepancy and poor ambulation. In these cases, reimplantation should be avoided and a prosthesis used for ambulation. Preservation attempts of amputated parts fail because of the presence of severe inflammation or infection, significant soft tissue necrosis, and severe functional deficit.

> ▶ **HINT:** Lower extremity reimplantation requires preservation of protective sensation for successful usage and ambulation.

■ *What body parts can tolerate a greater warm ischemia time?*

■ **Fingers**

Ischemic time begins at the time of injury, and muscle fibers are very sensitive to lack of oxygen, and demonstrate damage after 30 minutes of ischemia. Digits contain tendinous tissue and ligaments, which can tolerate a longer ischemic time than the more proximal limbs, which have a greater muscle mass. Digits can tolerate an increase in warm ischemic time to 24 hours and cold ischemic time to 48 hours.

> ▶ **HINT:** Candidates for reimplantation include amputation of scalp, hand, foot, nose, or penis (Box 8.2).

Box 8.2 Reimplantation: Indications and Contraindications

Indications for Reimplantation	Contraindications for Reimplantation
Proximal to distal interphalangeal of the digit	Severe crush or avulsion injuries
Younger age	Multiple levels of amputations
Occupational value of digit	Lower extremity with limb length discrepancy
Bilateral hands	
Multiple digits	
Thumb	

> ▶ **HINT:** Lower extremity reimplantations are less likely to be successful because of limb length discrepancies or loss of sensation of the sole of the foot.

■ *What pharmacological therapy is frequently utilized to prevent a decrease in perfusion to the reimplanted extremity?*

■ **Antiplatelet medication**

Aspirin or other antiplatelet medications are commonly administered following reimplantation to prevent platelet aggregation and loss of perfusion to the reimplanted part. Antiplatelet drugs improve arterial flow to the reimplanted extremity, lowering the incidence of procedures to revascularize the extremity.

▶ **HINT:** Instruct the patient to avoid smoking postoperatively because of the vasoconstrictive effects, which cause hypoperfusion.

■ *What is the primary surgical intervention for a compartment syndrome?*

■ **Fasciotomy**

A fasciotomy is the opening of the fascial compartment to decrease the pressure on surrounding structures.

▶ **HINT:** Each extremity has more than one compartment and the extremity may require more than one fasciotomy (Box 8.3).

Box 8.3 Extremity Compartments

Extremity	Number of Compartments
Thigh	2
Calves and feet	4
Upper extremity	3
Forearms	2
Hand	4

NURSING INTERVENTIONS

■ *What is the initial intervention for a trauma nurse to use to control bleeding from a wound?*

■ **Direct pressure**

A priority of care with musculoskeletal injuries is to control bleeding. It is recommended that direct pressure on an actively bleeding wound should be utilized first to control the blood loss. Tourniquet use may be recommended to prevent severe hemorrhage following a mangled extremity injury and, once placed, should be left on until surgical management is available.

▶ **HINT:** Improper or prolonged placement of a tourniquet can cause nerve paralysis and extremity ischemia.

■ *What is the recommended method to control severe blood loss following a traumatic extremity injury?*

■ **Tourniquet**

Applying direct pressure to a wound to control bleeding is the recommended first intervention to establish hemostasis. But severe bleeding that continues despite direct pressure may require a tourniquet to control blood loss and hemorrhagic shock. Bleeding may also be controlled with cautery and suturing.

> ▶ **HINT:** Scalp injuries typically require sutures to control blood loss.

■ *What does muscle spasms following a traumatic fracture cause in the patient?*

■ **Pain**

Pain management is a big concern for the trauma nurse caring for patients with traumatic fractures. Pain is caused by the bony fracture, tissue injury, tissue ischemia, and nerve injury. Muscle spasms can contribute to the pain and may be managed with muscle relaxants. Regional anesthesia with nerve blocks may be used to control pain following a fracture associated with a large amount of pain.

> ▶ **HINT:** Pain management is a big concern for the trauma nurse caring for patients with traumatic fractures throughout their hospitalization.

■ *Following a traumatic amputation, at what level should the extremity be positioned?*

■ **Elevated**

Elevating the stump or the remaining portion of the extremity limits edema.

> ▶ **HINT:** In compartment syndrome, the extremity should be placed level to the heart.

■ *Once an extremity part is reimplanted, what should the nurse assess for on the reimplanted part?*

■ **Perfusion**

Assessment of perfusion for the reimplanted extremity includes frequent neurovascular checks, Doppler tones, pulse oximetry, and surface temperature probes. A decrease in oxygen saturation or temperature of a reimplanted extremity indicates tissue hypoperfusion.

> ▶ **HINT:** A decrease of 2.5°C may indicate a decrease in perfusion to the limb.

■ *Following reimplantation of a hand, the nurse notes the fingers are cool to the touch, nail beds are pale, and there is a delay in capillary refill. What is the most likely complication?*

■ **Arterial congestion**

Arterial congestion is a potential complication following reimplantation of a body part. The reimplanted part appears mottled and pale, has a sluggish capillary refill, is cool to the touch, and the tissue turgor may appear "prune like" in arterial congestion. This indicates hypoperfusion and may require revascularization of the extremity.

> ▶ **HINT:** If the trauma nurse suspects arterial congestion in a reimplanted part, the extremity should be lowered to below the heart level, dressings loosened or removed, and the physician informed.

■ *During assessment of a reimplanted traumatically amputated extremity, the nurse notes the extremity appears to have a bluish discoloration, but a brisk capillary refill remains. What is the most likely complication?*

■ **Venous congestion**

Venous congestion of a reimplanted body part appears as cyanotic, is cool to the touch, with a brisk capillary refill, and tense skin turgor. The management of venous congestions is to elevate the affected extremity while maintaining alignment, and to change or remove tight dressings. Medical leeches are frequently used if the reimplanted body part develops venous congestion.

> ▶ **HINT:** Leech therapy is not indicated if the complication is impaired arterial flow. Leeches are used to assist with reestablishing venous outflow.

■ *What commonly used laboratory finding is used to assess for muscle injury following a crush mechanism of injury?*

■ **Creatinine kinase (CK)**

CK levels elevate in patients with crush injuries because of the release of CK from the muscle when injured. Potassium can also elevate following crush injuries because of the release of intracellular components, including potassium.

> ▶ **HINT:** Rhabdomyolysis is caused by the disruption of the muscle cell membrane, which releases myoglobin and other components (serum glutamic-oxaloacetic transaminase [SGOT], lactate dehydrogenase [LDH], CK, glucose, potassium) into the bloodstream.

■ *Which electrolyte abnormality is most commonly associated with crush injury and acute renal failure caused by rhabdomyolysis?*

■ **Hyperkalemia**

Potassium elevates following crush injuries because of the release of intracellular components following cellular injury. Potassium is primarily found intracellularly and is released with traumatic crush injuries. Hyperkalemia is most commonly found early and typically peaks within 12 to 36 hours after a crush injury. The hyperkalemia can be managed with kayexalate, insulin, and dextrose, bicarbonate infusion, or beta agonist. Calcium gluconate can be administered as a cardioprotectant in hyperkalemic cases.

> ▶ **HINT:** Hyperkalemia may be identified early by the presence of peaked T waves on the EKG.

■ *What is a sign commonly used to determine compartment syndrome in a patient unable to communicate abnormal sensation or pain in the affected extremity?*

■ **Tautness of skin**

A patient unable to communicate pain or abnormal sensation in the affected extremity can contribute to a missed compartment syndrome. Patients unable to verbalize pain following an extremity injury require frequent assessment of the affected extremity for firmness, tautness of skin, and the presence of skin blisters.

> ▶ **HINT:** The complication of an untreated compartment syndrome can be more severe than a fasciotomy.

■ *In what position should the nurse place the patient's extremity if compartment syndrome is suspected?*

■ **Neutral position**

An extremity suspected of having compartment syndrome should be maintained in a neutral position. Elevating the extremity may further compromise perfusion to the extremity. Allowing it to be lower than the level of the heart will increase edema and worsen compartment syndrome.

> ▶ **HINT:** Remove any constricting dressings or casts from the extremity suspected of developing compartment syndrome.

COMPLICATIONS

■ *What is a life-threatening complication of pelvic fractures?*

■ **Hemorrhage**

The pelvis contains a large vascular blood supply, including a large venous plexus, therefore injuries to the pelvis can result in significant blood loss and hemorrhagic shock. Posterior fractures of the pelvis have a greater incidence of hemorrhage complication than injuries to the anterior portion of the pelvis. A femur fracture may lose up to 1,500 mL of blood following an injury, and loss of about 700 to 750 mL can be attributed to tibial or humeral fractures.

> ▶ **HINT:** Assess for significant blood loss that may be associated with extremity trauma and bone fractures.

■ *What type of pelvic fracture has the greatest risk of complications and mortality?*

■ **Open pelvic fracture**

Complications associated with an open pelvic fracture include injury to the perineum, rectum, and genitourinary structure (especially the bladder).

■ *What is a complication of a hip dislocation?*

■ **Avascular necrosis**

A complication of a hip dislocation is avascular necrosis of the femoral head. Dislocation of the knee may cause damage to the peroneal nerve, and to the popliteal artery and vein. Posterior knee dislocation is associated with a higher incidence of vascular injury.

> ▶ **HINT:** Early surgical repair of hip dislocations may lower the incidence of avascular necrosis.

■ *What type of fracture most commonly develops the complication of an infection?*

■ **Open fracture**

Infections following fractures occur with the greatest incidence in open fractures. Infections may involve the wounds or bone. Complication of an infection leads to delayed wound healing, osteomyelitis, and even sepsis.

> ▶ **HINT:** Close observation by the trauma nurse for signs of sepsis is recommended following an open fracture and extremity wounds.

■ *What body system is most frequently involved with fat embolism syndrome?*

■ **Lungs**

Fat particles in the circulation cause damage to the capillaries and may involve eyes, skin, and heart, but the lungs are most commonly affected. An elevated intramedullary pressure following trauma causes fat to be released through open venous sinusoids and obstructs flow in the pulmonary capillaries. There is also a systemic response beyond the pulmonary capillaries, which may be a result of the release of free fatty acids, causing a release of inflammatory mediators.

> ▶ **HINT:** Fat embolism syndrome presents with signs of dyspnea and hypoxia.

■ *What is a complication of a crush syndrome following trauma to an extremity?*

■ **Rhabdomyolysis**

Crush syndrome is a condition in which prolonged muscle compression leads to muscle necrosis and the release of myoglobin. Rhabdomyolysis is a form of acute kidney injury in which there is a large amount of injured muscle releasing myoglobin in the blood (myoglobinemia), and is filtered through the kidneys (myoglobinurea).

> ▶ **HINT:** Rhabdomyolysis causes reddish to brownish urine, frequently described as "cola" or "tea" colored.

■ *An elevated pressure in the osteofascial compartment results in injury to which component of the bundle first?*

■ **Muscle**

An osteofascial compartment is a sheath of fascia that binds the muscle and the neurovascular bundles. Compartment syndrome is an elevated pressure within the osteofascial compartment that result in ischemic injury to muscle, nerve, and vascular structures. It occurs most commonly because of a compression or crush-type injury, but can also occur from an external source such as wraps, casts, or air splints.

▶ **HINT:** The onset of compartment syndrome is usually 6 to 8 hours after injury.

■ *What is considered a severe complication of an untreated compartment syndrome?*
■ **Amputation**

A severe complication of an untreated compartment syndrome is an amputation because of severe muscle damage and necrosis (Box 8.4).

▶ **HINT:** Performing a fasciotomy on an extremity with internal fixation can result in decreased stabilization of the fracture.

Box 8.4 Comparison of Complications: Compartment Syndrome and Fasciotomy

Complications of Compartment Syndrome	Complications of Fasciotomy
Crush syndrome	Bleeding
Foot drop	Damaged neurovascular structures
Gross muscle necrosis	Infection
Amputation	Inadequate decompression

▶ **HINT:** Crush syndrome as a result of a compartment syndrome causes myoglobinuria, hyperkalemia, metabolic acidosis, and acute kidney injury.

Questions

1. There are different types of pelvic fracture stabilization devices that can be utilized to manage unstable pelvic fractures. All of the following are appropriate stabilization methods except:

   A. Wrap the pelvis in a folded sheet clamped at the front
   B. Air splint device
   C. Pneumatic antishock garment
   D. External fixator

2. All of the following are forces applied to the pelvic region that can cause pelvic fracture except which of the following?

   A. Lateral compression
   B. Anteroposterior rotation
   C. Internal rotation
   D. Shear

3. An obvious open femur fracture should be addressed promptly once airway, breathing, and circulation are stable. This should include all of the following except:

   A. Sensory motor assessment
   B. Signs of infections and osteomyelitis
   C. Immobilization of extremity
   D. Application of a sterile dressing

4. The nurse performs an assessment of the extremity of a long-bone fracture. The nurse palpates and inspects the extremity, noting the extremity position and any open wounds or deformities. The nurse should assess for internal blood loss and estimate external blood loss. Which of the following examples best depicts a proper inspection and palpation of the injury?

   A. Inspect for ecchymosis, palpate for edema
   B. Inspect nail-bed color, palpate for crepitus
   C. Inspect for pain, palpate for muscle spasm
   D. Inspect for edema, palpate capillary refill

5. Proper immobilization of a traumatic long-bone injury is described as:

   A. Immobilization above the injury only
   B. Immobilization below the injury only
   C. Immobilization at the actual site of injury only
   D. Immobilization above and below the level of injury

6. The nurse receives a patient with an obvious open fracture to the arm. The extremity has glass and debris in the wound. Every time the nurse attempts to irrigate the wound, the patient screams in pain. What should the nurse do first to address this situation?

   A. Notify the physician of the patient's noncompliance
   B. Notify the physician for the need for analgesic orders

C. Inform the patient of the importance of removing the debris and attempt to irrigate the wound again

D. Cover the wound with a sterile dressing and administer the ordered antibiotics.

7. A 78-year-old woman fell and attempted to brace her fall by reaching out her arm. She is complaining of right shoulder pain. It is important not only to assess the site for obvious edema or hematoma, but also for capillary refill, motor function, and sensation because there may be vascular and nerve involvement with this injury. What structure is the most likely to be damaged?

A. Axillary artery
B. Brachial artery
C. Brachial plexus
D. Radial artery

8. The shoulder is the most mobile joint in the body. This leaves it susceptible to possible dislocation. What type of dislocation of the shoulder accounts for 80% of the injuries?

A. Inferior dislocation
B. Anterior dislocation
C. Posterior dislocation
D. Intrathoracic dislocation

9. A 60-year-old patient comes to the emergency room and is complaining of severe left shoulder and arm pain. The nurse suspects a possible axillary artery injury. Which of the following signs are not commonly found with axillary artery injury?

A. Axillary hematoma
B. Cool limb
C. Absent axillary pulses
D. Absence of distal pulses

10. All of the following are early complications of an open fracture except:

A. Altered sensation and mobility
B. Vascular compromise
C. Contractures
D. Pain

11. A 15-year-old boy was attempting to jump off a roof into a pool when he missed the pool and landed on the pavement. The patient has a calcaneus fracture and bilateral wrist fractures. What other injuries should the nurse suspect with this mechanism of injury?

A. Vertebral fractures
B. Sacral fractures
C. Pelvic fracture
D. Femur fracture

12. A 24-year-old female was involved in a motor vehicle collision (MVC). She was restrained and the airbag deployed. The patient's right patella came in contact with

the dashboard and caused a patellar fracture. Knowing that the impact of the injury was forceful enough to injure the patella, what other injuries may be associated?

A. Hip fracture
B. Popliteal artery injury
C. Femur fracture
D. All of the above

13. A patient has a radial fracture to the right arm. Which of the following is an associated injury with this type of injury?

A. Clavical fracture
B. Vertebral column injury
C. Cranial injury
D. Nerve damage to the right arm

14. A patient came to the emergency department with an open femur fracture. The bleeding has been controlled and the patient is hemodynamically stable. The nurse goes to splint the site. What splint would be recommended for this injury?

A. Rigid splint
B. Traction splint
C. Soft splint
D. Contraction splint

15. A patient presents with an ankle fracture and is very agitated in the emergency room. It is important for the nurse to instruct the patient of the need to avoid excessive movement to the injured foot because of all of the following except:

A. Manipulation can increase bleeding
B. Manipulation can convert an open to a displaced fracture
C. Manipulation can increase the risk of a fat embolus
D. Manipulation can convert a closed to an open fracture

16. A physician's orders for a patient with an open fracture include irrigation with normal saline, covering the open wound with a dry sterile dressing, performing dressing changes every 4 hours, routine site assessment, antibiotics, and a tetanus shot. These are all appropriate orders for an open fracture patient except which of the following?

A. Tetanus shot
B. Frequent dressing changes
C. Covering open wound with sterile dry dressing
D. Irrigating the site with normal saline

17. Assessing a patient's neurovascular status before and after splint application, removing constrictive clothing and jewelry, and initiating an infusion of isotonic intravenous solution are all interventions for which nursing diagnosis?

A. Altered tissue perfusion
B. Impaired physical mobility
C. Fluid volume deficit
D. Impaired skin integrity

18. Following musculoskeletal injuries, there is an activation of normal physiological responses to minimize the damage in the skeletal and muscle structures. All of the following are part of this repairing processes except:

    A. Shifting fluid to interstitial space
    B. Clotting system activation
    C. Cellular membrane renovation
    D. Collateral blood flow

19. Which of the following injuries can lose about 1,000 mL to 1,500 mL of blood?

    A. Vertebral fracture
    B. Femur fracture
    C. Hip dislocation
    D. Tibial fracture

20. This type of fracture has distal and proximal fracture sites wedged into each other:

    A. Displaced fracture
    B. Complete fracture
    C. Greenstick fracture
    D. Impacted fracture

21. The nurse receives a patient with a tibial open fracture. The wound is 3 cm and has the appearance of a crush injury. The risk of infection is greater with severe fractures, therefore the nurse should be aware of the grade of open fracture to modify treatment modalities. What grade of open fracture does this patient's injury describe?

    A. Grade I
    B. Grade II
    C. Grade III
    D. Grade IV

22. The patient in the emergency room (ER) with an extremity injury complains of a burning sensation and a throbbing pain to the extremity site. What does the nurse suspect to be the cause of this described pain?

    A. Nerve compression
    B. Ischemic pain
    C. Muscle spasm
    D. Crush injury

23. A patient who suffers a pelvic fracture may require the application of a pelvic binder to reduce bleeding, limit movement, and stabilize the fracture. What is the proper placement of a pelvic binder?

    A. At the level of the greater trochanters
    B. Over iliac crest
    C. Above the level of the greater trochanters
    D. Below the iliac crest

24. All of these terms are common classifications of pelvic fractures except which of the following?

    A. Straddle injury
    B. Open-book pelvic fracture
    C. Vertical shear
    D. Subtrochanteric fracture

25. Following a motor vehicle collision (MVC), the patient is complaining of back and pelvic pain. During the assessment, the trauma nurse notes instability and crepitus in the pelvis, and a hematoma is noted on the upper thigh. What is the medical term for the hematoma present in the upper thigh in a pelvic fracture patient?

    A. Murphy's sign
    B. Destot's sign
    C. Earle's sign
    D. Roux's sign

26. A patient with a fat embolism typically develops pulmonary interstitial edema. This places the patient at a high risk for:

    A. Pneumonia
    B. Chronic obstructive pulmonary disorder (COPD)
    C. Sepsis
    D. Acute respiratory distress syndrome (ARDS)

27. Fat emboli are usually caused by long-bone fractures and pelvic fractures. The patient typically has respiratory compromise, including tachypnea and hypoxia. Which of the following are the pulmonary signs of fat emboli?

    A. Productive cough with course crackles
    B. Dry cough with scattered rhonchi
    C. Productive cough with diminished breath sounds
    D. Dry cough with inspiratory wheezes

28. When a fat embolus is present, there are cardiac changes that may occur. Which of the following can be found on EKG with a fat embolus diagnosis?

    A. Depressed ST segments
    B. Left bundle branch block
    C. Inverted T waves
    D. All of the above

29. The presence of petechiae is a common symptom of fat embolus. All of the following are common areas for petechiae to appear except:

    A. Conjunctiva
    B. Upper extremities
    C. Axilla
    D. Upper trunk

30. Of the five Ps in the neurovascular assessment, which of the following is the most vital part of the assessment of a patient with compartment syndrome?

    A. Pain
    B. Pressure

C. Pulselessness
D. Paralysis

31. Ms. Long comes in to the emergency department (ED) because of a crush injury to the right arm. Her pain is rated a 10 on a 1 to 10 severity pain scale, and described it as pressure and throbbing. Blood pressure is 100/62 mmHg, pulse rate is 101 beats per minute (bpm), and the respiratory rate is 24 breaths per minute and regular. Compartmental pressure is obtained and the reading is 28 mmHg. What would be the suspected intervention for this patient?

A. Close observation and frequent assessment
B. Pain management and frequent assessment
C. Immediate surgical decompression
D. Elevate the extremity

32. The trauma nurse is caring for a patient with compartment syndrome. When reviewing orders, the nurse questions which of the following orders for this patient?

A. Hydromorphone
B. Serum creatine phosphokinase (CPK) every 2 hours
C. Urinary myoglobin every 12 hours
D. Both B and C

33. A nurse is precepting a new hire to the trauma emergency department (ED). The team receives a patient with signs of compartment syndrome. The experienced nurse questions the new orientee about the care for this patient. Which of the following statements would reveal an opportunity for further education about compartment syndrome and the management of care?

A. We need to elevate the extremity
B. We need to remove any constrictive clothing
C. The physician should remove constrictive casts if present
D. The extremity should be in a neutral position

34. Untreated compartment syndrome can result in all of the following complications except:

A. Amputation
B. Infection
C. Volkmann's ischemic contractures
D. Gross muscle necrosis

35. An increased blood flow to a previously ischemic muscle resulting in the washout of lipid-soluble intracellular metabolites causes which of the following complications of compartment syndrome?

A. Inadequate decompression
B. Reperfusion injury
C. Volkmann's ischemic contractures
D. Hypoperfusion

36. There are three major classifications for amputation injuries. Which of the following is the injury that can be best described as a result of forceful stretching and tearing away from tissue?

A. Guillotine
B. Avulsion

    C. Crush

    D. Cut

37. The trauma nurse in the emergency room (ER) receives an amputated extremity from the paramedics for a patient in a motorcycle collision. What is the proper way to handle an amputated extremity in the ER?

    A. Wash with hypertonic solution

    B. Wrap in penicillin-moistened sterile gauze

    C. Use iodine on the severed injury

    D. Place extremity directly on ice, or utilize dry ice

38. The management of a partial amputation differs somewhat from a complete amputation. The proper treatment for a partial amputation includes all but which of the following?

    A. Splint the attached part

    B. Apply saline-moistened sterile dressing

    C. Place the amputated portion on ice

    D. Pulse oximetry on distal extremity

39. A 65-year-old male comes into the emergency room with a severed finger from a knife incident while cooking. His blood pressure is 92/60 mmHg, heart rate is 98 beats per minute (bpm), respiratory rate is 22 breaths per minute, and oxygen saturation is 96% on 2 L via nasal cannula. The bleeding has stopped and a moist dressing is placed on the site. The amputated extremity was kept cool on ice prehospital. Which of the following is the most accurate statement?

    A. A finger is not a functional requirement and need not be reimplanted.

    B. A finger is a good candidate for reimplantation.

    C. Hands are more commonly reimplanted than a finger.

    D. Finger reimplants have a higher failure because of loss of tissue.

40. Ms. Rockwell was riding her bike when struck by a car. She was utilizing clip-pedal shoes and her one foot was severed from her leg. She is brought into the emergency department (ED) with her foot preserved by paramedics. However, she is bleeding profusely, the posterior tibial artery has been severely damaged, and there is significant tissue loss. Which of the following is the most accurate statement?

    A. Lower extremities are considered essential and are reimplanted in majority of patients.

    B. Significant tissue loss of vascular injury may prevent the reimplantation of the lower extremity.

    C. Loss of sensation to the reimplanted foot does not affect the ability to ambulate.

    D. Limb length discrepancies should not affect the decision to reimplant the lower extremity.

41. Which of the following amputated extremities is usually not a candidate for reimplantation?

    A. Scalp

    B. Penis

    C. Toe

    D. Nose

42. A patient suffered a guillotine-style bilateral hand amputation from a factory injury involving heavy machinery. This patient is a strong candidate for reimplantation because of the functional need of the extremity. Which of the following is typically considered an indication for reimplantation because of the function of the extremity?

A. Nondominate hand
B. Thumb
C. Fifth digit of hand
D. Sites distal to proximal interphalangeal

43. The nurse receives a trauma patient postoperatively after the right hand is reimplanted. While reviewing the orders, the nurse should question which of the following postoperative orders?

A. Intravenous heparin
B. Doppler tones every hour
C. Antibiotics for 14 days
D. Apply light-weight heating pad

44. Leech therapy is primarily indicated for venous circulation impairment. Arterial flow must be adequate for leeches to be effective. What is the proper method of leech therapy?

A. Puncture the site, allow the leech to attach, wrap with gauze, allow it to feed until it detaches on its own, then dispose with other waste material.
B. Puncture the site, attach the leech, and in 10 to 20 minutes detach the leech with forceps, and dispose with other waste material.
C. Puncture the site, attach the leech, and leave in place for 4 hours before disposing.
D. Puncture the site, attach leech, after the leech detaches, reapply the leech to another location.

45. A patient comes in with a crush injury to the right leg after being caught under the wheel of a truck. This soft tissue injury and muscle necrosis causes systemic complications to the patient. All of the following are possible associated complications except:

A. Compartment syndrome
B. Hypercoagulable state
C. Hypovolemia
D. Rhabdomyolysis

46. All of the following are anticipated treatments for crush syndrome and prevention of rhabdomyolysis except:

A. Mannitol
B. Diamox
C. Calcium gluconate
D. Sodium bicarbonate

47. Mr. Meek was involved in a motorcycle collision. His helmet was still intact, but he has a large area of partial-thickness wounds to his right thigh where the road caused

dermal friction, and there is a minimal amount of gravel debris to the area. What type of skin trauma is experienced?

A. Avulsion
B. Contusion
C. Traumatic tattooing
D. Abrasion

48. Which of the following mechanisms of injury is commonly associated with infection, scarring, devitalized tissue, and possibly even compartment syndrome?

A. Laceration
B. Avulsion
C. Puncture
D. Abrasion

49. A 17-year-old patient came to the emergency room after he got into an altercation with a classmate and received a deep bite wound to his left arm. What type of treatment is warranted with this injury?

A. An antibiotic that covers gram-positive infections
B. An antibiotic that covers gram-negative infections
C. An antibiotic that covers both gram-positive and gram-negative infections
D. Antiseptic wound care is recommended without antibiotics

50. Wound care promotes optimal healing in trauma patients. What is the most important primary intervention in wound care?

A. Wound cleansing
B. Wound irrigation
C. Hair clipping
D. Antibiotic administration

51. The application of antibiotic ointment and dressing, tetanus administration, and radiographic studies are part of what category of the four-step approach to wound care?

A. Hemostasis
B. Wound preparation
C. Wound closure
D. Aftercare

52. All of the following are wounds that may be treated by secondary intention, which includes leaving the wounds to heal by granulation and reepithelialization except:

A. Ulcerations
B. Lacerations
C. Punctures
D. Abrasions

Surface and Burn Trauma

MECHANISM OF INJURY

■ *What is the most common mechanism of injury for a burn in children between the ages of 2 and 4 years of age?*

■ **Scald injuries**

The age group of 2- to 4-year-olds (toddlers) is most commonly associated with scald injuries, whereas in adults injury is usually most commonly caused by a flammable liquid.

> ▶ **HINT:** Hot water from faucets, showers, and bathtubs is the leading source of scald burns in children.

■ *Which type of fire causes the majority of fire-related deaths?*

■ **Structural fires**

Structural fires are responsible for the majority of burn-related deaths but only account for 5% of the hospital admissions. Cigarette smoking and alcohol consumption are common factors in fatal structural fires.

> ▶ **HINT:** In elderly people, a significant number of burns are related to nightwear (i.e., robes, gowns).

■ *What complication of fire-related injuries is a common cause of fatality?*

■ **Smoke inhalation**

Most fire-related deaths have smoke inhalation as a major contributor to fatality.

> ▶ **HINT:** Inhalation of toxic substances (carbon monoxide, hydrogen cyanide, and other gases) in a structural fire is one of the leading causes of death.

■ *What is the usual cause of a thermal burn?*

■ **Flame**

Thermal burns are usually a result of events generating heat, flames, or both.

> ▶ **HINT:** An explosion increases the risk of the patient sustaining other trauma, especially penetrating injuries, in addition to flame or heat burns.

■ *What might a burn with well-demarcated lines and no splash patterns on a child indicate?*

■ **Child abuse**

Always assess whether the pattern of the burn is suspicious for abuse. A scald injury on a child with well-demarcated lines and no splash injuries may indicate child abuse.

▶ **HINT:** Children who pull pans of hot liquid on themselves commonly present with a burn pattern in the shape of Africa, with a large area of burn on top and a small area on the bottom.

■ *What is a common source of electrical burn injuries?*

■ **Lightning strikes**

Electrical burns can be a result of lightning strikes, or direct contact with an electrical current. The trauma nurse should determine the voltage, type of current, location of the electrical source contact, length of contact, and whether the patient sustained any loss of consciousness following a direct contact to the electrical source.

▶ **HINT:** Electrical current has a contact site, which is the point of entry and an exit site at a distal location.

■ *Which causes a more serious chemical burn, acid or alkaline chemicals?*

■ **Alkaline**

Caustic chemical agents, including acids, alkalies, and petroleum-based products, may produce chemical burns when in direct contact with skin or mucosal membranes (direct ingestion).

Alkaline chemical burns are usually more serious than acid burns because they penetrate the tissue more deeply. Alkaline chemicals are present in many household cleaning products and in wet cement.

▶ **HINT:** The extent of the tissue damage and injury from chemical burns may continue to progress after the initial exposure.

■ *A contaminated wound should be allowed to heal by what type of closure?*

■ **Tertiary**

Contaminated wounds should be cleaned, debrided, and left to close by tertiary healing. Closing a contaminated wound with primary closure increases the risk of infection. The advantage of a primary closure is less scarring but is used for clean cuts and lacerations. Primary intention closure can be accomplished by closure of the wound initially with sutures, staples, tape, or glue.

▶ **HINT:** Wounds that have minimal tissue loss and are cleaned can usually be closed by primary repair.

TRAUMATIC INJURIES

■ *What two components determine the extent of a burn injury?*

■ **Extent and depth**

Classification of burn severity is based on the extent and depth of the injury. The extent of injury depends on the intensity and strength of the causative agent, the duration of exposure, and the conductance of the tissue involved. An example is a ring that can continue to burn a finger because of the heat of the metal, which can produce severe tissue injury.

> ▶ **HINT:** Other contributing factors for determining the severity of injury in burn patients is preexisting illness and associated injuries.

■ *The zone of coagulation in a burn wound indicates what type of injury?*

■ **Irreversible injury**

Zone of coagulation is the area of irreversible cell death and involves the most severe area of the burn with the most intimate contact with the heat source (Box 9.1). This tissue is necrotic.

Box 9.1 Zones of Burn-Wound Injury

Zone of Hyperemia	Zone of Stasis	Zone of Coagulation
Involves peripheral and superficial area of the burn wound	Injury is less superficial.	Involves the most severe area of the burn with the most intimate contact with the heat source
The zone appears erythematous, indicating a first-degree burn.	Caused by vascular damage and the inflammatory response	Irreversible cell death
	Edema forms in the next 24 to 48 hours.	The tissue is necrotic.
	Reversible area of injury if treated in a timely manner	

> ▶ **HINT:** After 3 to 4 days, loss of tissue viability in the zone of stasis causes the burn wound to become larger and deeper.

■ *What is the phase of burn management that begins with hemodynamic instability and fluid shifts?*

■ **Resuscitative phase**

The resuscitative phase begins with an initial hemodynamic response and lasts until capillary integrity is restored and the plasma volume is replaced. The capillary leak allows for the loss of fluids, electrolytes (especially sodium), and plasma proteins extravascularly. The shift of fluids into the interstitial space causes intravascular volume loss and hypovolemia.

> ▶ **HINT:** Fluid is also lost through the wound, contributing to the hypovolemia.

■ *What is the clinical sign that signifies the onset of the acute phase of burns?*

■ **Diuresis**

Diuresis is the onset of the acute phase of burn injury. This onset of diuresis is caused by the fluid shifting from the interstitial space into the vascular space. The fluid loss also occurs from the burn wounds so the fluid shifts correct after the wound is closed.

> ▶ **HINT:** In partial-thickness wounds, the greatest fluid loss occurs on the day of injury although in full-thickness injuries the greatest fluid losses peak by day 4 postburn.

■ *Which of the layers of skin contain sweat glands and hair follicles?*
■ **Dermis layer**

The dermis layer, which is the second layer of skin, contains the sebaceous glands, sweat glands, vessels, nerves, and hair follicles. The dermis is not able to regenerate if completely damaged. Fat, muscle, and subcutaneous tissue are below the dermis layer and the outermost layer, the epidermis, is avascular.

> ▶ **HINT:** Injury to the dermis layer of skin may result in the loss of hair and inability to sweat in the previously damaged area.

■ *A burn wound that affects the epidermis only is called?*
■ **Partial-thickness burn**

A partial-thickness burn injury is superficial and involves the epidermis layer only. This used to be called a *first-degree burn* (Box 9.2).

> ▶ **HINT:** Epidermis and dermis layers are affected in second-degree burns.

Box 9.2 Burn Depth

Term	Layers Involved
Partial thickness (first degree)	Epidermis
Superficial partial thickness (second degree)	Epidermis and upper part of dermal layer
Deep partial thickness (second degree)	Epidermis and most dermis
Full thickness (third degree)	Epidermis, dermis, and underlying subcutaneous tissue
Full thickness (fourth degree)	Involves muscle and bone

■ *What is the typical extent of injury for electrical burns?*
■ **Deep muscle**

Electrical burns involve both cutaneous and deep muscle damage, commonly resulting in an amputation. The contact wound may not appear severe but can have extensive subfascial tissue damage (Box 9.3). The path of the electricity may follow along bone (bone does not conduct well), and transverse through internal organs and structures (nerves, tendons, blood vessels) to exit the skin in a location distal to the initial contact. The exit wound may have more extensive tissue injury and muscle necrosis.

> ▶ **HINT:** The external damage may not reflect the actual damage to the tissues. The average-size burn wound associated with electrical injury is approximately 5% of the total body surface area (TBSA).

Box 9.3 Determinants of Severity of Electrical Injuries

Voltage
Duration of contact to electrical source
Resistance of the tissue
Surface area of contact

▶ **HINT:** Tissue damage is determined by the current density, the smaller the area that comes in contact with the electricity, the greater the tissue damage.

■ *Besides the type of chemical, what is another variant that may determine the extent of injury with a chemical burn?*

■ **Duration of contact**

The amount of damage sustained to the skin and tissue depends on the chemical agent, the duration of contact with the skin or tissue, and the concentration of the chemical. Chemicals break down cell walls and destroy intracellular proteins, resulting in cellular death. The longer the chemical remains in contact with the tissue, the greater the damage to the tissue.

▶ **HINT:** Management of chemical burns is by copious irrigation for extended periods of time to wash the chemical away and decrease contact time.

■ *What type of injury causes a partial-thickness injury as a result of rubbing the skin across a hard surface?*

■ **Abrasion**

An abrasion is an injury caused by the friction of skin rubbing against a hard surface and typically is a partial- or full-thickness injury. A puncture is an open wound that is deeper than it is wide. Although an avulsion is typically a full-thickness injury caused by a ripping or tearing mechanism of injury. The wound edges do not approximate and are typically jagged, which requires debridement.

▶ **HINT:** When the skin is traumatically torn or pulled away from the soft tissue it is called a *degloving injury.*

ASSESSMENT/DIAGNOSIS

■ *What are the cardiovascular signs of burn shock?*

■ **Tachycardia and narrowed pulse pressure**

Burn shock results in hypovolemia and hypoperfusion. This triggers the autonomic nervous system and the release of catecholamines. The cardiovascular effects then include tachycardia and vasoconstriction. The hypotension that occurs is a result of the decrease in circulating blood flow.

▶ **HINT:** The initial sign of narrowed pulse pressure is a result of the vasoconstriction and occurs before onset of hypotension.

■ **What is the sign at the bedside frequently used to indicate correction of hypovolemia?**

■ **Increased urine output**

Signs of hypovolemia include decreased cardiac output, oliguria, and peripheral edema. These are characteristics of a burn shock. A sign frequently used at the bedside indicating adequate resuscitation of a hypovolemia is an increase in urine output or reversal of burn shock.

▶ **HINT:** Urine output reflects renal perfusion.

■ **A patient's burn wounds are described as mottled, red and "weeping." What is the most likely depth of burn?**

■ **Superficial partial thickness**

Superficial partial-thickness (second-degree) burns appear mottled, red to pale ivory, and are moist (weeping serous fluid) (Box 9.4). They form blisters and are very painful because of exposed nerve endings.

▶ **HINT:** A burn wound has different degrees of depth within the wound.

Box 9.4 Burn-Wound Classification

Depth of Wound	Appearance of Wound
Partial thickness	Local pain, erythema without blisters (bullae), dry, skin blanches
Superficial partial thickness	Mottled, red to pale ivory, moist, forms blisters and is very painful
Deep partial thickness	Mottled; large areas of waxy, white discoloration; decreased moisture; skin does not blanch or prolonged blanching exists
Full thickness	White, cherry red, brown, or black and dry, hard and leathery; may or may not have blisters and thrombosed veins

■ **In the rule of nines for an adult patient, the patient's palm represents how much of the patient's body surface area?**

■ **About 1%**

The patient's palm represents about 1% of the patient's body surface area and may be used to determine the surface area burned. This is called the *rule of palms*.

▶ **HINT:** The rule of palms is a quick and easy way to estimate the amount of body surface area burned but is not the most accurate method.

■ **What chart is considered a more accurate assessment of the amount of body surface area burned?**

■ **Lund and Browder chart**

The Lund and Browder chart may be used to estimate the amount of body surface area burned and is a more accurate assessment because it takes into account the changes in body surface area related to the growth of the individual. The size of the burn is a predictor of survival, with the greater body surface area burns having the highest predicted mortality.

> ▶ **HINT:** The presence of irregular or scattered burns can be estimated by using the palm of the patient's hand and can supplement the Lund and Browder chart in determining the size of the burn wound.

■ *A child's head counts as how much body surface area when doing the rule of nines to determine the extent of burns?*

■ **About 18%**

The rule of nines is used to estimate the extent of burn wounds. The rule of nines divides the TBSA into sections of 9% or multiples of 9, except for the perineum, which is equal to 1%. An adult's head counts for 9% of the TBSA, whereas a child's head is 18% (Box 9.5).

Box 9.5 Rule of Nines

Adult	Pediatric
Head: 9%	Head: 18%
Upper extremity: 9%	Upper extremity: 9%
Perineum: 1%	
Lower extremity: 18%	Lower extremity: 14%
Front: 18%	Front: 18%
Back: 18%	Back: 18%

> ▶ **HINT:** The rule of nines is an estimation of the body surface area involved and may be used in adults and children older than 10 years.

■ *What diagnostic test would the trauma nurse expect the physician to order for a burn patient with an altered level of consciousness?*

■ **A CT scan of the head**

A change or altered level consciousness requires a CT scan to assess for an associated brain injury. Burn trauma should not cause an altered level of consciousness.

> ▶ **HINT:** Associated traumatic injuries must be identified and managed in the same manner as any patient without a burn.

■ *What is an observational assessment finding that would provide the trauma nurse with a high suspicion of inhalation injury?*

■ **Singed nasal, facial, and eyebrow hairs**

In the initial assessment, the nurse assesses for soot; carbonaceous sputum; and singed nasal, facial and eyebrow hairs. These findings indicate the patient is at a high risk for inhalation injury.

> ▶ **HINT:** Early intubation in burn patients with the signs of inhalation injury may prevent a loss of airway when swelling occurs. Hoarseness, stridor, and audible breathing are indicative of partial obstruction and the potential for complete obstruction of the airway.

■ **What is the gold standard for diagnosing and evaluating the severity of inhalation injuries?**

■ **Bronchoscopy**

The gold standard diagnosis of inhalation injury includes bronchoscopy to identify carbonaceous debris in the tracheal and bronchial area as well as mucosal ulcerations.

> ▶ HINT: On the examination, a gold standard question is looking for the most specific or diagnostic answer, not necessarily what is performed the most frequently.

■ **What is a diagnostic test used to determine the presence of carbon monoxide poisoning following a house fire?**

■ **Serum test**

Serum levels of carbon monoxide can be measured to assess for exposure and toxicity. Toxic levels of carboxyhemoglobin are 25% to 35% and a lethal level is greater than 60%.

■ **What is a clinical sign of carbon monoxide poisoning and cyanide toxicity?**

■ **Altered level of consciousness**

Exposure to a large amount of carbon monoxide can cause an altered mental status and should be suspected in burn patients with a decrease in level of consciousness. Delayed sequelae of elevated carbon monoxide levels include headaches, irritability, personality changes, loss of memory, confusion, and gross motor deficits that presents within days to several weeks.

> ▶ HINT: Remember, a burn injury should not cause an altered level of consciousness. Any neurological abnormalities should clue the trauma nurse to the presence of a traumatic brain injury or toxicities.

MEDICAL/SURGICAL INTERVENTIONS

■ **What is a priority of care in a burn patient in the initial phase of resuscitation and fluid shifts?**

■ **Obtaining an airway**

Fluid shifts that occur with burn-injured patients cause significant peripheral edema, including in the region of the upper airway. Airway swelling can occur rapidly during the initial shock phase following burn injuries and an airway should be obtained before the airway swells.

> ▶ HINT: Patients with large burns, burns of the face and neck, or obvious inhalation injury should be intubated before the fluid resuscitation to prevent the loss of an airway.

■ **What is used to determine the amount of fluid resuscitation to administer to a burn patient within the first 24 hours?**

■ **Size of the burn**

The amount of fluid resuscitation is determined by the size of the burn, so estimation of surface area burned is very important to guide initial care for partial- and full-thickness burns. The extent of the burn wound is the percentage of TBSA burned.

▶ **HINT:** Superficial (first-degree) burns do not have open wounds through which plasma is lost so they do not require fluid resuscitation.

■ *What prehospital care should be done for the burn wound?*
■ **Cover with sterile sheet**

Covering burns that are greater than 10% of the TBSA with a dry, clean sheet can protect the wounds from contamination. At the scene, the prehospital personnel should not wait to clean the burn wounds.

▶ **HINT:** Do not apply any topical antimicrobial creams or ointments in the emergency stage before wound assessment can be performed in the hospital.

■ *What is a potential complication of cooling a burn wound in the field?*
■ **Hypothermia**

Cooling burn wounds should occur within the first 20 minutes to be most effective and should not be initiated or continued for greater than 20 to 30 minutes after the initial burn. Cooling burn wounds in patients with large body surface area wounds can cause hypothermia and may not be recommended. Attempt to keep the patient warm even if cooling the burn wound.

▶ **HINT:** Direct application of ice should not be used to cool burn wounds because of the potential of causing frostbite.

■ *With a burn wound larger than 15% of body surface area, what is a priority of care for the patient's stabilization?*
■ **Fluid resuscitation**

Patients with burn wounds will third-space large volumes of fluid resulting in hypovolemia. The fluid resuscitation is based on the percentage of body surface burned. The management of the fluid resuscitation in a burn patient requires the knowledge of the time of injury, careful estimation of burn size and depth, accurate patient weight, and a Foley catheter. Formulas are used to calculate the amount of fluids required in the first 24 hours following a burn trauma.

■ *What type of fluid should be added to the resuscitation of a pediatric burn patient?*
■ **Dextrose**

Infants and young children should receive intravenous fluid with 5% dextrose at a maintenance rate in addition to the fluid resuscitation with Lactated Ringer's solution or normal saline. Children have more limited glycogen storage than adults and frequently experience hypoglycemia in the early postburn stage.

▶ **HINT:** Monitor pediatric patients' blood glucose levels frequently during the early stages of their burn management.

■ *What is the most commonly used intravenous fluid for burn resuscitation in an adult patient?*
■ **Lactated Ringer's solution**

Lactated Ringer's is commonly used to resuscitate an adult burn patient during the resuscitation phase. Other isotonic solutions, such as normal saline and hypertonic, and colloids may also be used during resuscitation. The most commonly used formula to calculate fluid resuscitation needs in adult burn patients is the modified Parkland formula, but there are multiple different acceptable formulas to determine the volume required during resuscitation (Box 9.6).

> ▶ HINT: The fluid resuscitation of a burn patient occurs over 24 hours, with one half of the calculated amount being administered within the first 8 hours and the remaining half infused over the following 16 hours.

Box 9.6 Modified Parkland Formula

Volume of Lactated Ringer's solution = 2 mL × body weight (in kg) × % of TBSA burned (partial or full thickness only)

TBSA, total body surface area.

Box 9.7 Pediatric Fluid Calculation

Volume of Lactated Ringer's = 3 mL × body weight (in kg) × % of TBSA burned (partial or full thickness only)

TBSA, total body surface area.

> ▶ HINT: Children with burn injuries may require an increase in fluids during resuscitation compared with an adult with the same burn. The child requires more precise calculation and assessment of hemodynamics because of the limited reserve (Box 9.7).

■ *What is an indication for performing a chest wall escharotomy?*

■ **Elevating peak inspiratory pressures**

If the patient is on a mechanical ventilator, restriction of chest wall motion and elevating peak airway pressures are an indication for a chest wall escharotomy. Extremity escharotomy can also be performed with extremity circumferential burns. The incision of the escharotomy extends the entire length of the burn wound, down through the eschar and superficial fascia to a depth sufficient to allow the cut edges of the eschar to separate. The escharotomy site should be covered with topical antimicrobial agents.

> ▶ HINT: The most common type of burn requiring a fasciotomy is high-voltage electrical injury, or those patients with significant soft tissue, long-bone, or vascular injury.

■ *What is the initial intervention for a patient experiencing carbon monoxide poisoning?*

■ **Administer 100% oxygen**

Elevated carboxyhemoglobin or cyanide levels should be initially managed by placing the burn patient on 100% oxygen at the bedside. The administration of 100% oxygen in patients with elevated oxyhemoglobin levels can lower the half-life of carbon monoxide from 2.5 hours to 40 minutes.

> ▶ HINT: Accumulation of carbon monoxide is commonly found in patients burned in structural fires, so the question probably provides the hint in the scenario of a house fire.

■ *What is the initial intervention for most chemical contamination?*

■ **Irrigation**

The decontamination procedure is important to limit the amount of tissue injury that occurs following contact with a caustic chemical. The typical management of chemical burns is irrigation with water or normal saline until pain subsides. Alkaline chemical burns require more extensive and longer irrigation with water than acid burns. Dry or powdered chemicals should be brushed off the skin initially with a dry towel before water is applied. Substances containing lime can become corrosive to skin when water is added so the powdered substance must be brushed off before water irrigation is used (Box 9.8).

> ▶ **HINT:** The trauma nurse should attempt to identify the causative agent and contact a regional poison center to identify the characteristics of the substance and neutralization methods specific to the agent.

Box 9.8 Neutralization of Chemicals

Chemical	Neutralization in Addition Irrigation
Hydrofluoric acid	Calcium chloride gel
Tar and asphalt	Petroleum-based gels
Phenols	50% polyethylene glycol

■ *What can be applied to tar or asphalt on skin to decrease heat and burning?*

■ **Petroleum products**

Tar or asphalt on skin will continue to contain heat and burn. The tarred area needs to be cooled initially using petroleum products such as mineral oil or neomycin sulfate.

> ▶ **HINT:** Cooling hot tar-covered skin with water only will not stop the burning process.

■ *What is a priority for patients potentially contaminated with radiation?*

■ **Minimize contamination of others**

Patients presenting to the emergency room (ER) with the potential exposure to radiation should be placed in an area away from other patients to prevent contamination. Health care providers should protect themselves from exposure to the patient's clothing and skin. Appropriate protective gear should be worn when providing care to radiation-exposed patients.

> ▶ **HINT:** The patient exposed to radiation should not be undressed because of the potential of aerosolizing the contaminant; therefore, clothing should be saturated with water before being removed.

■ *What is the wound care recommended for nonviable skin and tissue?*

■ **Debridement**

Nonviable tissue is debrided to decrease the risk of infection and facilitate new tissue growth. Sharp debridement is commonly performed by the physician and nurses perform a more gentle debridement while cleansing burn wounds. Large blisters may be broken and gently debrided, but small blisters may be left intact.

▶ **HINT:** Gentle cleansing of the burn wound with tepid water and mild soap is used to remove debris, loose skin, and bacteria and cleanse the wound.

■ *Where is Sulfamylon cream usually applied for burn wound care?*

■ **Cartilage**

Sulfamylon is frequently used on ears and noses that are burned. It should not be used on burns on the body because of its potential to cause metabolic acidosis. Silvadene is a cream used more often on burns that cover a large body surface area. It is a broad-spectrum antibiotic that is painless.

▶ **HINT:** Silvadene is not effective against deep burn-wound infections.

NURSING INTERVENTIONS

■ *What is an important component of the initial current history the trauma nurse should obtain from the patient or emergency medical personnel?*

■ **Mechanism of injury**

It is important to determine the details of the injury in a burn patient. The cause of the burn, determining whether it occurred in a closed space, the time of injury, and whether any associated injuries or related trauma that occurred are the important answers for the trauma nurse to determine.

▶ **HINT:** The time of injury (as well as extent of burns) is used to determine adequacy of fluid resuscitation at the time of entry into the trauma hospital.

■ *A child is admitted to the trauma hospital with burns on his lower extremities. The scald burn wound is well demarcated. What should the trauma nurse suspect regarding this injury?*

■ **Child abuse**

Scald wounds on a child that are well demarcated indicate that the child was forcefully held in the hot water. If a child falls into hot water accidentally, he or she will splash around and the scald burn wounds will be irregular.

▶ **HINT:** Consider that the burn may be child abuse when treating a burned child, especially if the child is younger than the age of 2 years.

■ *While administering fluids during the initial resuscitation phase of a burn injury, what should the trauma nurse assess to assist with assuring adequate fluid resuscitation?*

■ **Urine output**

Urine output is frequently used to assess for adequate resuscitation following a burn injury. This is particularly important in electrical burns because the actual amount of body surface area involved is not visible and the typical formulas underestimate the fluid requirement. The goal for the urine output in an adult burn patient is a minimum of 30 to 50 mL/hr and 1 to 2 mL/kg/hr for children under 30 kg.

▶ **HINT:** On the test, a rate of 0.5 to 1 mL/kg/hr may be used as a minimum urine output in an adult patient.

■ *To maintain homeostasis, what is a nursing intervention that the trauma nurse should perform for a burn patient?*

■ **Keep the patient warm**

Burn patients will lose their body heat from the loss of skin. Hypothermia can affect other body systems, including potentiation of a coagulopathy. Maintaining a warm hospital room and resuscitating with warm fluid will assist with the warming of the burn patient. Patients with burns covering more than 50% of their total body surface require room temperatures higher than 86°F (30°C) (Box 9.9).

▶ **HINT:** One liter of room temperature fluid administered rapidly can lower the patient's body temperature by 1 degree.

Box 9.9 Nursing Interventions in the Emergency Room

Observe cardiac monitor for life-threatening arrhythmias
Administer warm fluids to avoid hypothermia
Place a gastric tube for gastric distension
Insert an indwelling bladder catheter to assess urine output
Remove all jewelry, especially jewelry that is circumferential such as rings and bracelets
Obtain peripheral access with large-gauge intravenous catheters
Avoid placing the intravenous catheter into the burn wound, if possible

▶ **HINT:** Common life-threatening arrhythmias following burn injuries include atrial fibrillation, ventricular fibrillation, and asystole.

■ *What type of assessment should be performed by the trauma nurse with circumferential extremity burns?*

■ **Palpation of pulses**

Assessment of a patient with burns to the extremities includes frequent palpation of pulses (radial, ulnar, posterior tibial, dorsalis pedis). The absence of flow or progressive diminishing of the pulse requires further assessment with a Doppler ultrasound.

▶ **HINT:** A Doppler ultrasound assessment of the distal palmar arch vessels in the upper limb and the posterior tibial artery in lower limbs are the most reliable locations to determine the need for an escharotomy.

■ *What should be a priority of care throughout the burn patient's course of wound healing?*

■ **Pain management**

Pain management is very important in the care of a burn patient, even with large amounts of full-thickness wounds. Areas of the burn wound that are full thickness do not have sensory or pain perception but surrounding the full-thickness injury are components of the burn that are less deep that maintain sensation and are very painful. Burn wounds have a combination of injury thickness so they are painful.

> ▶ **HINT:** When burns are severe, opioids should be administered via an intravenous route initially for better absorption, bioavailability, and improved pain management.

■ *What is the concern for the trauma team members when handling a patient with chemical contamination?*
■ **Exposure to the chemical**

When a patient with chemical skin contamination presents to the ER, the trauma nurse should determine whether the causative agent could pose a risk for health care providers and ensure appropriate protective gear and decontamination procedures are utilized.

The trauma team should be protected from contamination when handling a patient with chemical exposure or burns by using gloves, gowns, masks, and goggles.

> ▶ **HINT:** An example of a potential injury is phenol that gets absorbed through the skin, which can cause liver and kidney damage.

■ *When the physician is to suture a laceration of an ear, should the trauma nurse gather lidocaine with or without epinephrine for use as a local anesthetic?*
■ **Without epinephrine**

Epinephrine as a local anesthetic can help with some blood loss because of its vasoconstrictive properties, but in some smaller areas of the body, it may negatively affect perfusion. The suturing of the ears, digits, penis, and end of the nose should be done with a local anesthetic without epinephrine to prevent ischemia to these areas.

■ *What is the reason for suturing without prior shaving of hair?*
■ **Risk of infection**

Shaving hair can actually increase the risk of infection as a result of multiple skin cuts and is not routinely recommended. Any hair removal required for suturing or wound care should be done with scissors or clippers, and not a razor.

> ▶ **HINT:** Eyebrows should not be shaved when suturing the face.

COMPLICATIONS

■ *What is a potential complication of the initial fluid resuscitation in a burn-injured patient?*
■ **Volume overload**

Volume overload can occur as a result of the massive fluid resuscitation during the initial phase of a burn injury. Even though extravascular fluid shifts occur during the initial phase, the volume resuscitation can lead to complications of heart failure, acute respiratory distress syndrome (ARDS), and increased intracranial pressure in high-risk patients. The goal in fluid resuscitation with a burn patient is to provide enough to improve organ perfusion, but not too much to avoid volume overload complications. Therefore, assessment of hemodynamics is important.

> ▶ **HINT:** Adding hypertonic saline at some point in the fluid resuscitation can lower the total volume requirements and improve urine output by shifting fluid back into the vascular space.

■ *What electrolyte abnormalities are found with massive resuscitation of normal saline solution in the initial burn injury?*

■ **Hypernatremia and hyperchloremia**

Normal saline solution has a higher sodium and chloride content than blood, so large volumes administered can elevate the sodium and chloride levels. Lactated Ringer's replaces the sodium loss that occurs with burn shock with a sodium concentration of 130 mEq/L but does not cause hypernatremia. If hypertonic saline is used during resuscitation, the trauma nurse needs to frequently assess sodium levels, which should not be greater than 160 mEq/L.

> ▶ **HINT:** The hyperchloremia causes a nonanion gap metabolic acidosis.

■ *What is the primary complication of the fluid shift in the initial phase of burn injury?*

■ **Organ dysfunction**

In burn shock, fluid shifts out of the vascular space, resulting in hypovolemia. The hypovolemia results in hypoperfusion and affects all organs of the body.

> ▶ **HINT:** Organ dysfunction occurs in the resuscitative phase of burn shock because of hypoperfusion.

■ *What contributes to the tissue oxygen deficit in burn patients?*

■ **Increase in metabolism**

The hypermetabolic state following a burn injury is associated with an increase in oxygen demand and oxygen consumption. The patient is hypovolemic (because of third-spacing) with a decrease in tissue perfusion, therefore, the delivery is decreased and the demand is increased, further worsening the tissue-oxygen deficit. The hypermetabolism occurs within 24 to 48 hours postburn.

> ▶ **HINT:** Tachypnea, fever, and tachycardia are frequently present because of the hypermetabolic state of the severely burned patient.

■ *A circumferential burn to the chest can cause interference with what physiological function?*

■ **Ventilation**

A chest circumferential burn can cause difficulty with ventilation and the trauma nurse should be assessing for shortness of breath and increased work of breathing. If the patient is on a mechanical ventilator, the peak inspiratory pressures increase. The patient with circumferential burns frequently require an escharotomy to improve ventilation.

▶ **HINT:** Escharotomy of the chest may be required before transportation to a burn center to prevent ventilation complications during transport.

■ *What is a pulmonary complication that is found in victims of fires in small spaces?*
■ **Asphyxiation**

Asphyxiation occurs when the blood has a decreased amount of oxygen and there is an increase in the amount of carbon dioxide or toxic substances. Victims of fires in small spaces, such as a car or a house, frequently experience hypoxemia and asphyxia because the combustion of the fire consumes oxygen, leaving less than 21% of oxygen to breathe.

▶ **HINT:** Administer oxygen by a 100% nonrebreather mask at a flow rate of 12 to 15 L/min in the initial management of a patient with burns and carbon monoxide poisoning.

■ *Following a burn injury in a house fire, the patient has a pulse oximetry reading of 100% saturated, but the arterial blood gas comes back with a saturation of 82%. What is the most likely cause of this discrepancy?*
■ **Carbon monoxide poisoning**

Carbon monoxide, when inhaled, binds the oxygen receptor sites on the hemoglobin. It has a greater affinity for hemoglobin than oxygen. The affinity of hemoglobin to carbon monoxide is 200 to 300 times greater than oxygen and prolonged binding of hemoglobin decreases the oxygen-carrying capacity of the hemoglobin. Pulse oximetry monitors are unable to differentiate hemoglobin bound with oxygen from that bound with carbon monoxide. The arterial blood gas (SaO_2) is more accurate and shows the low oxygen saturation that occurs with carbon monoxide poisoning.

▶ **HINT:** When caring for a patient who has sustained burn injuries in closed-space fires, arterial blood gases should be monitored to identify oxygen saturation abnormalities.

■ *The upper airway can be injured in burn patients. What is the primary cause of injury?*
■ **Inhalation injury**

Direct inhalation injury is usually limited to the upper airway with the inhalation of superheated air. Inhalation of smoke and other toxins can damage the upper airway. Some gases formed during the fire combustion, when inhaled, produce harmful acids and alkali leading to edema and ulcerations in the lower airway. Inhalation injuries occur most commonly in patients trapped in a closed, smoke-filled space and not all inhalation injuries have associated facial cutaneous burns.

▶ **HINT:** Hot gases and steam can also directly injure the airways through direct thermal damage.

■ *What is the complication of smoke inhalation?*
■ **Respiratory failure**

Smoke inhalation extending into the alveoli leads to alveolar edema, loss of surfactant, and collapse of the lung units. ARDS is a complication of this alveolar damage. Other pulmonary complications include pulmonary edema, decreased lung compliance, tracheo-bronchitis, and pneumonia.

> ▶ **HINT:** The debris and secretions can overcome the airway's ability to clear the smoke and soot particles contributing to the atelectasis and alveolar collapse.

■ **Besides carbon monoxide poisoning, what is a common poisoning that occurs from inhalation of gases in a house fire?**

■ **Cyanide poisoning**

Cyanide poisoning is a result of inhalation of burning polyurethanes, silk, paper, and wool, and commonly is associated with house fires. Cyanide interferes with the ability to produce adenosine triphosphate (ATP) at the cellular level by binding cytochrome oxidase. The loss of ATP can eventually result in cellular death. The administration of inhaled amyl nitrate and intravenous sodium nitrate are used to treat cyanide poisoning in patients in house fires. The nitrates work by converting iron in the hemoglobin to methemoglobin. Methemoglobin attracts the cyanide molecules, unbinding the cyanide from the cytochrome oxidase, which is needed to produce ATP.

> ▶ **HINT:** The side effect of the nitrates is hypoxemia because methemoglobin interferes with the ability of hemoglobin to bind and carry oxygen.

■ **What laboratory value should the trauma nurse monitor in a patient with suspected cyanide poisoning?**

■ **pH**

A complication of elevated cyanide levels is a persistent metabolic acidosis and should be monitored in the clinical setting (Box 9.10). The arterial blood gas should be obtained to frequently evaluate the pH.

> ▶ **HINT:** Reminder, a patient with metabolic acidosis hyperventilates to lower the $PaCO_2$. So these patients show hyperventilation as a sign of cyanide toxicity.

Box 9.10 Complications of Smoke Inhalation

Complication	Onset
Acute pulmonary insufficiency	Immediate to early
Pulmonary edema	Occurs 48–72 hours after injury
Bronchial pneumonia	Occurs 48–72 hours after injury

> ▶ **HINT:** The examination may use questions about complications with the hint provided in the scenario as being the timing of onset of complications.

■ **What is a common cardiac complication following electrical burn injuries?**

■ **Cardiac arrhythmias**

Cardiac arrhythmias may be common because of the effects of the electrical current on the heart's intrinsic pacemaker. Cardiac arrhythmias can occur following any type of electrical current injury or burn (Box 9.11).

▶ **HINT:** Cardiac abnormalities may be evident on admission to the emergency department within several hours of the electrical burn.

Box 9.11 Complications of Electrical Burns

Rhabdomyolysis
Cardiac arrhythmias
Cataracts
Neurological injuries
Devitalized muscle and amputations
Bone fractures
Wound infections
Vascular disruption, hemorrhage, and thrombi
Cervical and spine injuries

■ *Following an electrical burn injury, the patient's urine is noted to be dark brown. What is the most likely cause?*

■ **Rhabdomyolysis**

Urine with myoglobin is a brownish red color, almost tea- or cola-colored. Extensive muscle damage from the electrical burn causes the release of myoglobin (protein pigment in muscle), which is then filtered and excreted in the urine (myoglobinuria). Myoglobinuria can cause acute renal failure, which is called *rhabdomyolysis*. If pigment (myoglobin or hemoglobin) is present, urine output of at least 100 to 150 mL/hr must be maintained.

▶ **HINT:** Sodium bicarbonate and mannitol may be administered in patients with myoglobinuria to alkalinize the urine and flush the myoglobin through the renal system.

■ *What is the term used to describe the complication of permanent marking of the skin following an abrasion?*

■ **Tattooing**

Dirt and debris can be grounded into the skin with an abrasion. If the abrasion is not thoroughly cleaned, it may leave a permanent stain or dark discoloration called a *tattoo*.

▶ **HINT:** Facial abrasions are most susceptible to tattooing.

■ *Following the loss of a large surface area of tissue, what is a potential complication the trauma nurse should be aware of?*

■ **Hypothermia**

Abrasions that cover greater than 40% of the TBSA are susceptible to heat loss and hypothermia. The trauma nurse should ensure the patient is being warmed, especially when large losses of skin and tissue have occurred.

▶ **HINT:** The trauma room temperature should be warm and intravenous fluids should be warmed prior to administration.

■ *What animal bite has the highest wound infection rates?*

■ **Cat bites**

Cat bites tend to have a greater risk of infection than dog bites because the fangs of cats are smaller and longer, causing a deeper puncture. Deep-puncture wounds carry a greater risk of infection because they are deeper wounds that can trap bacteria. Dog bites tend to have more of a tearing effect and bleed more than cat bites, thus clearing some of the bacteria from the wound.

> ▶ **HINT:** Puncture and lacerations of the hands carry a risk of wound infection and osteomyelitis because the bones are so close to the surface

■ *The management of contractures and correction of functional deficits occur during which phase of burn injury?*

■ **Rehabilitative phase**

The rehabilitative phase involves prevention of complications and treatment of contractures, job retraining, and correction of other functional deficits. Correct positioning of the patient's burned extremities prevents contractures in the acute period and prevents the need to correct a contracture.

> ▶ **HINT:** Rehabilitation begins on admission.

■ *To prevent contractures, what is the correct position of a hand with burns?*

■ **Fingers separated**

Patients with hand burns require a splint to keep the fingers separated and the wrist cocked-up to prevent contractures. Patients with burns to the neck area should have the neck maintained in a neutral position and avoid pillows being placed behind the head, which causes neck flexion and contractures.

> ▶ **HINT:** Splints should be assessed frequently for skin breakdown.

■ *Burns to the face may result in difficulty performing what activity of daily living?*

■ **Eating**

Burns on the face and head may cause problems with the patient's ability to talk, eat, swallow, or drink. Burns of the hands can interfere with many other activities of daily living and with many careers. Patients with burns on their feet may have difficulties with ambulation and running. Perineal area burns can result in urinary- and bowel-elimination difficulties, experience greater incidence of urinary tract infections, and may interfere with the patient's sexual activity.

> ▶ **HINT:** Burns on the arms require occupational therapy and burns on the feet and lower extremities need physical therapy.

■ *What complication can occur if the patient exposes the new skin following a burn to sun?*

■ **Altered pigmentation**

If the new skin is allowed to tan, this may cause it to have a permanently blotched appearance. Patients should be told to wear sunscreen with high sun protection on burned areas to prevent further thermal damage and pigmentation changes.

▶ **HINT:** Newly healed skin may be sensitive to heat and areas of the healed burn can be numb, therefore, instruct the patient to test the water of a bath or shower before entering.

■ *What are commonly used to prevent hypertrophic scarring on extremities during rehabilitation?*

■ **Pressure garments**

Pressure garments to the extremities can help limit the amount of hypertrophic scarring, which can develop during the wound-healing stages. To decrease the amount of scarring, silicone gel sheets and elastomer molds may also be used to soften and flatten skin.

▶ **HINT:** Pressure garments may be recommended for 2 to 3 hours a day over the next 1 to 2 years.

Questions

1. Which of the following is considered the number one cause of fatal fires?

   A. Cigarettes
   B. Cooking
   C. Candles
   D. Arson

2. Which of the following areas of the body is the most commonly involved burn area?

   A. Lower extremities
   B. Face
   C. Neck
   D. Upper extremities

3. There are three classification zones of burns based on the extent and depth of the injury. Which of the following zones is described as less superficial and is a result of vascular damage and inflammatory response resulting in compromised tissue perfusion?

   A. Zone of hyperemia
   B. Zone of stasis
   C. Zone of coagulation
   D. None of the above

4. Which of the following depths of burn wounds has thrombosed veins, muscle, and/or bone involvement?

   A. Superficial burn
   B. Partial-thickness burn
   C. Full-thickness burn
   D. None of the above

5. A patient came in with third-degree burns to the anterior torso sustained from a pot of boiling water. The patient is experiencing diuresis following the third-spacing and edematous tissue. What phase of burn shock is this patient presenting?

   A. Resuscitative phase
   B. Acute phase
   C. Recovery phase
   D. Rehabilitation phase

6. Following a partial-thickness burn, when would the greatest amount of fluid loss resulting in hypovolemia occur?

   A. 4 days postburn
   B. 3 days postburn
   C. 2 days postburn
   D. 1 day postburn

7. Within several hours after a burn, the edema and fluid shifts result in an intravascular volume deficit causing:

    A. Increase in cardiac output
    B. Hemodilution
    C. Hypercoagulopathy
    D. All of the above

8. Within 24 to 48 hours after a burn, there is an increase in metabolism, resulting in all of the following responses except:

    A. Hyperglycemia
    B. Hyperproteinemia
    C. Negative nitrogen balance
    D. Catabolism

9. This patient has been in the intensive care unit (ICU) for 2 days postburn to the right arm from a fire ignited by a cigarette in the living room. The patient's labs demonstrate a glomerular filtration rate of 30, red blood cell count of 3.8, platelet count of 500,000, and fibrinogen level of 150. All of the following are expected for this patient's diagnosis and stage of burn except:

    A. The glomerular filtration rate of 30
    B. The red blood cell count of 3.8
    C. The platelet count of 500,000
    D. The fibrinogen level of 150

10. Which of the following is not a systemic complication that may occur with burn-injured patients?

    A. Acute respiratory distress syndrome (ARDS)
    B. Acute kidney injury
    C. Peritonitis
    D. Sepsis

11. A patient came into the emergency room after receiving second-degree burns to the right hand from a hot liquid spill. The patient has a dressing applied to the site by the paramedic team; blood pressure is 119/82 mmHg, heart rate is 98 beats per minute, respiratory rate is 20 breaths per minute, oxygen saturation is 97% on room air, and pain is scored 8/10 on a 1 to 10 pain scale. What should the nurse do next?

    A. Place the patient on a nonrebreather facemask
    B. Administer ordered morphine sulfate
    C. Infuse intravenous normal saline
    D. Replace the dressing to the site

12. A 22-year-old patient was found unconscious in a running car inside a garage. The patient was brought to the emergency room. What would be the first intervention for this patient?

    A. 100% FiO_2 (fraction of inspired oxygen) via nonrebreather
    B. 50% FiO_2 via partial face mask
    C. 6 L oxygen via humidified nasal cannula
    D. 4 L oxygen via nasal cannula

13. Once an airway is established and the patient's primary and secondary assessments are completed, a history should be obtained from the burn patient. Which of the following would be the *least* important information to be obtained by the nurse?

    A. Cause of the burn
    B. Others involved
    C. Time of the injury
    D. Any noxious chemicals involved

14. Fluid resuscitation needs to be a priority in treating patients with greater than 20% total body surface area (TBSA) burned or greater than 10% in the pediatric or elderly populations. Using the Parkland formula for a 154-pound man with a 40% TBSA, what would be the amount of isotonic fluid that needs to be administered within 24 hours?

    A. 11,200 mL
    B. 2,800 mL
    C. 24,640 mL
    D. 6,160 mL

15. A burn patient is being resuscitated according to the Parkland formula and is determined to require 14,000 mL of fluid resuscitation within 24 hours. How much fluid should be administered in the first 8 hours?

    A. 7,000 mL
    B. 3,500 mL
    C. 14,000 mL
    D. 4,666 mL

16. A patient comes to the emergency room after being trapped in a burning house. While assessing the patient, the nurse notices a hoarse voice and stridor. What should the nurse request from the physician as a needed intervention to treat this patient?

    A. Keep the patient's head elevated at all times
    B. Racemic epinephrine every 2 to 4 hours
    C. Immediate intubation
    D. Bronchoscopy

17. A patient presents with cyanide poisoning after being exposed to burning plastics in a house fire. The patient is confused, dizzy, and is complaining of a headache. The patient's respiratory rate is 32 breaths per minute, pulse oximetry is 94% on a nonrebreather face mask, and heart rate is 121 beats per minute. All of the following are proper interventions for this patient except:

    A. Early intubation
    B. Amyl nitrate
    C. Sodium nitrate
    D. Sulfur nitrate

18. Patients who are victims of electrical burns typically experience multiple organ dysfunction and long-term complications. All of the following complications may be associated with an electrical injury except:

    A. Cataracts
    B. Hearing loss

C. Neurological injury
D. Cardiac abnormalities

19. A patient was struck by lightning while at a baseball game. The patient was stabilized and has been in the intensive care unit for 24 hours. Fluid resuscitation remains in progress and strict input and output monitoring has been ordered. The nurse notes dark pigmented urine. Which of the following would apply to this situation?

A. Keep the urine output at 50 to 100 mL/hr
B. Keep the urine output at least 30 mL/hr
C. Keep the urine output at 100 to 150 mL/hr
D. Keep the urine output between 150 and 200 mL/hr

20. An electrical burn patient has been stabilized and transferred to the intensive care unit for further monitoring. The patient is lethargic but hemodynamically stable. Six hours later, the patient is more alert, remains hemodynamically stable, and has clear amber urine. The nurse decreased the intravenous fluid administration as ordered. How much urine output should be maintained for this patient?

A. 1.5 to 2 mL/kg/hr
B. 30 mL/hr
C. 0.5 to 1 mL/kg/hr
D. 50 mL/hr

21. The initial treatment for a patient who experienced an electrical burn should ensure adequate ventilation and intravenous fluid administration. How much fluid should the nurse anticipate administering to the patient?

A. Maintain fluid intake at to keep open rate to prevent overload
B. 2-L fluid bolus followed by an infusion of 100 mL/hr for 24 hours
C. Administer fluid to maintain a urine output of 75 to 100 mL/hour
D. 4 mL/kg/body surface area burned administered for more than 24 hours

22. Wound care recommended for burns includes all of the following measures except:

A. Debridement
B. Silvadene
C. Sulfamylon
D. Bursting bullae/blisters

23. The intensive care nurse is precepting a new orientee to the burn unit. The preceptor asks the orientee to tell her about some complications commonly experienced by burn patients. Which of the following answers would be the *most* correct?

A. Hypokalemia
B. Pulmonary edema
C. Hyperthermia
D. Hypernatremia

24. What is the most useful clinical method to assess burn depth?

A. Thermography
B. Capillary refill
C. Palpation of the site
D. Laser Doppler

25. A patient comes into the emergency room with chemical burns to half of the face. The patient is experiencing respiratory compromise. Respiratory rate is 32 breaths per minute and the pulse oximetry reading is 90% on a nonrebreather facemask. The nurse prepares for advanced airway management. Which of the following is the *most* correct statement regarding the airway of a burn patient?

A. Secure the endotracheal tube with umbilical tape
B. Secure the endotracheal tube with adhesive tape
C. Endotracheal tube should not be used because of the facial burn
D. Prepare for cricothyroidotomy

26. Infants and young children are recommended to receive 4 mL of intravenous solution multiplied by their body weight in kilograms multiplied by the percentage of the total body surface area burned. An 18-month-old has been burned by a pot of boiling water. The infant weighs 10 kg and has burned 18% of his body surface area. How should the fluid resuscitation be administered?

A. 360 mL of Lactated Ringer's followed by 360 mL of 5% dextrose normal saline
B. 720 mL of Lactated Ringer's along with 5% dextrose at 45 mL/hr
C. 360 mL of normal saline followed by 360 mL of 5% dextrose
D. 720 mL of normal saline along with 720 mL of 5% dextrose normal saline

27. A 3-year-old boy comes into the emergency room with burn injuries to his bilateral feet. When obtaining the history of the situation, it was discovered that the patient obtained these burns when he got into the bathtub that was filling up with hot water. What would be the recommendation to the parents regarding this situation?

A. The water heater at home should be set below 120°F
B. Test the water before your child gets into the bathtub
C. Place a thermometer in the bathtub
D. Put safety mechanisms on the hot-water tap in the bathtub

28. Which of the following is a recommended measure that the nurse can take to aid in temperature regulation in a burn patient?

A. Apply ice to burn sites
B. Apply cool dressing to the burn
C. Increase the room temperature to 86°F
D. Apply topical lidocaine to the burn wound

29. Following a burn, alteration in capillary permeability occurs. All of the following are appropriate nursing interventions for this patient except:

A. Administer Lactated Ringer's or normal saline boluses
B. Position the patient in reverse Trendelenburg position
C. Administer blood transfusions
D. Position the patient with the legs elevated

30. Burn patients experience a disruption in the integrity of capillary membranes. There are four forces that contribute to the fluid movement across capillary membranes and control the pressures contributing to capillary flow. What force is responsible for pulling fluid into the capillary at the venule end?

    A. Hydrostatic pressure
    B. Plasma colloid osmotic pressure
    C. Interstitial free fluid pressure
    D. Interstitial fluid osmotic pressure

31. A patient who has been electrocuted by a live electrical wire on the ground presents to the emergency room. After the patient's airway is secured and the patient is hemodynamically stabilized, the nurse should know that affiliated injuries from the electrical current may be present and should assess for all of the following except:

    A. Spinal fracture
    B. Long-bone fracture
    C. Laryngospasm
    D. Vertebral compression fractures

32. Which of the following mechanisms of injury would result in an inhalation injury below the level of the glottis?

    A. Direct thermal injury
    B. Chemical exposure
    C. Superheated air
    D. Steam inhalation

33. The body's inflammatory response is activated with burn trauma injuries and releases several substances. What is the substance that leads to vasodilation and increased capillary permeability?

    A. Thromboxane A
    B. Leukotrienes
    C. Bradykinin
    D. Histamine

34. The pathophysiological response to burn trauma patients is a change in the vascular system. Hemoconcentration of the blood occurs because of the loss of plasma volume, which elevates hematocrit levels. All of the following are vascular responses to the fluid shifts except:

    A. Increased blood viscosity
    B. Decreased peripheral vascular resistance
    C. Greater percentage of red blood cells
    D. Decreased red blood cell count

35. A 20-year-old patient has suffered a traumatic burn to his left leg from a fireworks injury. The following are his vital signs:

30 breaths per minute
Oxygen saturation of 94%
Heart rate of 122 beats per minute
Temperature of 100.2°F

This patient is displaying symptoms of which of the following?

A. Carbon monoxide poisoning
B. Hypermetabolic response
C. Hypometabolism
D. Hypoxemia

36. An electrical injury was sustained by a 14-year-old boy at home through an electric socket, which is an alternating-current electrical injury. Which of the following statements is true regarding this type of injury?

A. A direct-current injury causes tetany
B. An alternating-current injury is more dangerous than a direct-current injury
C. A direct-current injury is the most dangerous
D. An alternating current passes in one direction straight through the body

37. Electrical currents follow a specific pathway in the body. Which of the following is the correct pathway that electricity travels through the body?

A. Nerves, muscles, blood vessels, skin, tendons, bone, fat
B. Nerves, blood vessels, muscles, skin, tendons, fat, bone
C. Nerves, tendons, blood vessels, muscles, skin, fat, bone
D. Nerves, blood vessels, tendons, muscles, bone, skin, fat

38. Following an inhalation injury, the primary goal is to ensure adequate oxygenation. This can be accomplished best by which of the following?

A. Warmed and humidified oxygen delivery via facemask
B. Positive end-expiratory pressure (PEEP) with mechanical ventilation
C. Continuous positive airway pressure (CPAP)
D. Nonrebreather mask at 12 to 15 L/min

39. A patient with 13% body surface area burns is in the burn intensive care unit (ICU). Each of the following burn wound management practices is appropriate for burn wound care except:

A. Cleansing wound with mild soap and lukewarm water
B. Shaving eyebrows and hair surrounding the wound
C. Applying a topical antimicrobial agent with silver
D. Debriding nonviable tissue

40. Hyperbaric oxygen therapy may be considered for the treatment of all of the following injuries except:

A. Carbon monoxide inhalation injury
B. Cyanide poisoning
C. Carbon tetrachloride poisoning
D. Sodium thiosulfate inhalation injury

41. A textile factory caught fire with two factory workers trapped inside the building. The fire rescue team recovered the victims and brought them into the emergency room. The receiving nurse obtains the reports and expects to administer which of the following medications to the patients, based on the mechanism of injury?

    A. Inhaled amyl nitrate
    B. Sodium nitrate intravenously
    C. None of the above
    D. Both A and B

42. Patients with surface burns involving phenol contamination should be treated with attention to other capacities that can be affected by this substance. Which of the following should be evaluated?

    A. Serum calcium levels
    B. Blood urea nitrogen (BUN) levels
    C. Myoglobin level
    D. Serum bicarbonate level

43. Family members of burn patients need to be part of the care for the patient. All of the following are proper ways to reduce the fear and anxiety of patients and their families except:

    A. Facilitate family presence during procedures
    B. Encourage patients and families to express concerns
    C. Obtain a referral for social services
    D. Monitoring vital signs for indicators such as tachycardia

44. All of the following are proper nursing interventions for a patient with an alteration in tissue perfusion from a burn except:

    A. Avoiding unnecessary exposure
    B. Maintain warmer room temperature
    C. Monitor for possible compartment syndrome
    D. Perform escharotomies on circumferential burns

Part IV

Clinical Practice: Special Considerations

Psychosocial Issues of Trauma

■ *What is one of the biggest reason patients and families may have a difficult response to the traumatic event?*

■ **Unexpected event**

A traumatic or sudden event results in patients and families being unprepared for the injury (Box 10.1). The unexpected injury disrupts the normal routine and is not expected.

▶ **HINT:** Trauma is frequently seen as something that "happens to other people."

Box 10.1 Common Psychological Responses of Patient to Trauma

Anxiety
Fear
Pain
Isolation
Grief
Embarrassment (lack of privacy)

■ *What happens to normal coping mechanisms during a crisis?*

■ **Become ineffective**

A crisis is a sudden unexpected threat or loss of the basic resources of life and occurs when people's normal coping mechanism become ineffective. Trauma patients and their families frequently experience crisis immediately following the trauma and during periods throughout their hospitalization.

▶ **HINT:** Normal coping mechanisms may not be sustained for long periods of time during a crisis because of mental exhaustion.

■ *All of the unfamiliar sounds, sights, and constant stimulation can lead to what sensory abnormality?*

■ **Sensory overload**

Sensory overload is a common experience that occurs following severe trauma. It involves abnormal sounds such as unfamiliar voices and alarms, unfamiliar lines and tubes, unpleasant and unusual smells, and constant stimulation.

▶ **HINT:** The loss of day and night routines, and associated sleep deprivation contribute to the sensory overload (Box 10.2).

Box 10.2 Prevention of Sleep Deprivation

Dim lighting at night
Sleep masks for patients to limit light
Grouping nursing interventions

■ *What is a premorbid condition that influences the response of the patient to the traumatic event?*

■ **Preexisting mental illness and/or personality disorder**

A preexisting emotional, mental illness or personality disorder influences the patient's perception and response to the traumatic event. The patient's past experiences with health care and hospitalizations, either negative or positive, may also influence the patient's response to the trauma.

▶ **HINT:** Other influences of patient's reactions to a traumatic event include religious, spiritual, and philosophical beliefs as well as educational level and socioeconomic status.

■ *During the resuscitative phase of a trauma, what is the most common concern or fear of the patient?*

■ **Fear of death**

The fear of death or disability is a common concern of the patient during the initial resuscitation in the prehospital and emergency department. Severe pain is commonly associated with death.

▶ **HINT:** The patient may initially only focus on the loss and not what is still intact. They may be unable to see any part of their life not affected by the injury.

■ *During resuscitation of a patient following a severe traumatic injury, the patient may exhibit behaviors of agitation. This may be a fear of what?*

■ **Loss of self-control**

The trauma patient may exhibit avoidance behavior, agitation, and/or verbal and physical hostility. This is typically a result of their experience of a loss of self-control and fear of what is happening.

▶ **HINT:** An intervention to assist the patient in this phase is to get the patient's attention and have the patient listen to your voice as you provide instructions or explanation.

■ *What is the major concern for patients during the critical-care stage?*

■ **Pain**

The patient's focus begins to shift from fear of dying to fear of altered function or appearance. One of the biggest concerns or fears is of pain during this stage. Other issues include sleep deprivation, development of delirium, and anxiety. These can negatively affect outcomes.

▶ **HINT:** Many of the patients have no recall of their experience in the intensive care unit (ICU).

■ *Following a traumatic injury, during the recovery phase the patient displays periods of anger and guilt. What are these signs of?*

■ **Grief**

Grief may be experienced following a trauma as a result of the loss of a body part, function, or even a loss of control. Grief is commonly displayed in stages of anger, guilt, bargaining, and depression. Patients may experience all of these stages or only some of them.

▶ **HINT:** These are the same stages of grief following a loss of one's loved one.

■ *No matter how critical the situation, the family needs to maintain a sense of what?*

■ **Hope**

Hope can be for improvement of their loved one's status or for recovery (Box 10.3). Hope can also be for their loved one not to suffer at the end of life.

▶ **HINT:** Hope can be the only positive emotion the patient or family may experience.

Box 10.3 Psychosocial Needs of Patient

Need for information
Need for compassionate care
Maintenance of hope

■ *Frequently, what is the initial response of family members when receiving bad news regarding loved ones?*

■ **Shock and denial**

Most people are unprepared for the impact of a sudden injury or loss, and react with shock and denial. They may also exhibit anger at the person relaying the information about their loved ones. Family reactions are dependent on past coping mechanisms, past experience with loss, and current situations (Box 10.4).

▶ **HINT:** Family members also move through the stages of grief and may not be at the same stage as the patient.

Box 10.4 Common Reactions of Family Members

Anxiety
Shock
Fright
Denial
Hostility

(continued)

Box 10.4 Common Reactions of Family Members   *(continued)*

Distrust
Guilt
Remorse
Bargaining
Depression
Denial
Hope

■ *Families commonly go through phases in regard to interactions with their loved one and staff members in the hospital. What is the primary reaction in the vigilance phase?*

■ **Wanting to be at the bedside 24/7**

The typical initial response of family members following a traumatic injury to their loved one is to feel the need to be at the patient's bedside every minute of the day. This is commonly called *vigilance*. They express concerns about being gone because of their fear of something bad happening in their absence, fear that they may miss speaking to the physician, or that their loved one may "wake up" while they are gone.

> ▶ **HINT:** Nurses need to take the initiative and call family frequently with updates of the patient's status, which establishes a trusting relationship.

■ *The trauma ICU nurse has been receiving frequent calls from different family members regarding the status of the patient. What would be the best response by the nurse?*

■ **Establish a contact person**

This is a common issue with patients in the ICU. The constant calls from family and friends seeking updates can be distracting and interfere with nursing care of the patients. Setting up a contact person within the family to whom health care staff can provide information regarding the updated status of the patient alleviates some of the calls.

> ▶ **HINT:** Phone calls to the contact person from other family members and friends can also overwhelm the contact person. Nurses need to recommend methods for handling the calls (Box 10.5).

Box 10.5 Suggestions for Dissemination of Information

Establish a website with updated information, status, and progress
Establish chain of calls to deliver information to a larger number of people
Develop an updated outgoing message daily on the phone
E-mail updates as a group
Text updates as a group

> ▶ **HINT:** Encourage immediate family members to have down time. "Allow" them to screen their calls.

■ *The husband of a trauma patient in the ICU is found standing by his wife's bedside without talking to her. What would be an appropriate response by the nurse?*

■ **Encourage the husband to talk to her**

Families frequently do not know what to say to the patient or to talk about at the bedside. The nurse should encourage family and friends to normalize their conversations, for example, talk about daily happenings at work and home. Avoid only talking about the illness, injury, or treatments. If the patient is unresponsive, then talk about his or her hobbies, likes, or favorite activities. This is a component of a coma stimulation program.

> ▶ **HINT:** Encourage family members to keep a diary at home and then talk to the patient from the diary. A role of the nurse is to assist with finding things to talk about when with their loved ones.

■ *A physician enters the room of a comatose patient and begins to talk to the family about the prognosis over the patient's bed. What would be the best response of the nurse?*

■ **Ask them to step outside the patient's room**

Asking the physician and the family member to step away from the patient's bedside is the best response of the nurse. Avoiding talking over the patient's bed about the patient's medical condition is the best practice.

> ▶ **HINT:** The last thing to go on a comatose patient is believed to be hearing.

■ *During family conferences, what is a common problem encountered when medical health care providers are informing the family of the patient's diagnosis and treatments?*

■ **Use of medical jargon**

When speaking with patients and family members, health care providers should avoid the use of medical jargon. Health care providers are frequently perceived as "speaking a different language." Nurses frequently play the role of "interpreter" for the physicians.

> ▶ **HINT:** Nurses should regularly attend family conferences to help the family interpret, clarify, and continue cohesive discussions regarding the patient's medical illness and treatments.

■ *What should the nurse do if the patient has repeated the story about the traumatic event several times during the shift?*

■ **Listen**

A step toward acceptance of a traumatic event is to verbally reconstruct the event. Allow the patient to reconstruct the event of the trauma. He or she may repeat the story or talk about the event repetitively but the nurse should actively listen each time to assist with validation of the event.

▶ **HINT:** Posttraumatic distress syndrome has been found to lessen the more the person involved in the traumatic event tells the story of the event.

■ **What has been found to be the number one need of the family during the hospitalization of their loved one?**

■ **Information**

The number one identified need of the family of a hospitalized loved one is the need for information. They frequently want to know everything that is going on with their loved one and often ask for lab results, vital signs, or watch the monitor. There are three information-seeking reactions by family: monitoring, vigilance, and learning (Box 10.6).

▶ **HINT:** Family commonly fixate or focus on certain things about their loved ones such as the blood pressure, heart rate, or temperature.

Box 10.6 Information-Seeking Reactions

Monitoring	Ask general questions about their loved ones
Vigilance	Seek information to ensure necessary tasks are being carried out ("I thought they were going to do CT this morning." "Has she had her dinner yet?")
Learning	Use the information to understand aspects of the care

■ **What is the primary benefit of assigning the same nurse to the patient every day when possible?**

■ **Continuity of care**

Continuity of nursing assignments provides consistency for patient and family. The nurse is more aware of family needs and is better able to reinforce teaching already provided to the family.

▶ **HINT:** Family and patient's comfort level increases when they know who is providing the care.

■ **What type of visitation in the ICU has been shown to be more effective for the patient and family?**

■ **Open visitation**

Families allowed to remain at the bedside with their loved one express feeling more assured about the care their loved one is receiving. They are more aware of any changes being made in the patient's care and this provides a sense of control for the family.

▶ **HINT:** Not knowing what is happening on the "other side" of the doors when not allowed to visit produces anxiety.

■ **What is an advantage of allowing a family member to remain at the bedside during the trauma resuscitation?**

■ **Family knows everything possible has been done for their loved one.**

Currently, many institutions allow a family member to remain with their loved ones during the trauma resuscitation in the emergency room or during major invasive procedures. One of the most frequently found advantage is that the family is able to see the resuscitation and know that everything possible has been done for their loved one (Box 10.7).

> ▶ **HINT:** An important aspect for the success of family presence during resuscitation is identifying a support person to be with the family to explain the events during the resuscitation and provide clear family guidelines.

Box 10.7 Advantages of Family Presence During Resuscitation

Facilitation of bonding between patients' family members and health care providers
Family members observe the efforts of the health care providers; know everything possible has been done
Family members can provide comfort and words of encouragement to the patient
Ability of the family to have closure
Acceptance of the outcome is facilitated
Families perceive they are actively involved in the resuscitation of their loved one
Family members can touch the patient while the patient is still "alive" or warm to say their goodbyes
Staff can view patient as part of a loving family; perceived as a "real" person
The mystery of activities behind "closed doors" is reduced
Assist the family's comprehension of the seriousness of the condition
Allows the family to become a part of the decision making on when to stop a resuscitation
Reminds staff of the patient being a person
Encourages professional behavior of the health care team

■ *What is the approach that is used to improve the quality of life at the time of a life-threatening illness?*

■ **Palliative care**

Palliative care is an approach that improves the quality of life of patients and families facing problems associated with life-threatening illness (Box 10.8). It involves the integration of physical, psychological, spiritual, cultural, and social needs of all those involved. It takes a significant role at end of life, but may be administered concurrently with curative therapy.

> ▶ **HINT:** Palliative care uses a multidisciplinary approach.

Box 10.8 Measures Provided by Palliative Care

Humanity
Dignity
Respect
Good communication
Clear information
Comfort
Pain management

■ *What is the ethical principle that is used to justify the administration of medication to relieve pain even though it may lead to the unintended, although foreseen, consequence of hastening death by causing respiratory depression?*

■ **Principle of double effect**

The principle of double effect provides that an action with both a good and a bad effect is ethically permissible if the following conditions are met:

1. The action itself must be morally good or at least indifferent.
2. Only the good effect must be intended (even though the bad or secondary effect is foreseen).
3. The good effect must not be achieved by way of the bad effect.
4. The good result must outweigh the bad result.

> ▶ **HINT:** There is no debate among specialists in palliative care regarding pain control, and the belief is that it is unethical to withhold pain medication at the end of life.

■ *A patient has recovered from a gunshot wound and is discharged home. At the 3-month follow-up clinic visit, the patient states he is beginning to experience nightmares and the family reports the person is easily angered and has heightened sensitivity. What is the most likely diagnosis?*

■ **Posttraumatic stress disorder (PTSD)**

PTSD occurs when an individual witnesses, experiences, or learns indirectly about a life-threatening event that endangers self or others. Trauma and critically ill patients can experience PTSD after the event and hospitalization. The onset of nightmares and being easily angered with heightened sensitivity are both signs of PTSD (Box 10.9).

> ▶ **HINT:** Following a critical care illness, patients may develop PTSD 3 to 6 months after discharge.

Box 10.9 Symptoms of Posttraumatic Stress Disorder

Hyperarousal	Anger, irritability, hypervigilance, difficulty concentrating, heightened startle response
Intrusive recollection	Intrusive thoughts, nightmares, feelings and imagery, dissociative-like reexperiencing of trauma
Avoidance	Numbing of responsiveness; avoidance of feelings, situations, and ideas
Reliving the event	Mentally and emotionally
Flashbacks	
Avoiding people and situations	
Developing heightened sensitivity to changes in environment	Constantly on guard, "jumpy," easily startled
Severe anxiety	
Nightmares	
Intense emotions	Guilt, helplessness, hopelessness, or shame
Anhedonia	Loss of interest in former enjoyable activities

Questions

1. The trauma patient, Mrs. Jack, is experiencing sleep deprivation, anxiety, and frequently complains of pain. Knowing the phase cycle of trauma patients, Mrs. Jack is in what phase?

   A. Resuscitative phase
   B. Critical care phase
   C. Recovery phase
   D. Community phase

2. It is important that the trauma nurse understands the stages of grief and the grieving process to better recognize a trauma patient's behavior in grief. Which of the following is *not* included in the stages of grief?

   A. Anger
   B. Depression
   C. Bargaining
   D. Frustration

3. The family members of a trauma patient want to be there 24 hours a day and are frequently asking questions, many of which are unanswerable. The family members are afraid to leave and miss seeing the physician. The nurse can perform a number of interventions to aid the family in this process. Which intervention is *least* effective in dealing with this situation?

   A. Obtain their phone numbers to keep at bedside for the physician when he comes to the bedside or when an emergency arises.
   B. Encourage family to take breaks and rest to conserve their energy for when the patient leaves the intensive care unit (ICU).
   C. Promise them that they will not miss anything and encourage them to leave and take a break.
   D. Set up family/physician visits.

4. Patients with traumatic brain injuries exhibit different personalities, which can be painful for the family to witness. This adds stress on a family and the nurse should intervene and aid the family by doing all of the following except:

   A. Teaching the family to communicate slowly, calmly, and with short sentences.
   B. Distract the patient to change subjects.
   C. Encourage the family to correct the patient.
   D. Encourage the patient to talk about older memories.

5. Which of the following medications may be prescribed at the time of discharge following hospitalization for a major trauma?

   A. Protonix
   B. Vitamin B_{12}
   C. Vitamin D
   D. Lexapro

6. The spouse of a patient who has just physically recovered from a traumatic injury and has been diagnosed with depression reports that the patient is often writing about death and talking about guns. The spouse should be informed to:

   A. Make an appointment with a psychologist
   B. Follow-up with the primary physician treating the patient
   C. Call emergency services or 911
   D. Find a trauma support group

7. Which of the following is not found in posttraumatic stress disorder (PTSD)?

   A. Reexperiencing the traumatic event
   B. Avoiding reminders of the event
   C. Denial of the event
   D. Increased anxiety and emotional arousal

8. A 5-year-old girl was witness to a domestic dispute between her mother and father. The event concluded with her father physically attacking the mother and shooting her in the head. All of the following are behaviors of a child who is suffering from posttraumatic stress disorder (PTSD) except:

   A. Bed wetting
   B. Being disrespectful
   C. Being unable to talk
   D. Clinging behavior

9. All of the following are approved and recommended methods of treatment for a patient with posttraumatic stress disorder (PTSD) with the exclusion of:

   A. Prazosin
   B. Fluoxetine
   C. Cognitive restructuring
   D. Exposure therapy

10. Which best describes a patient reconstructing the traumatic event and telling it to multiple people frequently?

    A. This is a step toward acceptance
    B. Dealing with the anger about the event
    C. Reconstructing the event so others will have empathy with them
    D. Allows them to tell their side of the story

11. The family member of a trauma patient makes the following comment to the nurse, "I noticed the heart rate went down to 96 when it once was 113, is this okay?" This question is directly related to the number one identified need for the family of a trauma patient:

    A. Learning
    B. Information
    C. Vigilance
    D. Hope

12. There is a point during a prolonged hospitalization stay that they family begins to "pitch in" on the patient's care. Which of the following is the *best* example of the "pitching in" stage, which occurs frequently with families?

A. The family member demonstrates fear of touching the tubing
B. The family member suctions the patient
C. The family member performs bathing and skin care alone
D. The family member brings treats for the nurses

13. The spouse of a trauma patient is pacing around the room; the nurse goes in to speak with her about starting tube feedings. The spouse immediately becomes frustrated and responds by saying, "I don't know what to do, I don't know whether I want him to have a feeding tube, I can't make any decisions right now." What does this best exemplify?

A. Stages of grief
B. Ineffective coping
C. Crisis intervention
D. Stress response

14. It is recommended that family presence be implemented during resuscitation. A key role in making this successful is appointing a support person. The role of the support person during the resuscitation is being responsible for all of the following except:

A. Limiting the number of family members/visitors in the resuscitation room
B. Allowing the family to come and go throughout the resuscitation
C. Maintaining communication with the family member
D. Allowing them to make the decision to be present or not

Shock

ANAPHYLAXIS

■ *How is anaphylaxis different than anaphylactoid reaction?*

■ **It is immunoglobulin E (IgE) mediated**

Anaphylaxis and anaphylactoid reactions are both acute life-threatening hypersensitivity reaction but anaphylaxis is immune related, whereas anaphylactoid reaction is not. Anaphylaxis involves IgE binding to an antigen to which the person was previously exposed. Anaphylactoid reactions do not have the immune component but are similar in assessment, diagnosis, and treatment.

> ▶ **HINT:** Anaphylaxis and anaphylactoid are called life-threatening hypersensitivity reactions.

■ *How quickly can symptoms of hypersensitivity reactions occur following exposure to the provoking agent?*

■ **Within minutes**

Onset of symptoms can occur within minutes to hours. Typically, symptoms will peak in severity within 5 to 30 minutes. The episode frequently lasts less than 24 hours but can be protracted or reoccur after an initial resolution.

> ▶ **HINT:** Rapid intervention to hypersensitivity reactions is required to maintain airway and circulation.

■ *In both hypersensitivity reactions, what is triggered causing the release of chemical mediators?*

■ **Mast cells**

Mast cells are activated in both anaphylaxis and anaphylactoid reactions, releasing several chemical mediators (Box 11.1). Overall, the mediators increase capillary permeability and cause peripheral vasodilation. The increased capillary permeability can cause airway swelling and angioedema. Peripheral vasodilation results in hypotension, which is considered a distributive shock.

> ▶ **HINT:** The most life-threatening component of a hypersensitivity reaction is angioedema.

Box 11.1 Chemical Mediators

Bradykinin
Platelet-activating factor
Prostaglandins
Leukotrienes

■ *What are the two most common causes of anaphylaxis?*

■ **Food allergies and insect stings**

Food sensitivities (Box 11.2), insect stings, and antibiotics are the most common causes of an IgE-mediated anaphylaxis reaction (Box 11.3). These occur after previous exposure to the provoking agent. Stinging insects, such as bees, wasps, and fire ants, contain a substance in their venom that initiates the IgE antibody response. Penicillin is the most common antibiotic to cause an anaphylaxis reaction. Other common antibiotics include cephalosporin and sulfonamides (Box 11.4).

▶ **HINT:** Some food allergens are so severe that just touching or inhaling the odor of the food can cause the hypersensitivity reaction.

Box 11.2 Common Food Allergies Causing Anaphylaxis

Peanuts
Shellfish
Fish
Tree nuts
Milk
Eggs
Seeds

Box 11.3 Causes of IgE-Mediated Hypersensitivity Reactions

Food allergies
Insect stings
Pollen
Antibiotics
Muscle relaxants
Latex
Snake bites

Box 11.4 Causes of Nonimmunological Hypersensitivity

Contrast media
Opioids
ASA and NSAIDs

ASA, acetylsalicylic acid; NSAIDs, nonsteroidal anti-inflammatory drugs.

■ *What is the most life-threatening symptom of anaphylaxis reactions?*

■ **Angioedema**

Angioedema can cause the loss of airway from edema and is the most life-threatening symptom of anaphylaxis. Symptoms include wheezing and dyspnea. Urticaria is a common associated symptom. Sudden loss of consciousness can also be an initial sign and patients may report a feeling of "impending" doom (Box 11.5).

▶ **HINT:** Airway issues should be considered the most life-threatening complication of an anaphylaxis reaction.

Box 11.5 Symptoms of Anaphylaxis

Airway swelling
Urticaria and pruritus
Dyspnea
Wheezing
Nausea and vomiting
Diarrhea
Abdominal pain
Hypotension
Dizziness and syncope
Chest tightness and pain
Headache
Seizure
Flushing

■ *What is the initial drug used to treat an anaphylaxis reaction?*

■ **Epinephrine**

Epinephrine is administered in a 1:1,000 dilution 0.2- to 0.5-mg dose subcutaneously or intramuscularly. If severe hypotension, administer epinephrine via continuous infusion. It is an alpha and beta agonist, but will also decrease release of mast cells. Hypotension is treated with fluid resuscitation and vasopressors, and supplemental oxygen is supplied. Steroids and antihistamines (Benadryl) sometimes provide even greater relief of symptoms.

▶ **HINT:** Antihistamines block the H1 receptor; adding an H2 receptor blocker (Ranitidine) can enhance effectiveness.

■ *What drug can limit effectiveness of epinephrine?*

■ **Beta-blockers**

Patients taking beta-blockers may be resistant to epinephrine, demonstrating continued hypotension and bradycardia. Atropine may be required to manage the bradycardia.

▶ **HINT:** Other drugs that may interfere with the effectiveness of epinephrine include angiotensin-converting enzyme (ACE) inhibitors and monoamine oxidase (MAO) inhibitors.

■ *If a patient states that she has an allergic reaction to contrast dye but still requires the diagnostic procedure, what can be given prior to the administration of contrast dye to decrease its allergic reaction?*

■ **Steroids and antihistamines**

Pretreatment can be performed with steroid and antihistamine prior to giving contrast dye in a sensitive patient requiring a diagnostic procedure.

> ▶ HINT: Pretreatment with steroids and antihistamines does not guarantee that the patient will not have hypersensitivity reactions; therefore, the patient requires close monitoring.

CARDIOGENIC SHOCK

■ *What type of shock is the most severe form of heart failure?*

■ **Cardiogenic shock**

Cardiogenic shock is the most severe form of heart failure and requires emergency management. It is a life-threatening condition.

> ▶ HINT: Cardiac tamponade can also result in shock and is called an *obstructive shock.*

■ *What is the primary cause of cardiogenic shock?*

■ **Ischemia**

Cardiogenic shock remains the leading cause of mortality in acute myocardial infarctions. Ischemic cardiomyopathies are the primary causes of cardiogenic shock (Box 11.6). Cardiogenic shock is defined as hypoperfusion caused by cardiac failure.

> ▶ HINT: Blunt trauma to the chest can cause myocardial contusion resulting in cardiogenic shock.

Box 11.6 Other Causes of Cardiogenic Shock

Hypertrophied cardiomyopathy
Aortic dissection with aortic insufficiency
Aortic or mitral stenosis (increases myocardial stress)
Acute myopericarditis
Stress-induced cardiomyopathy (Takotsubo cardiomyopathy)
Acute valvular regurgitation (endocarditis or chordal rupture)
Cardiac tamponade
Massive pulmonary embolism

■ *What are the characteristic hemodynamic parameters of cardiogenic shock?*

■ **Low cardiac output (CO)/cardiac index (CI), high systemic vascular resistance (SVR), and high filling pressures**

Cardiogenic shock demonstrates persistent hypotension with severe reduction in CI and adequate or elevated filling pressures (Box 11.7). Compensatory mechanisms for low CO include vasoconstriction (elevates SVR) and tachycardia, which actually worsen the CO because of the high resistance and increased workload of the heart, causing a vicious cycle to develop.

▶ **HINT:** Severe reduction of CI is defined as less than 1.8 L/min/m² without support, and less than 2.0 to 2.2 L/min/m² with support.

Box 11.7 Other Symptoms of Cardiogenic Shock

Tachycardia
Cool, clammy skin
Pale nail beds with delayed capillary refill
Decreased urine output
Altered mental status
Tachypnea
Presence of arrhythmias

■ *What monitoring device may be used to assist with the diagnosis of cardiogenic shock?*

■ **Pulmonary artery catheter (PAC)**

The PAC provides information on the CO/CI, filling pressures, and calculates the SVR. These readings are used to define and recognize cardiogenic shock. Newer hemodynamic monitors that are minimally invasive and use the arterial waveform may also be used to assist with the diagnosis.

▶ **HINT:** Echocardiogram may be used to confirm the diagnosis of high filling pressures and rule out other causes of hypotension following blunt chest trauma.

■ *What is the greatest concern when administering an inotropic agent to a patient in cardiogenic shock?*

■ **Increased myocardial workload and oxygen consumption**

Inotropic agents are frequently needed to increase CO and reduce filling pressures in the right and left ventricles, but they can increase the oxygen demand in the heart with limited oxygen supply. This may increase the ischemic injuries to the myocardium. Inotropes are recommended in hypoperfusion states with or without pulmonary congestion, but may be initiated at a lower dose in cardiogenic shock to limit complications.

▶ **HINT:** Inotropes can also induce arrhythmias in ischemic hearts and should be closely monitored.

■ *What is a first-line intervention in managing hypotension in cardiogenic shock?*

■ **Inotropes**

Vasoconstrictors (i.e., norepinephrine) should not be used initially to treat hypotension in cardiogenic shock because of the presence of increased SVR. Other interventions for managing hypotension in cardiogenic shock include a combination of inotropic agents with vasodilators, fluid challenges with inotropic agents, and mechanical assistance (intra-aortic balloon pump [IABP], left ventricular assist device [LVAD]).

> ▶ HINT: If vasoconstrictors are needed, cautious use of norepinephrine is recommended instead of dopamine.

HEMORRHAGIC/HYPOVOLEMIC SHOCK

■ *What is the major component in defining shock?*

■ **Hypoperfusion**

Shock is the pathophysiological state in which there is defective vascular perfusion of tissues and organs. It is a state of inadequacies between delivery of oxygen and the removal of end products of metabolism from peripheral tissues. This results in widespread reduction in tissue perfusion, hypoxia, and conversion of cellular respiration to an anaerobic form of metabolism that produces lactate as a by-product. Rapid restoration of oxygen delivery can be a major factor in preventing the development of multiple organ dysfunction syndrome.

> ▶ HINT: Remember, shock is defined by hypoperfusion not hypotension.

■ *During hypovolemic shock, which compensatory mechanism decreases urine output in an attempt to restore circulating blood volume?*

■ **Renin–angiotensin system**

During periods of hypovolemia and hypoperfusion, the kidneys release renin, which converts angiotensin I to angiotensin II. Angiotensin II is a potent vasoconstrictor that shunts blood away from nonvital organs. Angiotensin II stimulates the release of aldosterone, which results in sodium and water reabsorption. This decreases the urine output while increasing vascular volume. The sympathetic nervous system is another compensatory system activated during hypovolemic shock. It results in tachycardia, increased myocardial contractility, and vasoconstriction.

> ▶ HINT: Vasoconstriction may maintain a blood pressure (BP) during hypovolemic shock. Vital signs may not reflect presence or severity of shock.

■ *What are the hemodynamic findings of hypovolemic shock that differentiate it from other types of shock?*

■ **Low filling pressures and high SVR**

Hypovolemic shock is caused by a decrease in circulating blood volume, causing a low stroke volume/CO. Hypovolemia can be caused by blood loss, poor intake, increased fluid losses, or redistribution of fluid (third-spacing).

> ▶ HINT: Both the central venous pressure (CVP) and pulmonary capillary wedge pressure (PCWP) are low.

■ *What compartmental fluid shift occurs with hemorrhagic shock?*

■ **Fluid shifts from extravascular space to intravascular space**

In hemorrhagic shock, fluid shifts from the extravascular spaces into the intravascular space in an attempt to replace volume caused by acute blood loss. In disease states in which plasma volume is lost, fluid shifts from the intravascular to the interstitial space.

> ▶ **HINT:** This is frequently called *third-spacing* and can result in hypovolemic shock. Examples include peritonitis, burns, and crush injuries.

■ *Following a trauma, the patient presents with the following vital signs on admission:*

Heart rate (HR): 124 beats per minute
Respiration rate: 32 breaths per minute
BP: 94/60 mmHg
Urinary output: 15 mL/hr

Based on these vital signs, what is the class of hemorrhagic shock?

■ **Class III hemorrhagic shock**

The American College of Surgeons (ACS) has developed a classification of hemorrhagic shock based on vital signs to indicate the severity of blood loss. This is not exact and patient presentation can vary.

> ▶ **HINT:** Elderly patients may not become tachycardic because of limited response to catecholamines.

■ *A class III hemorrhagic shock would indicate what percentage of blood loss?*

■ **About 30% to 40%**

The classification is based on percentage of total blood volume (TBV) loss. The estimated amount of blood volume loss is based on a 70-kg male (TBV approximately 5 L). A 30% to 40% TBV loss (class III) would be approximately 1,500 to 2,000 mL (Box 11.8).

Box 11.8 ACS Classification of Hemorrhage

	Class I	Class II	Class III	Class IV
Blood loss (mL)	Less than 750	750–1,500	1,500–2,000	Greater than 2,000
Blood loss (%)	Less than 15	15–30	30–40	Greater than 40
Systolic BP	Normal	Normal	Decreased	Decreased
Heart rate (beats/min)	Less than 100	Greater than 100	Greater than 120	Greater than 140
Respiratory rate (breaths/min)	14–20	20–30	30–40	Greater than 35
Mental status	Anxious	Agitated	Confused	Lethargic

ACS, American College of Surgeons, BP, blood pressure.

> ▶ **HINT:** Because of the effectiveness of their compensatory mechanisms, young patients may have a normal BP/HR even in the presence of significant blood loss. Elderly patients may be hypotensive even with minimal blood loss.

■ *What classification of drugs limits the tachycardic response that occurs during hemorrhagic shock?*

■ **Beta-blockers**

Blocking the beta-receptors of the heart results in limited ability to respond to the sympathetic nervous system with tachycardia. The lack of tachycardia does not rule out hemorrhagic shock in patients taking beta-blockers. Other signs of hypovolemic shock include pale, cool, and clammy skin. The urine output will progressively decrease as shock worsens.

▶ **HINT:** Hypovolemic or hemorrhagic shock patients may narrow the pulse pressure before decreasing systolic BP.

■ *Which laboratory studies may be used to identify the presence of shock in a normotensive patient?*

■ **Lactate and base deficit**

Vital signs are not reliable in identifying all patients in shock. Cellular metabolism is limited by inadequate tissue hypoperfusion and results in mandatory changes from an aerobic to an anaerobic metabolism. In anaerobic metabolism, the production of lactic acid is an end product that creates lactic acidosis.

▶ **HINT:** Elevated lactate levels and presence of a base deficit are used to identify anaerobic metabolism.

■ *What is a base deficit?*

■ **Amount of base needed to titrate 1 L of whole blood to pH of 7.40**

The base deficit reflects the extent of anaerobic metabolism and severity of the metabolic acidosis. This value is obtained from an arterial blood gas. The normal base is +2 to −2 mEq/L, with positive numbers indicating a base excess and negative numbers indicating a base deficit.

▶ **HINT:** Base deficit is used as an end point of resuscitation (Box 11.9).

Box 11.9 Base Deficit Determines Severity of Hypovolemia

Severity of Hypovolemia	Base Deficit
Mild	−3 to −5
Moderate	−6 to −14
Severe	Greater than −15

■ *Why does the hemoglobin (Hgb)/hematocrit (Hct) not accurately reflect the red blood cell (RBC) mass during an acute hemorrhage?*

■ **Equal loss of all blood components**

Hematocrit and hemoglobin concentrations are indices of balance between loss of blood and movement of extravascular fluid to intravascular space. During an acute hemorrhage, a loss of whole blood occurs with a decrease of all blood components in a similar ratio. If the initial Hgb is low, it is caused by fluid administration and hemodilution. The rate of change in Hgb over time is more predictive of the severity of bleeding.

▶ **HINT:** A normal Hgb/Hct does not rule out active bleeding.

■ *What is the primary treatment for hypovolemic/hemorrhagic shock?*

■ **Intravenous (IV) fluids**

IV fluids are the mainstay treatment for hypovolemia. In the case of trauma or acute bleeding, finding the source of blood loss and stopping the bleeding surgically may be required. If the patient is hypothermic, the resuscitation fluids should be warmed prior to or during infusion.

▶ **HINT:** Remember that airway and breathing are still priority of care in hemorrhagic shock patient.

■ *What is the greatest disadvantage of resuscitating with crystalloids?*

■ **Fluid shifts from intravascular to interstitial space**

Crystalloids are electrolyte solutions with small molecules, which can shift across the spaces. A large amount of infused crystalloids will shift from the intravascular to the interstitial space within minutes of administration. This requires larger volumes of fluids to be administered to replace the vascular losses. Frequently used crystalloids for resuscitation include isotonic solutions such as Lactated Ringer's and normal saline (NS).

▶ **HINT:** A 3:1 replacement rule has been used to determine the amount required for crystalloid resuscitation.

■ *Large-volume infusions of NS can cause which acid–base imbalance?*

■ **Metabolic acidosis**

A 1-L bag of NS contains 154 mEq/L of sodium and chloride. Large amounts of NS administered during resuscitation can cause a hyperchloremic metabolic acidosis. Lactated Ringer's solution is a more balanced salt solution and may be used in large-volume resuscitations to prevent metabolic acidosis (Box 11.10).

▶ **HINT:** Patient's respiratory rate may be rapid to compensate for metabolic acidosis.

Box 11.10 Crystalloids Versus Colloids

	Crystalloids	Colloids
Advantages	Replaces interstitial fluid losses that may have occurred Cheaper Easier to store	Use less fluid to resuscitate May draw fluid into the vascular space from interstitial Albumin may have anti-inflammatory effects
Disadvantages	Uses larger amounts of fluid to resuscitate	During altered capillary permeability, albumin shifts extravascularly Synthetic colloids (i.e., dextran) activate immune response May cause hypersensitivity reaction Synthetic colloids increase bleeding tendencies More expensive Difficult to store

■ *Which crystalloid is used to increase serum osmolality and rapidly expands the intravascular space?*

■ **Hypertonic saline**

Small amounts of hypertonic saline (4 to 5 mL/kg) can decrease the total amount of crystalloids used during resuscitation. Hypertonic saline increases serum osmolality and draws fluid from the extravascular into the intravascular space. It may improve blood flow to organs and has been found to lower intracranial pressure (Box 11.11).

> ▶ **HINT:** Metabolic acidosis and hypernatremia are complications of hypertonic saline caused by the large amount of chloride, even greater than normal saline.

Box 11.11 Hypertonic Saline

Na⁺ (sodium) in 3% saline is 513 with Cl⁻ (chloride) of 513
Na⁺ in 7.5% saline is 1,283 with Cl⁻ of 1,283

■ *When giving multiple units of packed red blood cells (PRBCs), what other blood products need to be administered?*

■ **Fresh frozen plasma (FFP) and platelets**

Administering PRBCs and fluid causes a dilutional coagulopathy. PRBCs are void of clotting factors and platelets. Transfusion practice is changing by adding more FFP and platelet transfusions into the resuscitation. Some practitioners are using a 1:1 replacement rule. For every one unit of blood, administer a unit of FFP.

> ▶ **HINT:** Whole blood does have platelets and clotting factors and can be used instead of PRBCs to resuscitate a trauma patient.

■ *What is a benefit of hypotensive resuscitation in a bleeding patient?*

■ **Limits blood loss**

Avoiding aggressive fluid resuscitation to increase the BP may limit the amount of blood volume loss in a bleeding patient prior to surgery. Hypotensive resuscitation aims to maintain the systolic BP between 80 to 90 mmHg with smaller boluses of fluid (200 mL bolus). Higher systolic BP increase intravascular hydrostatic pressure, worsening blood loss in a bleeding patient. The risk of this strategy is hypoperfusion.

> ▶ **HINT:** Maintain the systolic BP greater than 90 mmHg for those with traumatic brain injury.

Questions

1. A shock patient experiences vasoconstriction, tachycardia, and increased myocardial contractility. This is because of which system being activated?

   A. Parasympathetic nervous system
   B. Sympathetic nervous system
   C. Renin–angiotensin system
   D. Angiotensin system

2. What is the fluid shift that occurs with hemorrhagic shock?

   A. Fluid shifts from the extravascular to the intravascular space
   B. Fluid shifts from the intravascular to the extravascular space
   C. Fluids shifts into the brain parenchyma
   D. Fluid shifts out of the renal tubules

3. A patient comes into the emergency room after an accidental saw injury to the right arm. The patient is anxious and confused to time and situation. The following vital signs are obtained:

   Respiratory rate is 33 breaths per minute
   Heart rate is 135 beats per minute (bpm)
   Blood pressure is 92/56 mmHg
   Oxygen saturation is 92% on 2-L via nasal cannula

   What classification of hemorrhagic shock is the patient most likely experiencing?

   A. Class I
   B. Class II
   C. Class III
   D. Class IV

4. All of the following statements are true regarding hypertonic solutions except:

   A. Osmotically draws fluid into the extravascular space
   B. Improves myocardial activity
   C. Increases renal, splanchic, and coronary blood flow
   D. Smaller volumes are required for adequate resuscitation

5. A bleeding patient comes into the emergency room. The health care team is administering blood products. There is no cross-match; so this patient will receive the universal donor blood, O negative, until a cross-match can be obtained. A new cross-match should be sent after multiple blood transfusions. Which of the following statements is incorrect?

   A. A new cross-match needs to be sent after multiple universal blood transfusions.
   B. The universal donor blood type is AB negative.
   C. Massive transfusion patients are defined as 10 units or more in a 24-hour period.
   D. O-positive blood can be administered to a male patient as uncross-matched blood.

6. Which of the following is *not* considered a sequelae of massive fluid resuscitation following a trauma?

   A. Hypothermia
   B. Coagulopathy
   C. Acidosis
   D. Hemodynamic instability

7. Which of the following is *not* the first-line treatment to limit acidosis and improve perfusion during hemorrhagic shock and massive resuscitation?

   A. Administer fluids
   B. Administer vasopressin
   C. Transfuse with packed red blood cells (PRBCs)
   D. Transfuse with fresh frozen plasma (FFP)

Systemic Inflammatory Response Syndrome/Multiple Organ Dysfunction

■ **What is the presence of bacteria in the bloodstream called?**

■ **Bacteremia**

Bacteremia is the viable presence of bacteria in the bloodstream as determined by blood cultures being positive for bacteria. Fungemia is the presence of a fungus in the bloodstream. A positive culture is one of the signs of an infection. An infection initiates the inflammatory response and onset of sepsis (Box 12.1).

Box 12.1 Signs of an Infection

Presence of white blood cells in normally sterile body fluid
Positive culture (urine, blood, sputum)
Perforated viscous
Radiographic evidence of pneumonia in association with purulent sputum

■ **What is the white blood cell (WBC) criterion used to define sepsis?**

■ **WBC count of more than 12,000, or less than 4,000, or band cells of more than 10%**

Sepsis is the inflammatory response to a known infection. Sepsis is defined as the presence of two or more of the stipulated criteria (Box 12.2). Systemic inflammatory response syndrome (SIRS) is a systemic inflammatory response to a variety of severe clinical insults. SIRS is defined by the same criteria used to determine sepsis, but without signs of infection and a negative blood culture.

> ▶ **HINT:** Sepsis is a disease process managed in all areas of the hospital and is not exclusive to critical care.

Box 12.2 Criteria That Defines Sepsis

Temperature > 38.3°C (101°F) or < 36°C
Heart rate > 90 beats/min
Respiratory rate > 20 breaths/min or $PaCO_2$ < 32 mmHg
WBC > 12,000 cells/mm^3 or < 4,000 mm^3 , or > 10% immature granulocytes (bands)

WBC, white blood cells.

> ▶ **HINT:** SIRS frequently has negative blood cultures.

■ *What is present in septic shock?*

■ **Hypotension and hypoperfusion**

Septic shock is a subset of sepsis, and is accompanied by profound hypotension and hypoperfusion. It is also called sepsis-induced tissue hypoperfusion or organ dysfunction. Hypotension is defined as a systolic blood pressure (SBP) less than 90 mmHg, mean arterial pressure (MAP) less than 70 mmHg, or a decrease in blood pressure (BP) by greater than 40 mmHg from baseline, or MAP less than 70 mmHg. Hypoperfusion may include but is not limited to oliguria, increased lactate levels greater than 4 mmol/L or acute alteration in mental status (Box 12.3). The sepsis bundles use a lactate level greater than 2 mmol/L to recognize hypoperfusion.

> ▶ **HINTS:** Definitions and therapeutic goals may be different when managing sepsis. The definition of hypotension in sepsis is an MAP less than 70 mmHg, but the goal or therapeutic threshold is to maintain an MAP greater than 65 mmHg.

Box 12.3 Signs of Hypoperfusion

Acute altered mental status
Blood glucose > 140 mg/dL in patients without diabetes
Arterial hypoxemia (PaO_2/FiO_2 ratio < 300)
Acute oliguria (< 0.5 mL/kg/hr for at least 2 hours)
Creatinine increase > 0.5 mg/dL above baseline
Coagulation abnormalities (INR > 1.5 or a PTT > 60 sec)
Ileus
Thrombocytopenia (platelet count < 100,000)
Hyperbilirubinemia (total bilirubin > 2 mg/dL)

INR, international normalized ratio, PTT, partial thromboplastin time.

> ▶ **HINT:** Septic shock is hypotension and hypoperfusion despite adequate resuscitation.

■ *What is multiple organ dysfunction syndrome (MODS) in sepsis caused by?*

■ **Hypoperfusion**

MODS is the presence of altered organ function in two or more organs in an acutely ill patient such that homeostasis cannot be maintained without intervention. It is progressive but potentially reversible, and is a result of hypoperfusion and injury to the organs (Box 12.4).

> ▶ **HINT:** Mortality is related to the number of organs involved and the severity of organ dysfunction.

Box 12.4 Signs of Organ Dysfunction

System	Major Sign
Pulmonary	PaO_2/FiO_2 ratio < 300
Renal	Increased serum creatinine > 2.0 or creatinine increase > 0.5 mg/dL or 44.2 mmol/L

(continued)

Box 12.4 Signs of Organ Dysfunction (*continued*)

System	Major Sign
Hepatic	Increased bilirubin levels > 4 mg/dL
Hematology	Decreased platelet counts < 100,000/µL INR > 1.5 PTT > 60s
Central nervous system	Altered GCS

GCS, Glasgow Coma Scale; INR, international normalized ratio; PTT, partial thromboplastin time.

■ *What is the most common microorganism that causes sepsis?*

■ **Gram-positive bacteria**

Gram-positive bacteria have surpassed the gram-negative bacteria in causing sepsis (Box 12.5). A common gram-positive bacteria is methicillin-resistant *Staphylococcus aureus* (MRSA) (Box 12.6).

Box 12.5 Types of Gram-Negative Bacteria

Escherichia coli
Klebsiella pneumonia
Pseudomonas aeruginosa
Enterobacter
Serratia
Proteus

▶ **HINT:** Gram-negative bacteria colonize the gastrointestinal (GI) tract and oral secretions.

Box 12.6 Types of Gram-Positive Bacteria

Staphylococcus
Streptococcus

▶ **HINT:** Central-line sepsis is caused by gram-positive bacteremia.

■ *Which microorganism is the most common cause of a secondary infection?*

■ **Fungus (*Candida*)**

Fungal infections are found to cause a second episode of infection. This is because the use of antibiotics to treat the first infection alters the normal flora, thereby allowing opportunistic infections to develop. Immunosuppressed patients are also at high risk for secondary infections. Fungal sepsis (fungemia) has a higher mortality than bacteremia and is harder to diagnose. Presence of fungemia may not result in a positive blood culture. Management is typically based on presumptive therapy, which is to "presume" fungemia is present and treat with antifungal medication. New tests may be used to assist with diagnosis of *Candida* (1,3 beta-D-glucan assay [grade 2B], mannan, and antimannan antibody assays). SIRS is frequently caused by a fungal infection because of an inflammatory response without a known infection or positive blood culture.

■ *An increase in bands greater than what percentage indicates severe sepsis?*

■ **Greater than 10%**

Bands are immature WBCs. When more than 10% of the circulating WBCs are bands, an over whelming infection and sepsis are indicated. Other WBC changes that potentially indicate sepsis are a WBC count greater than 12,000 or less than 4,000.

> ▶ **HINT:** For example, if a complete blood count (CBC) differential finds 45% bands, this indicates 45% of the circulating WBCs are immature and not functional.

■ *In severe sepsis or septic shock, does the left ventricle (LV) ejection fraction (EF) increase or decrease?*

■ **Decrease**

Proinflammatory cytokine and tumor necrosis factor (TNF) are released following the presence of a microorganism and initiate the inflammatory response. Sepsis has also been found to have a negative contractility effect on the myocardium and results in a decrease in EF. The cardiac output is usually high in sepsis because systemic vasodilation lowers the resistance (Box 12.7).

> ▶ **HINT:** Use of a right ventricular ejection fraction (RVEF) pulmonary artery catheter in sepsis patients has shown a decrease in EF even during periods of high cardiac output. RVEF commonly ranges between 30% and 40% during early sepsis.

Box 12.7 Symptoms of Sepsis or Septic Shock

Tachycardia
Tachypnea
Leukocytosis, leukopenia, or increase in bands
Fever
Decreased systemic vascular resistance
Hypotension (vasodilation)
Increased cardiac output
Decreased ejection fraction
Left ventricular dilation
Metabolic acidosis
Respiratory alkalosis
Pulmonary artery hypertension
Altered mental status
Edema or positive fluid balance
Hyperglycemia (> 140 mg/dL or 7.7 mmol/L) in nondiabetic patients
Signs of organ dysfunction

> ▶ **HINT:** A significant positive fluid balance is defined as greater than 20 mL/kg over 24 hours.

■ *What is used to determine the microorganism(s) involved in causing the infection and the best antibiotics needed to treat the infection?*

■ **Culture and sensitivity**

Diagnosis of sepsis is based on the presence of two or more of the defining criteria for sepsis. Once sepsis is recognized, cultures are sent for testing to determine the causative microorganisms and their susceptibility to certain antibiotics. Recommendation is at least two sets of blood cultures (both anaerobic and aerobic bottles) with at least one drawn percutaneously; one can be drawn with a vascular access device if the device was inserted no less than 48 hours prior to the draw. Both blood cultures can be drawn at the same time if obtained from two different sites. Cultures from other potential sites of infection (urine, sputum, cerebrospinal fluid [CSF], wounds) should also be obtained and sent with blood cultures.

▶ **HINT:** If the same organism is recovered from both samples, there is a better likelihood that the organism is responsible for the sepsis.

■ *What other lab tests besides the CBC can be used to determine the presence of an infection?*

■ **Plasma C-reactive protein and prolactin**

Plasma C-reactive proteins and prolactin are biomarkers for diagnosis of infection. They may be used as additional information but at this time are not shown to distinguish from infection and other causes of inflammation.

▶ **HINT:** Procalcitonin levels may be beneficial in determining when to discontinue the antibiotics.

■ *What is the overall best management goal for sepsis?*

■ **Prevention**

Prevention of an infection or sepsis is still the best management. Handwashing is the main area of prevention found to lower incidence of infections across the continuum of patient types and ages (Box 12.8).

Box 12.8 Sources of Hospital-Associated Infections

Catheter-associated urinary tract infection
Central line-associated bloodstream infections
Ventilator-associated pneumonia
Hospital-acquired pneumonia
Intra-abdominal source

■ *What is the current recommendation to prevent a catheter-associated urinary tract infection (CAUTI)?*

■ **Minimize use and duration of a urinary catheter**

Urinary tract infections are the most common type of health care–associated infections. The most current practice is to avoid a Foley catheter insertion, if possible. If a bladder catheter is required in surgery, the goal is to discontinue it within 24 hours. Removing the indwelling catheter as soon as possible lowers the incidence of urinary tract infections (Box 12.9). The most common causative microorganisms are *E. coli* and *Candida* (Box 12.10).

▶ **HINT:** Remember all lines and tubes in the patient are a source of infection and should be removed as soon as possible.

Box 12.9 Appropriate Reasons for Urinary Catheter Use

Accurate I & O in critically ill patients – Need to monitor urine output
Unable to use bedpan or urinal – Coma – Sedation and paralytics
Large volume of fluid infusions or diuretics
Urological surgery patients
Urinary retention or obstruction

I & O, input and output.

Box 12.10 Prevention of Urinary Tract Infections

Aseptic insertion technique and use of sterile equipment
Keep bag off the floor
Keep bag lower than the bladder
Properly secure the collecting bag to prevent movement in the bladder
Maintain a closed drainage system
Empty collecting bag regularly
Use catheters impregnated with antiseptic or antimicrobial agents

▶ **HINT:** Changing bags or indwelling catheters on a routine basis is not recommended. It is suggested that clinical indications to change a catheter include infection or contamination of the system.

■ *What is a nursing intervention found to lower the incidence of ventilator-associated pneumonia (VAP)?*

■ **Oral care with chlorhexidine**

Oropharyngeal decontamination with chlorhexidine gluconate is recommended to lower the incidence of VAP. Selective digestive decontamination has also been proposed to lower the risk of VAP (Box 12.11).

Box 12.11 Methods of Preventing VAP

Proper handwashing
Oral decontamination
Digestive decontamination
Elevated HOB
Subglottic suctioning
Prevent unplanned extubations/ reintubations
Avoid saline lavages

HOB, head of bed; VAP, ventilator-associated pneumonia.

■ *How quickly should antibiotics be started following the diagnosis of sepsis?*

■ **Within 1 hour**

Antibiotics are the main treatment of sepsis, and may halt the progression of sepsis and improve outcomes if administered early in the course of sepsis. Cultures should be obtained before the administration of antibiotics, unless this causes a significant delay in the administration of antibiotics. Antibiotics can result in sterilization of the cultures within a few hours, making identification of the causative organism more difficult. Broad-spectrum antibiotics should be used to be effective against all likely organisms. Once culture results are obtained, antibiotics should be changed to be more specific to the organism's susceptibility (within 3 to 5 days).

> ▶ **HINT:** The recommendation is to maintain on a 5- to 7-day course of antibiotic therapy. The number of days may increase if there is a slow clinical response or continued presence of infection.

■ *In early goal-directed therapy of severe sepsis, what is the central venous pressure (CVP) goal of the initial fluid resuscitation in a spontaneously breathing patient?*

■ **CVP of 8 to 12 mmHg**

Severe sepsis is persistent hypotension or hypoperfusion after an initial bolus of fluid. An early goal-directed strategy includes monitoring CVP and central venous oxygen saturation ($ScvO_2$) to determine the adequacy of resuscitation. CVP of 8 to 12 mmHg is recommended for spontaneously breathing patients, and slightly higher on ventilated patients (12 to 15 mmHg) because of the positive pressure effects in the chest. The $ScvO_2$ can be monitored intermittently or continuously. The goals should be obtained within 6 hours on recognition of sepsis. Goals can be obtained with fluid administration, blood products, dobutamine infusion, or lower oxygen demands with sedation or paralysis. Another parameter used to monitor hemodynamics is stroke volume variance (SVV), which is used to determine fluid responsiveness (Box 12.12).

> ▶ **HINT:** Lactate levels may also be monitored with the goal to normalize serum lactate.

Box 12.12 Goals of Resuscitation of Severe Sepsis

CVP 8–12 mmHg in spontaneous breathing CVP 12–15 mmHg ventilated
MAP $\geq$ 65 mmHg
Urine output $\geq$ 0.5 mL/kg/hr
$ScvO_2$ 70% or SvO_2 65%

CVP, central venous pressure; MAP, mean arterial pressure; $ScvO_2$ central venous oxygen saturation; SvO_2, mixed venous oxygen saturation.

> ▶ **HINT:** A decrease in heart rate is also a good indication of successful resuscitation.

■ *What fluids are recommended for the initial resuscitation in sepsis?*

■ **Crystalloids**

The current recommendation for fluid resuscitation in severe sepsis or sepsis-induced hypoperfusion is crystalloids. They are recommended because of the lack of benefit if albumin is used initially, coupled with albumin's greater expense. If the patient requires a substantial amount of fluid to meet the goals of volume resuscitation, then albumin administration is recommended with crystalloids. The fluid challenge initially should be a minimum of 30 mL/kg bolus with more fluids if needed to meet the predetermined goals of volume resuscitation.

> ▶ **HINT:** Hydroxyethyl starches (hetastarch) are not recommended in resuscitation of sepsis patients because of the worsening effect on kidneys.

■ *What vasopressor is considered the first choice to maintain MAP more than 65 mmHg?*

■ **Norepinephrine (Levophed)**

Vasopressor therapy is recommended to maintain the MAP at 65 mmHg or greater. Below this perfusion pressure, the autoregulation in the critical vascular beds is lost. Norepinephrine is the recommended first-line vasopressor. If an additional vasopressor is required, epinephrine or vasopressin may be added to maintain pressure or to lower the dose of norepinephrine. Vasopressin is not recommended as a single first-line vasopressor in sepsis. Dopamine may be an alternative vasopressor to norepinephrine, but only in certain patients at very low risk for tachyarrhythmias. Low-dose dopamine should not be used as renal protection. A patient with absolute or refractory bradycardia may receive dopamine as the first-line vasopressor. Phenylephrine is not recommended in the treatment of septic shock unless associated with serious arrhythmias, or cardiac output is known to be high, or when other vasopressor agents have failed to achieve the targeted MAP.

> ▶ **HINT:** An arterial line is recommended for continuous and more accurate BP readings. Central venous access is required for administration of vasopressors.

■ *When should corticosteroid therapy be considered in a patient with sepsis?*

■ **When refractory to vasopressors**

A patient who responds to fluids or vasopressor therapy by improving hemodynamic parameters (BP) and lactate levels does not require corticosteroid treatment. If hemodynamic stability cannot be achieved, even after resuscitation and vasopressor administration, 200 mg/day of hydrocortisone as a continuous infusion is recommended. Continuous infusions may control blood glucose more effectively than intermittent boluses with less significant hyperglycemia. Once vasopressors are not required, hydrocortisone may be tapered and discontinued. The adrenocorticotropic hormone (ACTH) test is not recommended to determine an indication for corticosteroid therapy.

> ▶ **HINT:** Side effects of hydrocortisone are hypernatremia and hyperglycemia.

■ *According to the Sepsis Campaign guidelines, when should the insulin protocol be initiated in a sepsis patient?*

■ **When two consecutive blood glucose levels are greater than 180 mg/dL**

The current recommendation for glucose control is to treat with sliding-scale insulin if blood glucose levels are greater than 180 mg/dL two consecutive times. Maintain glucose less than 180 mg/dL while avoiding hypoglycemia. Blood glucose levels may be checked every 4 hours when stable and every 1 to 2 hours while elevated. Maintaining strict glucose levels of less than 110 mg/dL is not recommended because of the incidences of hypoglycemia.

> ▶ **HINT:** Point-of-care glucose tests may not be as accurate as plasma glucose levels from the laboratory and should be interpreted cautiously.

■ *At what serum pH would sodium bicarbonate therapy be administered in septic shock patients with lactic acidosis?*
■ **Less than 7.15**

There is no benefit of treating a pH with sodium bicarbonate until pH decreases to less than 7.15. The side effects of sodium bicarbonate cause the risks of administration to be greater than the benefit (Box 12.13).

Box 12.13 Complications of Sodium Bicarbonate

Fluid overload
Hypernatremia
Increased lactate levels
Hypercarbia
Decreased serum ionized calcium
Greater affinity of Hgb to RBCs

Hgb, hemoglobin; RBCs, red blood cells.

■ *What is the best management if there is a known source of infection?*
■ **Remove the source of infection**

Radiographics are frequently used to find the location of the infection. If the infectious source is amendable to drainage, percutaneous drainage or surgical excision may be required. Source control as rapid as possible can lower the incidence of mortality (within 12 hours).

> ▶ **HINT:** If the source is determined to be an intravenous access source, the catheter needs to be removed promptly after obtaining other access.

Box 12.14 Surgically Amendable Focal Infections

Abscesses (including intra-abdominal)
Gastrointestinal perforation
Cholangitis
Pyelonephritis
Intestinal ischemia
Necrotizing soft tissue
Empyema
Septic arthritis

■ *What is the primary physiology for the hypoperfused state in sepsis?*

■ **Inability of cells to utilize oxygen**

Initial hypoperfusion is a result of distributive shock (vasodilation) and hypovolemia (increased vascular permeability). Even after fluid volume is restored, hypoperfusion may persist. This is largely attributed to an inability of the cells to utilize the oxygen delivered to the tissues. Another major contributing factor is that maldistribution of blood flow occurs at the regional level (splanchnic, renal, and mesenteric) as well as the microvascular level (Box 12.15).

> ▶ **HINT:** Remember the saying, "You can lead a horse to water but you can't make it drink." In sepsis, you can optimize delivery of oxygen to the tissues or cells but you can't make them take the oxygen.

Box 12.15 Causes for Inadequate Tissue Oxygenation

Decreased oxygen delivery
Inability to extract oxygen
Blockage of normal cellular metabolism
Greater distance between vessels and tissue (edema)
Inability to offload O_2 from Hgb
Arteriovenous shunt
Endothelial injury
Loss of vascular tone

Hgb, hemoglobin.

■ *What is a gastrointestinal (GI) complication that occurs because of the use of multiple antibiotics in treating sepsis?*

■ *Clostridium difficile*

C. difficile is a superinfection that may occur as a result of using multiple, broad spectrum antibiotics for a prolonged period of treatment. Narrowing the spectrum and shortening the time of antibiotic therapy may lower the risk of acquiring opportunistic infections such as *Candida*, or superinfections such as *C. difficile*, and resistant bacteria (vancomycin-resistant *Enterococcus faecium*).

> ▶ **HINT:** Antibiotics can change the normal gastrointestinal flora. Probiotics may be used to prevent this altered flora.

■ *What is the most common cause of death in septic shock?*

■ **MODS**

MODS is a complication of the tissue and organ hypoperfusion that occurs in severe sepsis and septic shock. MODS is defined as the presence of altered organ function in acutely ill patients such that homeostasis cannot be obtained without intervention (Box 12.16). The number of organs affected predicts mortality. Any organ can be affected by sepsis-induced hypoperfusion.

▶ **HINT:** This is also commonly called *multisystem organ failure (MSOF)*.

Box 12.16 Common Types or Organ Failures

Acute respiratory distress syndrome
Acute kidney injury
Hepatic failure
Gastrointestinal tract
Septic encephalopathy
Systolic and diastolic dysfunction myocardium
Disseminated intravascular coagulation
Metabolic dysfunction with hyperglycemia

■ *What plays a central role when microvascular dysfunction occurs in MODS?*
■ **Endothelium**

The endothelium regulates vasomotor tone, coagulation, vascular permeability, and balance between pro- and anti-inflammatory cytokines. Biomarkers that measure endothelial activity (plasminogen activator inhibitor-1) demonstrate increased levels following activation of the inflammatory system and correlate with the severity of MODS.

■ *What tool can be used to determine the rate and extent of organ failure?*
■ **Sequential organ failure assessment (SOFA)**

The SOFA scoring system is used to determine the extent of organ function or rate of failure (Boxes 12.17–12.22).

▶ **HINT:** When scoring, if none match the patient, the score is 0 for that organ. If more than one matches, use the highest score.

Box 12.17 SOFA Scoring: Respiratory System

PaO_2/FiO_2	SOFA Score
< 400	1
< 300	2
< 200 and mechanically ventilated	3
< 100 and mechanically ventilated	4

Box 12.18 SOFA Scoring: Nervous System

Glasgow Coma Scale	SOFA Score
13–14	1
10–12	2
6–9	3
< 6	4

Box 12.19 SOFA Scoring: Cardiovascular System

MAP or Vasopressor Requirement	SOFA Score
MAP < 70 mmHg	1
Dopamine < 5 OR dobutamine (any dose)	2
Dopamine > 5 OR epi ≤ 0.1 OR norepi ≤ 0.1	3
Dopamine > 15 OR epi > 0.1 OR norepi > 0.1	4

Epi, epinephrine; MAP, mean arterial pressure; norepi, norepinephrine.

Box 12.20 SOFA Scoring: Liver

Bilirubin	SOFA Score
1.2–1.9	1
2.0–5.9	2
6.0–11.9	3
> 12	4

Box 12.21 SOFA Scoring: Coagulation

Platelets × 10^3	SOFA Score
< 150	1
< 100	2
< 50	3
< 20	4

Box 12.22 SOFA Scoring: Renal System

Creatinine or Urine Output	SOFA Score
1.2–1.9	1
2.0–3.4	2
3.5–4.9	3
> 5	4

Questions

1. A trauma patient has been on a ventilator in the intensive care unit for 2 weeks. The patient is tachycardic, has been spiking fevers, and now has decreased urine output. The nurse notes that the white blood cell (WBC) count is 25,000 and the sputum cultures reveal gram-positive cocci. Which of the following is responsible for this systemic inflammatory response as demonstrated by the elevated WBC count?

   A. Cytokines
   B. Interleukins
   C. Procalcitonin
   D. Lactate

2. Dr. Hughes has come into the emergency room with a fever of 102.1°F and is tachycardic with a heart rate of 110. The nurse draws two sets of blood cultures, administers antibiotics, and then transfers the patient to the unit. The preliminary result of the cultures reveal gram-negative bacteria. Which of the following is *not* a type of gram-negative bacteria?

   A. Pneumococci
   B. *Escherichia coli*
   C. *Klebsiella pneumonia*
   D. *Serratia*

3. A trauma patient remains awake and alert, urine output is sustained at greater than 1 mL/kg/hr, and is absent of fever, tachypnea, and tachycardia. This indicates that this patient:

   A. Has not sustained a traumatic injury
   B. Is without signs of an infection
   C. Has optimal cerebral tissue perfusion
   D. Has adequate gas exchange

4. Pulmonary artery pressure will run higher in all of the following patients except those with:

   A. Mitral valve regurgitation
   B. Pulmonary emboli
   C. Hypoxia
   D. Low arterial pressure

5. A patient came into the emergency room 48 hours ago presenting with tachycardia, hypotension, vomiting, and a large foot wound with purulent drainage. The patient's lactate level on arrival was 3.1. The patient was diagnosed with sepsis and has been started on antibiotics, fluid resuscitation, and vasopressors. The repeat lactate today is 1.8. What statement would be most accurate about this patient's plan of care?

   A. The patient's lactate level is now normal.
   B. The patient is demonstrating signs of improvement.
   C. The lactate level is not used to predict outcomes.
   D. The patient has a high predictive mortality risk.

6. Which would be considered an endpoint of resuscitation in a septic patient?

    A. Mixed or central venous oxygen saturation of 72%
    B. Central venous pressure (CVP) of 10 mmHg
    C. Urine output of 35 mL/hr
    D. All of the above

7. A sepsis patient came into the emergency room yesterday and now remains in the intensive care unit (ICU) on a ventilator. The sepsis management bundle is in progress. The patient is on hydrocortisone 200 mg/d, glucose control parameters of 80 to 110 mg/dL, and inspiratory pressures of less than 30 cm H_2O on the ventilator. Which of these treatment modalities is *not* recommended?

    A. Hydrocortisone 200 mg/d
    B. Glucose control of 80 to 110 mg/dL
    C. Inspiratory pressures less than 30 cm H_2O
    D. All are recommended

Part V

Continuum of Care for Trauma

Injury Prevention and Public Education

■ *What is the first step of trauma prevention?*

■ **Identify risks**

When risks for trauma or injury are identified, then prediction of an injury and prevention are possible. Injuries follow patterns, therefore, they are frequently preventable. Analysis of risk factors leads toward identifying steps that may be used to prevent the injury. Injury surveillance systems may be used on the national level to determine trends of injuries (Box 13.1).

▶ **HINT:** The word "accident" is no longer recommended when referring to a trauma because an accident would not be preventable.

Box 13.1 Steps to Injury Prevention Programs

Collect data
Analyze data
Identify specific concerns or problems
Identify the population at risk
Develop preventive strategies or countermeasures
Implement the prevention plan
Evaluate the effectiveness of the plan

▶ **HINT:** Identifying risk factors include answering the questions of where, who, and with whom.

■ *What does the physical damage caused by the transfer of energy cause?*

■ **Injury**

Injury is physical damage caused by the transfer of energy, which can include kinetic, chemical, thermal, or electrical energy. Linking the mechanism of injury to the trauma is one step in identifying potential prevention strategies.

▶ **HINT:** The word *injury* has replaced *accident* because most injuries are preventable and an accident, by definition, is not preventable.

■ *When identifying the biomechanics of a trauma, a commonly used physics law states that force equals mass multiplied by what?*

■ **Acceleration**

Force is mass multiplied by the rate of acceleration or deceleration. A mechanism of injury is the transfer of energy from an external source to the human body. Energy is defined in trauma as the source of the physical injury (Box 13.2).

> ▶ **HINT:** *Kinematics* refers to motion and is used to study trauma mechanisms by looking primarily at the motion involved.

Box 13.2 Agents of Trauma

Mechanical	Blunt trauma
	Penetrating trauma
	Bites
	Assault and battery
	Machines
	Falls
Chemical	Poisons
	Snake bites
	Gases
	Drugs
Thermal	Burns
Lack of oxygen	Drowning
	Smoke inhalation
	Carbon monoxide poisoning
	Asphyxiation
Electrical	Electrical burns
	Lightning
Radiant	Sunburn
	Explosions
	X-ray exposures
	Radiation
	Nuclear exposure

■ *What level of injury prevention actually prevents the trauma from occurring?*

■ **Primary prevention**

Primary prevention is the least commonly used and most difficult form of prevention to accomplish. It is designed to prevent the occurrence of the injury. The goal is to reduce the number of traumas, or totally eliminate the incident from occurring.

> ▶ **HINT:** An example of primary prevention is the placement of a stoplight at a dangerous intersection. The goal is to prevent collisions.

■ *What does secondary injury prevention focus on?*

■ **Decreasing the severity of injury**

Secondary prevention is designed to reduce the severity of the injury once the trauma has occurred. This is the most common form of prevention (Box 13.3).

> ▶ **HINT:** An example of secondary prevention is the use of seat belts and air bags. They do not prevent collisions, but if a collision occurs they decrease the severity of the injury.

Box 13.3 Examples of Primary and Secondary Prevention

Primary Prevention	Secondary Prevention
DUI checkpoints	Use of safety belts
Stoplights at dangerous intersections	Air bags
Limited access to weapons	
Rumble strips on side of and center of road	
Bike paths	
Animal barriers along highways	

DUI, driving under the influence.

■ *When one initiates a bundle of care to improve outcomes following a trauma, what level of injury prevention is this?*

■ **Tertiary**

Tertiary prevention is the improvement in outcomes after a trauma has occurred.

> ▶ **HINT:** An example of tertiary prevention is the initiation of a sepsis protocol for early recognition and treatment of sepsis. This lowers the risk of mortality, improving outcomes.

■ *What type of injury-prevention strategy is being used when a bicycle helmet safety talk is being given to young children?*

■ **Education**

Education is one of the most common methods of trauma prevention. Education can be targeted at high-risk populations or general populations.

> ▶ **HINT:** The education method typically relies heavily on behavior modification to prevent trauma.

■ *What type of injury-prevention strategy is being used when a person is ticketed for texting while driving?*

■ **Enforcement**

Enforcement strategies are injury-prevention techniques that can be legally mandated or legislated to protect the people. These involve laws or regulations.

> ▶ **HINT:** Seat belt laws are an example of enforcement.

■ *The placement of air bags in car doors in response to the high morbidity and mortality of lateral impacts is what type of injury-prevention strategy?*

■ **Engineering**

Engineering is an effective way to reduce the degree of injury from a traumatic event. It involves redesigning products and vehicles to improve safety. This involves modification of the environment or of products. In this case, engineering was used to determine how to reduce the impact of energy.

> ▶ **HINT:** The development of air bags for car doors to lower the severity of injury in a lateral impact is an example of using engineering in prevention.

■ *When a person is speeding and is ticketed, what type of injury-prevention strategy is being used?*

■ **Economic**

This uses money as an impetus for behavioral modification. Therefore, economic prevention involves a financial impact, such as paying fines for speeding, to discourage certain behaviors (Box 13.4).

Box 13.4 Examples of the Four Es of Injury-Prevention Strategies

Engineering	Air bags Seat belts Automated collision notification Athletic safety gear
Enforcement	Laws (local)—seat belts, helmets, DUI, no cell phones while driving, no texting while driving Legislation (Federal)—gun safety
Education	School-based injury-prevention programs Multimedia—newspapers, Internet, billboards, commercials Education for health care providers
Economic	Fines Loss of license to drive

DUI, driving under the influence.

■ *Preventive interventions that occur automatically and do not require an action from an individual are an active or passive approach?*

■ **Passive**

Preventive measures are categorized as either passive or active approaches. Passive approaches are interventions that occur automatically without an individual having to do anything. An active approach involves an individual having to make a choice for a particular action for the intervention to be effective (Box 13.5).

> ▶ **HINT:** The most successful intervention for prevention is one that requires a minimal amount of effort. Air bags are an example. They deploy automatically and do not require an effort as compared to putting on a seat belt, which requires effort.

Box 13.5 Examples of Active and Passive Interventions

Active Intervention	Passive Intervention
Seat belt	Air bag
Life vest	Smoke detector
Child car seats	Antilock brakes
Helmet	Guard rail
Safety glasses	Antiscald device

▶ **HINT:** Engineering and environmental strategies to prevent trauma tend to be passive interventions, whereas education usually involves an active intervention.

■ *When developing a countermeasure to prevent an identified risk for injury, what should be determined about the intervention before initiating it?*
■ **Proven effectiveness**

This is based on the concept of evidence-based practice. When developing an intervention in an attempt to prevent an injury, the data on effectiveness of the intervention should be reviewed. A countermeasure should either have already been proven to be successful or have a reasonable potential to be effective at preventing the identified injury.

▶ **HINT:** The countermeasure needs to have acceptable side effects and be cost-effective.

■ *A person drinks at a party and then while driving home becomes involved in a collision. What is identified as the risk factor for this injury?*
■ **Human factor**

The human factor was the person drinking alcohol before driving a motor vehicle. When considering risk factors for an injury, there are several factors to be considered, including the human factor. This is usually the behavior that needs to be modified to prevent an injury (Box 13.6).

Box 13.6 Considerations in Identifying Risk Factors

Human factor contributes to the event or injury
Agent involved in the injury
Environmental factors
Social factors

■ *Which of the following would be considered a priority for developing a countermeasure to prevent the injury: high frequency or low mortality?*
■ **High frequency**

The highest priority for developing injury-prevention programs is for those injuries that have either a high frequency or a high mortality.

▶ **HINT:** A data analysis finds out of the four intersections with stop signs, one has had 10 crashes within a month. That intersection would be the priority for placement of a traffic light, as it has a higher frequency of injury.

Questions

1. Trauma nurses need to be aware that trauma prevention can reduce the risk of trauma-injury events. All of the following are methods that enhance injury-prevention research and health care science research to achieve the common goal of trauma prevention except:

   A. Using animal and cadaver models for testing
   B. Enhancing the national intentional injury surveillance system
   C. Increasing awareness of biological warfare
   D. Developing a national policy addressing prevention of firearm injuries

2. Calculating an annual estimate of costs for fatal and nonfatal injuries is a challenging undertaking. Which of the following is *not* associated with evaluating these annual costs?

   A. Indirect morbidity
   B. Medical care
   C. Indirect mortality
   D. Direct mortality

3. Which of the following is not a component of the four Es for injury-prevention programs?

   A. Elective
   B. Education
   C. Enforcement
   D. Engineering

4. Which is the best example of enforcement of an injury-prevention program?

   A. Mandatory seat belt law
   B. Fines for infractions of laws
   C. Development of air bags
   D. Instruction in high school regarding drunk driving

5. A pediatric patient in the emergency department is suspected of being abused. Notifying child protective services is which type of prevention?

   A. Primary trauma prevention
   B. Secondary trauma prevention
   C. Educational trauma prevention
   D. Engineering trauma prevention

6. The utilization of best practices and guidelines when managing trauma patients in the acute care setting is which of the following type of prevention?

   A. Educational prevention
   B. Secondary prevention
   C. Tertiary prevention
   D. Enforcement prevention

7. Which of the following trauma prevention techniques is the *least* successful technique for preventing trauma?

   A. Engineering
   B. Education
   C. Enforcement
   D. Ergonomics

Prehospital Care

■ *A patient has a fall from second-floor balcony. Which one of the four recommendations for field triage by prehospital personnel would be considered in transporting this patient to a level 1 trauma center?*

■ **Mechanism of injury**

The recommendation for field triage of a trauma patient utilizes a four-step process to evaluate the severity of injury in the field. The four components are physiologic, anatomical, mechanism of injury, and special considerations.

> ▶ **HINT:** In rural areas, it is not always possible to transport trauma patients to level 1 or 2 trauma centers because of the distance, and level 3 or 4 trauma centers must be used until air transport can be arranged.

■ *What is considered a hemodynamic criteria used by emergency medical services (EMS) to triage a trauma patient to a level 1 trauma center?*

■ **Systolic blood pressure (SBP) less than 90 mmHg**

EMS attempts to identify the most seriously injured patient in the field to assure transportation to the most appropriate level of care. An SBP less than 90 mmHg is one criteria used by the prehospital emergency personnel to decide to transport a trauma patient to a specialized trauma center such as a level 1 trauma center. Physiologic criteria have been found to be a good predictor of severity of injury and mortality (Box 14.1).

> ▶ **HINT:** A trauma patient with an SBP less than 90 mmHg with tachycardia has typically lost 30% to 40% of his or her blood volume.

Box 14.1 Examples of Physiologic Criteria

GCS < 13
SBP < 90 mmHg
Respiratory rate > 29 or < 10
Cool, diaphoretic skin

GCS, Glasgow Coma Scale; SBP, systolic blood pressure.

HINT: If the patient is younger than 15 years of age, the EMS is usually directed to transport the patient to a pediatric unit designated as level 1 or 2.

■ *What type of trauma is more likely going to be transported to a level 1 or 2 trauma facility, blunt or penetrating?*

■ **Penetrating**

All penetrating trauma to the head, neck, torso, or proximal extremities should be transported to a level 1 or 2 trauma center, if available. High-impact blunt trauma also requires a higher level of trauma care, but some blunt trauma is considered low impact and less likely to incur injuries (Box 14.2).

▶ **HINT:** Burn patients may require transportation to designated burn centers depending on the degree and location of the burn.

Box 14.2 Examples of Anatomical Criteria

Penetrating injury to head, neck, torso, and proximal extremities
Flail chest
Pelvic fractures
Paralysis
Open or depressed skull fractures
Two or more proximal long bone fractures
Amputation
Crushed or mangled extremity
Severe facial injuries

▶ **HINT:** Some patients with lethal injuries may have normal vital signs, therefore, using physiologic criteria only may result in undertriage.

■ *What type of impact is involved if the patient was an unrestrained passenger in a 45-mile-per-hour motor vehicle collision (MVC)?*

■ **High-energy impact**

A high impact event is described as a patient involved in a rapid acceleration–deceleration event who absorbs large amounts of energy. Determinants of high- versus low-energy impact include direction, velocity of impact, and the use of personal protective devices. Following a high-energy impact, the trauma victim is considered severely injured until proven otherwise.

▶ **HINT:** Use of personal protective devices can lower the energy of the impact by dissipating the energy. The previous scenario involved an unrestrained person, so the impact would be considered one with high energy.

■ *What mechanism of injury in an MVC requires transporting the patient to a level 1 trauma center if available?*

■ **Ejection**

There are certain mechanisms of injury that are associated with greater severity of injuries and require a higher level of care. High-speed MVCs and ejection from the vehicle are two types of mechanisms that indicate the need for a higher level of trauma care (Box 14.3).

▶ **HINT:** The goal of prehospital triage is to get the right patient to the right place in the right amount of time.

Box 14.3 Examples of Mechanism-of-Injury Criteria

Significant intrusion of doors (> 12" occupant side and > 18" any side)
Ejection (complete or incomplete) from the vehicle
Vehicle rollover
Death at the scene
Motor vehicle/pedestrian injuries
High-speed MVC (> 20 mph)
Automobile versus bicycle, especially if victim is thrown or run over
Falls (> 20 ft in adults)
Burns > 10%

MVC, motor vehicle collision.

■ *Following a low-speed MVC, the patient is determined to be on Coumadin for atrial fibrillation. Which is the more appropriate center to transport the patient, level 2 or level 3 trauma center?*

■ **Level 2**

A level 2 trauma center is more equipped to care for a complicated trauma patient. Although this patient was involved in a low-speed MVC, the patient is on Coumadin, an anticoagulant. The anticoagulant places the patient at a higher risk for bleeding and would increase this patient's potential for a greater severity of injury (Box 14.4).

> ▶ **HINT:** The clinical judgment of the EMS personnel on the predicted severity of injury is also considered.

Box 14.4 Examples of Special Considerations

Anticoagulation therapy or bleeding disorders
Elderly (age > 55 years)
Pediatrics (age < 15 years)
Burns
End-stage renal disease needing dialysis
Pregnancy > 20 weeks
Insulin-dependent diabetes
Morbid obesity
Immunosuppression

> ▶ **HINT:** Geriatric patients commonly have occult injuries that are more difficult to recognize and rapid deterioration can occur unexpectedly.

■ *When EMS transports a large number of patients to a level 1 trauma center that could have been easily managed in a level 3 trauma center, what is this called?*

■ **Overtriage**

When looking at the patients transported to trauma centers, their acuity level and appropriateness of the facility are reviewed. Overtriage occurs when a large number of patients who could have been treated in outlying hospitals are transported to a level 1 or 2 trauma center. This causes overcrowding of those centers and can adversely affect the care of those with higher acuity levels. Undertriage occurs when patients who do require a higher level of trauma care are not transported to level 1 or 2 trauma centers.

▶ **HINT:** Of the two, overtriage is preferred. Undertriage of potentially severe trauma patients to facilities unable to provide appropriate interventions can result in greater morbidity and mortality.

■ *What is the goal for transport from the time of arrival on the scene?*
■ **About 10 minutes**

The goal of EMS, from the time of arrival at the scene to initiation of transport, is 10 minutes. This is frequently called "scoop and run" to facilitate getting the patient to definitive care quickly, but some effort toward stabilization is recommended at the scene (following Prehospital Trauma Life Support protocol). Transportation should be to the nearest most appropriate facility. A notification to the receiving hospital of the estimated time of arrival facilitates the care of the trauma patient on arrival at the emergency room (Box 14.5).

▶ **HINT:** Trauma injuries are time sensitive. Trauma has always used the "golden hour" to stress the need for early intervention.

Box 14.5 Interventions at the Scene

Airway control
Oxygen or ventilatory support
Hemorrhage control
Spinal immobilization

▶ **HINT:** Intravenous (IV) catheters may be placed enroute to the trauma facility.

■ *Should a trauma patient always be transported to the nearest hospital for stabilization because of the time factor?*
■ **No**

Trauma centers are designed to recognize, stabilize, and provide definitive care to the trauma patient in the shortest amount of time. Therefore, even if the transport of the trauma patient might take 10 minutes longer for a designated trauma center, the overall time to definitive treatment may still be lower.

▶ **HINT:** Prehospital personnel should match the needs of the injured patients to the closest hospital with the capability to provide definitive care within an appropriate time frame.

■ *What would be the best mode of transportation to a trauma center in an MVC occurring in a rural area with a prolonged extrication?*
■ **Air transport**

In prolonged extrications with serious injuries, especially in a rural area, air transportation should be considered to reduce transport time as well as the ability to administer blood.

▶ **HINT:** Air transport may be limited in bad weather conditions.

■ *EMS arrives at the scene of an MVC involving two vehicles. What important information should the prehospital personnel obtain regarding the collision?*

■ **Speed and details of the collision**

Mechanism of injury can guide the care provided for a trauma patient, both in appropriate diagnostic testing and interventions. Information deemed important about an MVC includes the speed of vehicles at time of impact and the details (front- or rear-end collision, or lateral impact; Box 14.6).

> ▶ **HINT:** Photographs of the involved vehicle at the scene have been found to assist the emergency care providers in the trauma center with understanding the mechanism of injury.

Box 14.6 Pertinent Information EMS Obtain at the Scene

MVC	Falls	Gunshot Wounds	Knife Wounds
Speed of impact	Height of fall	Distance from perpetrator	Type of weapon
Damage to vehicle	Which body part impacted first	Caliber of weapon	Angle of penetration
Type of impact	Surface of impact		
Death within vehicle			
Ejection (complete or partial)			
Rollover			
Restraints or air bag deployed			

EMS, emergency medical services; MVC, motor vehicle collision.

■ *A patient is noted to have a wood sliver impaled in his eye. What would be the best intervention by the EMS in the field?*

■ **Eye shield**

The prehospital care of a patient with an impaled object in the eye is to place an eye shied to protect the eye. The removal of the object should not be attempted in the field.

> ▶ **HINT:** Chemical injuries to the eye require copious irrigation of the eye prehospital.

■ *The EMS arrive at the scene to find a complete amputation of the patient's hand. What would be the best intervention for the amputated part?*

■ **Place on ice**

The ice cools the extremity and allows for a greater time to reimplant it. The limb should not be buried in the ice because of the tissue damage that occurs when frozen and during the defrosting of the limb.

> ▶ **HINT:** Do not clean, scrub, or apply an antiseptic to the wound or amputated extremity part in the prehospital setting.

■ *What type of injury should have limited fluids provided in the prehospital?*
■ **Penetrating injury to torso**

IV fluids should be limited or withheld in the prehospital setting for patients with penetrating trauma to the torso, chest, and abdomen. Administration of IV fluids before definitive treatment of the injuries may increase the blood loss, and the patient may require more blood transfusions. Limiting fluid intake until active bleeding is controlled is recommended. IV fluids in the prehospital setting should be titrated for palpable radial pulse using small boluses of fluid (250 cc). Aggressive rapid fluid resuscitation should not be used in the prehospital setting.

> ▶ **HINT:** This practice of minimal to no fluids before definitive care is sometimes referred to as *permissive hypotension* or *delayed fluid resuscitation.*

Questions

1. Which of the following is defined by the number of affected persons with a particular injury present in a population at a specified time divided by the number of persons in the population at that time?

   A. Incidence of injury
   B. Mechanism of injury
   C. Prevalence of injury
   D. Morbidity following injury

2. Which of the following is the most accurate statement regarding time of emergency response at the scene of trauma of a patient?

   A. Emergency medical services (EMS) should remain at the scene until the trauma patient is stabilized.
   B. Rapid transport to the nearest appropriate trauma center with minimal interventions except basic ABCs (airway, breathing, circulation) being performed in the field.
   C. The trauma patient should be transported to the nearest hospital for stabilization.
   D. All trauma patients should be taken to a level 1 trauma center.

3. A family member wants to follow the ambulance from the scene to the hospital. Which of the following would be the best response by the paramedic?

   A. "Yes, stay right behind us all the way to the hospital."
   B. "The police can provide you a lead through the intersections."
   C. "Please do not try to follow the ambulance. You need to obey all speed limits and traffic lights."
   D. "There is no hurry to get to the hospital since the patient will need to be stabilized in the emergency room first before you can visit."

4. What is the optimal time for emergency medical services (EMS) to remain at the trauma scene before transport?

   A. 30 minutes
   B. 1 hour
   C. 10 minutes
   D. Less than 2 minutes

5. Which of the following is considered the best rapid assessment of the hemodynamics of the trauma patient in the field during primary survey?

   A. Pulse assessment to include slow, fast, or normal
   B. Obtain the actual heart rate
   C. Obtain a blood pressure
   D. Determine a pulse pressure

Patient Safety and Patient Transfers

- *What does EMTALA stand for?*
- **Emergency Medical Treatment and Active Labor Act**

EMTALA is a statute that governs when and how a patient may be refused treatment or transferred from one hospital to another when in an unstable medical condition. This was passed as a part of the Consolidated Omnibus Budget Reconciliation Act (COBRA). The purpose of EMTALA is to assure that patients with an emergency condition are assessed and treated at any hospital providing emergency services without any consideration to the ability to pay.

> ▶ **HINT:** This statute is intended to prevent hospitals from refusing emergency care to patients who are unable to pay for their care.

- *What does EMTALA require the hospital to provide for a patient seeking medical assistance?*
- **Medical screening examination**

Any patient who comes to the emergency room seeking medical assistance must be provided with an appropriate medical screening examination to determine whether the patient is suffering from an emergency medical condition. If he or she is, the hospital is obligated to provide treatment until stable, or provide transfer to another hospital in accordance with the statute.

> ▶ **HINT:** The person doing the medical screening must be a qualified medical person as determined by the hospital's bylaws.

- *When should a hospital inquire about the patient's ability to pay for the emergency room services?*
- **After the screening examination**

The patient should not be asked to pay for, or the hospital should not try to elicit payment for the medical screening covered by the EMTALA. The emergency room staff should be trained to respond to the patient's questions about costs in an effort to make sure the patient realizes the extent to which EMTALA procedures are available without cost.

> ▶ **HINT:** The ability to pay should not interfere with the medical screening of the patient presenting for an emergency condition.

■ *When can a patient be transferred to another facility?*

■ **After being stabilized**

When the patient is stabilized, or the emergency medical condition is resolved, then the patient can be transferred to another facility. A patient can be transferred to another facility before he is stabilized only if the patients meet certain standards and the transfer is appropriate.

▶ **HINT:** A hospital that does not specialize in trauma may transfer a trauma patient to a trauma facility even if the patient is not stabilized.

■ *What is the best description of the patient's condition if no deterioration of the patient's condition is likely to result from the transfer or is likely to occur during the transfer?*

■ **Stabilized**

A stabilized condition allows for the patient to be transferred and is often considered a clinical judgment. The definition frequently used is that no material deterioration in the patient's condition is likely to result from the transfer or to occur during the transfer.

▶ **HINT:** If the trauma patient is in active labor, she is stabilized only after the baby and placenta are delivered.

■ *When would it be appropriate to transfer a trauma patient who is unstable to a level 1 trauma center?*

■ **When the patient requires treatment only the receiving hospital can provide**

If a patient requires a treatment that can only be provided by the receiving trauma center and the medical benefits outweigh the risks, then a transfer would be appropriate even if the patient is deemed unstable. The transferring hospital stabilizes the patient as best as possible within its limits. Transfer of the patient for definitive care in a trauma center should occur as early as possible. If the patient is deemed to need a higher level of trauma care, the transferring hospital should not complete all of the diagnostic studies.

▶ **HINT:** All trauma patients should have a chest x-ray (CXR) before transfer to identify presence of pneumothorax or hemothorax.

■ *What is the priority of care for the referring hospital before transporting a patient to a trauma center?*

■ **Airway management**

The primary role of the referring hospital is to assure that the patient's airway, breathing, and circulation (ABCs) are checked before the transfer. Obtaining and securing the airway is the priority of the transferring hospital. If the patient has a pneumo- or hemothorax, a chest tube should be placed before transfer. Adequate intravenous (IV) fluids should be obtained and fluid resuscitation initiated, including administering blood transfusions if required. Bleeding should be controlled before transfer.

▶ **HINT:** When in doubt, secure the airway before transport. A lower threshold for intubation should be used when transporting a trauma patient from one facility to another.

- **Which hospital is responsible for arranging transportation, the transferring or receiving hospital?**
- **Transferring**

The transferring hospital is responsible for securing the appropriate transportation based on the acuity of the patient. The transferring hospital must assure the transport is with qualified personnel and equipment as required by the patient's circumstances, including appropriate life-support measures during transfer. The transferring hospital is ultimately responsible for decisions made in modes of transfer.

> ▶ **HINT:** A copy of the medical records and a summary of the treatment that was provided to the transferring hospital must accompany the patient to the receiving hospital.

- **A patient in the emergency room following a motor vehicle collision (MVC) is refusing care and wants to leave the hospital without care. What does EMTALA require the hospital to document?**
- **Discussion of risks**

If a patient is refusing treatment or transfer, EMTALA requires certain documentation, which includes that the patient was properly informed of the risks of leaving and the benefits of the treatment or transfer.

> ▶ **HINT:** If an emergency medical condition is recognized by the hospital, it is required to provide transfer to another hospital if unable to provide the care required by the patient's condition.

- **What is the risk or penalty if a hospital is found to have violated EMTALA?**
- **Medicare provider agreement is revoked**

The regulation of the EMTALA statute is enforced on hospitals although individual physicians may be making the decisions in the emergency room. The Medicare provider agreement can be revoked by the Centers for Medicare & Medicaid Services (CMS) as a penalty for violation of the EMTALA statute. Smaller penalties, typically monetary, may also be utilized during violations of the statute.

> ▶ **HINT:** A transfer of the patient from the emergency room to another hospital cannot be based on the patient's inability to pay for services.

- **What is the primary obligation of a burn center or shock trauma center?**
- **Accept the transfer**

Most of the responsibilities for a transfer belong to the transferring hospital, and not the burn centers or shock trauma centers. The primary obligation of these centers is to accept the transfer if it they have the capacity to treat the patient. In most cases, if the receiving hospital's capabilities exceed the transferring hospital's capabilities, the specialized center is obligated to accept the transfer.

> ▶ **HINT:** This obligation may stand even if there is a temporary overcrowding or staff are unavailable.

■ *A patient is brought to the emergency room in a rural hospital without a trauma designation and is noted to have a widened mediastinum on CXR. What would be the most appropriate intervention?*

■ **Transfer to trauma center**

A patient with a widened mediastinum on CXR is likely to have an aortic injury. This would be an indication for a rural hospital to transfer the patient to a designated trauma center after initial stabilization (Box 15.1).

> ▶ **HINT:** Patients with severe injuries or multiple traumatic injuries may require stabilization and transportation to a designated trauma center.

Box 15.1 Examples of Indications for Transfer to Trauma Center

Major vessel injuries (e.g., carotid or vertebral dissection)
Thoracic aortic dissection
Severe traumatic brain injuries
Spinal cord injuries
Severe facial injuries
Pelvic ring disruption (unstable pelvis)
Extremity injury with loss of pulse
Multiple injuries
Severe single-organ injury
Hemodynamic instability
Abdominal trauma patient requiring multiple blood transfusions
Serious eye injury
De-gloving injuries
Bilateral pulmonary contusions

■ *What is an anatomical scoring system that provides an overall score for patients with multiple traumatic injuries?*

■ **Injury Severity Score (ISS)**

The ISS is used to determine the severity of injury in patients with multiple trauma. The ISS can be used to determine the need to transfer to a higher level of trauma care or determine predicted outcomes. The ISS uses six body regions and the Abbreviated Injury Scale (AIS) in each region (Box 15.2).

> ▶ **HINT:** The ISS cannot be calculated in a prehospital setting and is used in the hospital primarily for motor vehicle collisions.

Box 15.2 Six Regions of ISS

Head and neck
Face
Chest
Abdomen
Extremity
External

ISS, Injury Severity Score.

■ *What is the highest score a patient can get on the ISS?*

■ **75**

The scoring system uses a range of 0 to 75. The higher number correlates to a greater severity of injury. This scoring system correlates with mortality, morbidity, length of hospital stay, and other severity scores (Box 15.3).

▶ **HINT:** A patient who scores a 6 on the AIS for a body region (indicates nonsurvivable injury) automatically scores 75 on the ISS.

Box 15.3 Other Trauma Scores

Trauma index
Trauma score or revised trauma score
CRAMS scale
Prehospital index

CRAMS, circulation, respiration, abdomen, motor, speech.

■ *How is a hospital declared a trauma center by the state: designation or verification?*

■ **Designation**

Trauma center designation is a process that is developed at the state or local level. The process and requirements vary from state to state, although the verification is a process performed by the American College of Surgeons (ACS). The ACS verifies the presence of resources outlined by the ACS, including the hospital's commitment, readiness, resources, policies, and performance improvements. This occurs at a national level and is standardized.

▶ **HINT:** The verification by ACS lasts for 3 years, and then the trauma center needs to be reverified.

■ *A trauma center that has 24-hour in-house coverage by general surgeons and prompt availability of specialized services meets which level of trauma designation or verification?*

■ **Level 1**

A level 1 trauma center has the general surgeons in-house 24-hours a day, whereas the level 2 trauma center has 24-hour immediate coverage by general surgeons. The level 1 trauma centers are able to provide trauma care from prevention to rehabilitation.

> ▶ **HINT:** Transferring to level 1 from level 2 trauma centers improves outcomes and lowers mortality.

■ *How many levels of trauma designation or verifications are there?*

■ **Four (ACS verification)**

The trauma center verification by ACS has four levels. Some state-designated systems have five levels. Level 1 is the specialized trauma center, going all the way to level 4 or 5 in which the hospital wants to provide the best trauma care but does not have the capabilities to provide complete trauma care (Box 15.4).

> ▶ **HINT:** Severely injured trauma patients are frequently transported by emergency medical services (EMS) or air transport to a level 1 or 2 trauma center for definitive care.

Box 15.4 Coverage in the Designated or Verified Levels

Level 1	Level 2	Level 3	Level 4
24-hour in-house coverage by general surgeon	24-hour immediate coverage by general surgeon	24-hour immediate coverage by ER physician with prompt availability of general surgeon	Basic ER coverage with ER physician and nurse available on patient's arrival
In-house OR and SICU service	24-hour OR availability desirable	24-hour x-ray, CT scan, and PACU required	24-hour ED and lab; does not need 24-hour emergency medicine
Level 2 requirements plus cardiac and microvascular surgery	Level 3 requirements plus hand, neurosurgery, OB/GYN, ophthalmic, thoracic care	Orthopedics, plastic surgery, radiology, and anesthesia staff available 24 hours	
Teaching center and research	Injury-prevention outreach		

ED, emergency department; ER, emergency room; OB/GYN, obstetrics and gynecology; OR, operation room; PACU, postanesthesia care unit; SICU, surgical intensive care unit.

> ▶ **HINT:** A level 3 hospital may have to provide emergency surgery to stabilize the patient before transfer (e.g., splenic rupture).

Questions

1. Transfer agreements with other facilities outline treatment and transfer protocols that can accurately address and treat special trauma conditions. Which of the following would *not* be an appropriate trauma condition to use for a transfer agreement?

   A. Burns
   B. Amputations
   C. Fractures
   D. Brain injuries

2. A trauma facility receives a burn patient in the emergency department (ED). Upon assessment of the patient, it is noted that this patient would be a candidate for transfer to a burn center. Which of the following criteria supports this assessment as correct?

   A. Partial-thickness burn less than 20% total body surface area (TBSA)
   B. Partial-thickness burns to the thighs
   C. Inhalation injuries
   D. Full-thickness burns on 3% TBSA

3. Which of the following is incorrect regarding the nurse's responsibilities for the trauma patient who is being transferred?

   A. Have the patient's family remain until the patient departs
   B. Call report to the receiving facility
   C. Copy radiographs to go with the patient
   D. Bedside report from transferring facility to receiving facility

4. Which of the following is the most accurate statement regarding discharge planning?

   A. All patients are candidates for rehabilitation following a trauma.
   B. Discharge planning should occur once the patient is stabilized.
   C. Arranging for transportation is the final step in transfer to a rehabilitation center.
   D. Discharge planning should involve both the patient and family and include completion of tests before transfer.

5. Which is considered the most important step in the intrafacility transfer of a trauma patient?

   A. A transport team is important for transferring patients in the facility.
   B. Nurse-to-nurse report is provided.
   C. Sending unit should send extra intravenous fluid.
   D. All tests should be completed before transfer.

6. Which of the following is *not* an example of interfacility transfer?

   A. Hospital to hospital
   B. Hospital to dialysis department
   C. Hospital to rehabilitation
   D. Hospital to long-term care facility

7. A nurse on the trauma floor is providing discharge instructions for a patient being discharged home. The patient primarily speaks Spanish with limited English. Which of the following is the most correct statement regarding the discharge instructions?

   A. Provide the patient with written discharge instructions in Spanish in place of the discharge instructions.
   B. The patient is able to understand some English and should be okay with the instructions.
   C. The nurse can use a family member to assist with the translation.
   D. The nurse should use a hospital-provided translator.

8. Which of the following would *not* be indicated before transfer from the initial hospital to a trauma center?

   A. Chest tube placed for pneumothorax
   B. Intravenous (IV) fluid resuscitation
   C. Intubation to secure an airway
   D. Full set of radiographs

16

Forensic Issues

■ *Following a violent crime, who is a candidate for evidence collection, the victim or the perpetrator?*

■ **Both**

Both the victims and perpetrators of violent crimes or accidental injuries should have evidence collected in the emergency room. It is essential for trauma nurses to have basic skills in the preservation of evidence. During resuscitations or treatment, evidence can be overlooked, lost, or destroyed.

> ▶ **HINT:** Trauma nurses need to be aware of potential cases for the forensic and medical examiner (Box 16.1).

Box 16.1 Examples of Medical Examiner Cases

Domestic violence (child, spouse, partner, elder abuse)
Trauma (nonaccidental or suspicious and accidental injuries)
Motor/vehicle pedestrian Injury
Substance abuse
Attempted suicide or homicide
Environmental hazard incidents (fire, smoke, toxins, chemicals)
Occupational injuries
Victims of terrorism or violent crimes
Illegal abortion practices
Supervised care injuries

■ *What type of trauma should be considered a potential forensic case with the need for evidence collection?*

■ **All trauma**

All trauma cases are potential forensic cases until ruled out. All nonvehicular trauma should be considered abuse until ruled out.

> ▶ **HINT:** For evidence to be used in court, the evidence must be properly collected and preserved (Box 16.2).

Box 16.2 Types of Evidence

Clothing
Hair
Nails
Bullets
Lacerations
Contusions
Any wounds

■ *What belongings can the trauma nurse give to the family following a traumatic death in the emergency room?*

■ **Only valuables**

In any trauma death, whether dead on arrival or death in emergency room or hospital, the patient's belongings, except for valuables, should not be returned to the family in case the death may require the medical examiner (Box 16.3).

▶ **HINT:** The valuables returned should be accurately documented in the medical records.

Box 16.3 Care of Trauma Death

Do not wash body
Do not remove any lines or tubes
All appliances should be left in place
Personal clothing should be carefully packaged and retained with the body
Do not return belongings to the family (except valuables)

■ *Evidence collected from a trauma patient should be placed in what type of bag?*

■ **Paper bag**

Place evidence collected from a trauma patient in a paper bag or an envelope. Always use paper to prevent breakdown of biological evidence (semen, blood, or saliva). If evidence is placed in plastic containers, it may decay or mildew because of moisture inherent in the plastic, so holes would need to be punched in the lid. If an envelope is used, seal the envelope with evidence tape and initial, indicating the date and time on the patient label. Do not use gummed envelopes or staple to seal (Box 16.4).

▶ **HINT:** The hands of a patient with a potential self-inflicted gunshot wound should be covered with paper bags to preserve residue.

Box 16.4 Method for Folding Paper Containing Evidence

Step 1	Place evidence on a white piece of paper while wearing gloves
Step 2	Fold the paper in thirds with evidence in the center
Step 3	Turn paper 90°
Step 4	Fold the paper again into thirds

(continued)

Box 16.4 Method for Folding Paper Containing Evidence (*continued*)

Step 5	Tuck the upper third into the lower third of the second folding
Step 6	Place paper in an envelope
Step 7	Tape the envelope and label

- **When cutting the clothing off of a gunshot or stabbing victim, what does the trauma nurse need to avoid?**
- **Avoid defects in clothing**

When cutting clothes, do not cut through defects in clothing such as bullet holes, tears, or stab entry. Cutting through a tear in the clothing can destroy evidence.

> ▶ **HINT:** Document the description of all defects in the clothing, including defects such as tears, holes, residue, burns, or stains.

- **How can gunpowder around a wound best be preserved?**
- **With tape**

The gunpowder can be preserved from around a wound with tape pressed on the wound then placed on a glass slide. This is then preserved in an envelope in the appropriate manner.

> ▶ **HINT:** If gunpowder is present on a wound, photograph the wound prior to cleansing it.

- **A bullet is found in the clothing of a trauma patient during resuscitation. What is the best method to use to handle the bullet?**
- **Rubber-tipped forceps**

Rubber-tipped forceps are used to handle a bullet in a trauma patient. The use of metal forceps can alter the markings on the outside of the bullet, thereby damaging evidence. The bullet should then be wrapped in gauze and secured in a container.

> ▶ **HINT:** Do not shake clothing after removal from a patient. This can potentially cause loss of evidence.

- **What is the priority when a victim of an intentional trauma is being resuscitated?**
- **The patient**

The collection of evidence should never take priority over lifesaving interventions.

- **What should be placed on the floor when removing the clothing of a victim of an intentional trauma?**
- **Clean, white sheet**

Place a clean, white sheet on the floor, under the gurney or for the patient to stand on while undressing. This sheet will collect any evidence that may be shed from the clothing or victim's body. Once the clothing is removed, place the clothing on the sheet away from traffic. After the crisis, take the clothing from the sheet and place each garment in a paper bag and label appropriately.

> ▶ **HINT:** Never just throw clothes on the emergency room floor because this may lead to gross contamination of critical evidence.

■ *How is evidence collected from under the fingernails?*
■ Scraping

Scraping or swabbing under the fingernails can preserve evidence. The scrapings should be allowed to fall on clean, white paper. Any broken nails should be clipped.

> ▶ **HINT:** Separate evidence and nail clippings by right and left hand.

■ *When handling clothing of a patient that requires forensic management, what should the nurse change frequently?*
■ Gloves

Frequently changing the gloves during the handling of the clothing prevents cross-contamination of the evidence being handled. The trauma nurse should also use powder-free gloves when handling the evidence.

> ▶ **HINT:** Minimizing the handling of the evidence also helps prevent contaminating the evidence.

■ *What should be obtained to document a wound prior to suturing victims of a traumatic crime?*
■ Photographs

Good-quality photos should be taken of the location of injury or traumatic wounds in victims of crime. The photo of the injury should be with and without a scale to judge the size of the wounds. If possible, photograph before suturing or other procedures are performed in the area of injury.

> ▶ **HINT:** Bruises and bite marks may require the use of ultraviolet or infrared photos, if available.

■ *When should body fluids be obtained for forensics on a trauma victim?*
■ As early as possible

The earlier the fluids are drawn or obtained, the greater the forensic value of the fluids. Blood work includes sending one red-, purple-, and gray-topped tube, each for a different lab. Do not use alcohol to prepare a venipuncture site if blood alcohol levels are being obtained. Cleanse with povidone-iodine followed by saline. Place evidence tape across the top of the tubes, label and initial them, then wrap the tubes with protective material and package, label, seal, and store in a secure location.

> ▶ **HINT:** Body fluids that may be obtained include blood, urine, gastric secretion, peritoneal fluid, or spinal fluid.

■ *How should a gunshot wound be described in the medical records?*

■ **Exact description**

All physical findings should be precisely documented using correct terminology. Traumatic wounds, such as gunshot and stab wounds, should be described using exact location, size, and character of the wound. To be most accurate, the use of both narrative descriptions and body diagrams are recommended.

> ▶ **HINT:** Refrain from forensic statements, such as "entry" or "exit" wound, when documenting in the medical record.

■ *What needs to be generated every time evidence changes hands?*

■ **A receipt**

There needs to be a documented trail of who handled the evidence and where the evidence was located. Minimizing the number of people handling the evidence assists with securing the evidence and minimizes tampering or destroying the evidence. Each time the evidence changes hands, a receipt should be generated and signed by both people involved in the transfer of the evidence.

> ▶ **HINT:** Ensure the evidence is well secured to prevent tampering.

Questions

1. The trauma nurse received a patient who sustained a gunshot wound to the head. He is covered in blood and presents to the emergency room dead on arrival. The family comes into the emergency room crying and upset, they think that suicide may be a factor for consideration and they want to see the patient's body. Which of the following is the best response by the nurse?

   A. Tell the family that you are sorry for their loss and that they can go see the patient once he is cleaned up so that they do not see him covered in blood.
   B. Let them see the patient after the nurse removes all of the invasive lines that emergency medical personal placed so that it is not so traumatic for them.
   C. Prepare the family for how the patient looks and allow the family into the room.
   D. Cover the patient with a blanket, comfort the family, and give the clothes to the family in a sealed bag.

2. There was a severe motor vehicle accident and the trauma team is currently treating the driver of one car and the passenger of the car that the driver hit. While assessing the driver, he begins to display belligerent behavior and the nurse notes a strong alcohol smell on his breath. Which of the following actions is the proper way of addressing these findings?

   A. Then nurse gets an order for a toxicology screen on the patient and collects the sample.
   B. The nurse documents the patient's behavior as "agitated" and notes the "smell of alcohol in his breath."
   C. The nurse personally does not feel any sympathy for the patient because this is a clear drinking-and-driving situation; so the nurse tells the patient, "Next time, call a cab."
   D. The nurse reorients the patient to the surroundings and treatment modalities and then tells him that she will provide him with information on an Alcoholics Anonymous program.

3. When collecting biological evidence from a victim of a violent crime, which of the following is *not* collected in the emergency room?

   A. Semen
   B. Saliva
   C. Blood
   D. Nails

4. A patient is brought into the emergency room following an altercation in a bar. The patient was attacked by several men in the parking lot and the police have not been able to locate the men. Which of the following is the *most* accurate statement regarding the emergency care of this patient?

   A. Emergency medical care should not be delayed to collect forensic data.
   B. Evidence must be collected as soon as the patient is in the emergency room.
   C. The patient's clothes are too soiled to be useful as forensic data.
   D. The police need to be present during resuscitation to assure the data is secured.

5. Following a trauma, where would the forensic data/evidence collection occur?

   A. Emergency room only
   B. Prehospital during transport
   C. Emergency room, operating room, and intensive care unit
   D. Only after the patient is stabilized and in intensive care

6. Which of the following procedures to protect forensic evidence is recommended when the patient is noted to have gunshot residue on the hands following a gunshot to the head?

   A. Use paper bags to cover the hands.
   B. Wash the patient's hands before the family is allowed to visit.
   C. Do nothing; patient care comes first.
   D. Wrap hands in plastic bags.

7. A patient who has sustained a gunshot wound to the abdomen is brought in by emergency medical services (EMS). Which of the following is the *best* action by the trauma nurse?

   A. Do not damage the shirt when removing to prevent loss of forensic evidence.
   B. Cut around the bullet hole when cutting the patient's clothes off.
   C. Document the wound as being either an entrance or an exit wound.
   D. Circle the hole on the shirt with a marker.

17

End-of-Life Issues

■ *When a person participates in making arrangements for end-of-life care, this is called?*

■ **Advance planning**

Advance planning refers to a person's preferences regarding care at the end of life. The health care provider should follow this arrangement when the person is unable to make his or her own decisions or to communicate his or her wishes.

> ▶ **HINT:** Living wills and advance directives are the legal documents of advance planning.

■ *What is it called when you identify a person to make your health care decisions at a time when you are unable to make them yourself?*

■ **Durable power of attorney for health care**

Advance directives, determining a durable power of attorney for health care, and living wills are the patient's opportunity to inform health care providers of his or her preferences regarding critical illness and end of life. The Patient Self-Determination Act (PSDA) requires health care providers (primarily hospitals, nursing homes, and home health agencies) to give patients information about their rights to make advance directives under state law (Box 17.1).

> ▶ **HINT:** Living wills may include an individual's desire for analgesia, antibiotics, hydration, feeding, and the use of ventilators or cardiopulmonary resuscitation.

Box 17.1 Advance Directives

| Durable power of attorney for health care | The person authorizes someone to make decisions on his or her behalf when incapacitated. |
| Living wills | Allow one to document his or her wishes concerning medical treatments at the end of life. |

■ *What is the best method for health care providers to share information with family members in an organized fashion?*

■ **Family conferences**

Family conferences allow for a scheduled time, away from the bedside, for health care providers to meet with the family. Family conferences are used to provide information about the patient, discuss the prognosis, and make joint decisions about treatments. Family members should be encouraged to be active participants in the family conference.

▶ **HINT:** Obtaining a consensus among health care providers is recommended before presenting treatment options and goals.

■ *What is the frequent role of the nurse in the family conference and after family meetings with the physician?*
■ **Translator**

The nurse frequently assumes the role of the translator of medical jargon. Medical terminology is a language that frequently requires interpretation by nurses. Physicians may be in a hurry when speaking with patients and family, and are not always sensitive to the fact that the family may not understand the terminology. Explaining the information to the family in a different way can facilitate the communication.

▶ **HINT:** Nurses are advocates when taking on the role of communicator and medical translator.

■ *What is the best practice for visitation of family with loved ones at the end of life?*
■ **No restrictions**

Family and patients need the time at the end of life to be together without restrictions. The ability to see, touch, and talk with the patient is reassuring to both the patient and the family members at the end of life. Not allowing the family to be there and say their good-byes can complicate the grieving process.

▶ **HINT:** Patients do not usually want to experience the process of dying alone and benefit from the presence of others.

■ *What does "DNR" stand for?*
■ **Do not resuscitate**

A DNR order can vary in the content of the order, including requesting no resuscitative efforts to limited efforts (medications or defibrillation only) if cardiac arrest occurs. A "do not resuscitate" does not mean "do not treat." The degree and amount of interventions initiated to "save" the patient should be determined separately from the decision to enact a DNR, which involves the decision of what to do if cardiac or respiratory arrest occurs.

▶ **HINT:** Another phrase being used to replace *DNR* is *allow a natural death.*

■ *When discussing withdrawal of specific life-supporting therapies, what is the assurance the family needs to have from the health care providers?*
■ **Continued care**

It is essential when working with patients and families that they understand withdrawal of specific life supports does not mean withdrawal of care. Palliative measures continue to be performed and interventions to provide comfort and relief of pain continue to be important in the care.

▶ **HINT:** Patients and family should be treated with compassion and dignity during these times of decision.

■ *After a decision is made to withhold or withdraw life-sustaining therapies, what type of care is provided for the patient?*

■ **Comfort care**

After the decision has been made to decrease the intensity of interventions, to withhold or withdraw life-sustaining therapies, and a DNR order is written, the focus shifts from saving the patient's life to providing comfort care to the patient. Comfort care may involve discontinuing any invasive diagnostic tests or therapeutic interventions, which do not contribute to comfort.

> ▶ **HINT:** Providing comfort care focuses heavily on relieving any pain or discomfort the patient may be experiencing with the use of analgesics, sedatives, and alternative methods (Box 17.2).

Box 17.2 Discomfort at End of Life

Pain
Breathing problems
Skin irritations
Digestive problems
Temperature sensitivities
Fatigue

■ *What is the primary goal of hospice or palliative care?*

■ **Relief of suffering**

The primary goal of hospice and palliative care is to improve the quality of life, for patients and family, through the relief of suffering during the end of life, and into the bereavement period for the family. Hospice care begins when decisions are made to move away from curative medical care to supportive care and a peaceful death, although palliative care can be initiated at the same time as curative interventions are being performed.

> ▶ **HINT:** Hospice is not the end of hope, but is a change in goals to maximize quality of life.

■ *Honoring a patient's refusal of treatment uses which ethical principle?*

■ **Autonomy**

Autonomy is the patient's ability to make his or her own decisions regarding treatments, and is legally and ethically required.

> ▶ **HINT:** In some situations, a patient may need to be evaluated to determine whether he or she is able to make his or her own decisions.

■ *A patient at the end of life begins to make "gurgling" sounds or breathe noisily. What would be the best intervention to provide comfort to the patient?*

■ **Provide analgesia**

Very near death, patients frequently develop noisy breathing and this is often called a *death rattle.* This gurgling sound or noisy breathing is a result of fluids collecting in the throat and by the throat muscles relaxing. Suctioning would increase discomfort and administering a diuretic is ineffective. Providing analgesia is the best intervention to provide comfort at end of life.

> ▶ **HINT:** Administration of oxygen does not necessarily improve dyspnea at end of life, may prolong life, and can actually increase discomfort.

■ *A patient at the end of life expresses behaviors of not wanting to eat. What would be the best response of the nurse?*

■ **Do not force eating**

Nausea, vomiting, constipation, and loss of appetite are common at the end of life. Encouraging eating by offering favorite foods in small amounts until the point at which the patient refuses to eat is acceptable. Do not force a person to eat. Going without food and/or water is generally not painful and losing one's appetite is a common and normal part of dying (Box 17.3).

> ▶ **HINT:** Preparing the family for a patient's loss of appetite is important for acceptance.

Box 17.3 Interventions to Provide Comfort Measures

Breathing issues	Raise the head of the bed Use a vaporizer Have a fan circulating air in the room
Skin irritation	Gently applying alcohol-free lotion
Face and mouth dryness	Apply lip balm Apply a damp cloth over closed eyes Offer ice chips if the person is conscious Wipe the inside of the mouth with a damp cloth, cotton ball, or a specially treated swab
Digestive problems	Limit intake Provide anticholinergics Provide antiemetics Agents to decrease oral secretions
Pain	Use the WHO ladder for pain management Administer scheduled pain medications Administer long-acting or slow-release opioids with short time to action for breakthrough pain

WHO, World Health Organization.

■ *If symptoms of pain and discomfort are intractable at the end of life and cannot be relieved despite appropriate interventions, what should be considered?*

■ **Terminal sedation**

Terminal sedation is used at the end of life when the patient is experiencing unbearable and unmanageable pain. The goal of end-of-life sedation is to obtund pain sufficient to relieve suffering, but not to hasten death.

> ▶ **HINT:** Multidisciplinary care (palliative care, psychosocial support, spiritual counseling) is to be tried first before terminal sedation.

■ **What is the ethical principle that is commonly applied to the administration of opioids at the end of life even if the known risk of the opioids is respiratory depression?**

■ **Principle of double effect**

The principle of double effect distinguishes between consequences of intent and consequences that are unintended but foreseen. This principle is commonly applied to the administration of opioids at the end of life. The intent in administering opioids to a dying patient is to relieve pain and suffering, but opioids can depress breathing. The intent is pain management, but the unintended and foreseen effect is respiratory depression.

▶ **HINT:** If the intent is for pain relief but respiratory depression occurs, this is both legal and ethical.

■ **What is it called when a nurse knows the proper course of action to take, but family interpersonal constraints make it impossible to do so?**

■ **Moral distress**

Moral distress occurs when the nurse is unable to turn moral choices into moral actions, typically because of constraints from family or physicians. Nurses who identify that invasive procedures are only prolonging the inevitable may experience moral distress when the family continues to insist on all potential interventions.

▶ **HINT:** The American Association of Critical-Care Nurses (AACN) has developed the 4 As of moral distress: ask, affirm, assess, and act.

■ **When a family states that they promise to be more attentive if their loved one survives this injury, what stage of grief are they experiencing?**

■ **Bargaining**

In the bargaining stage, the person is looking for ways to postpone the inevitable death. Most of the time, the bargaining of the family is for a change in a certain lifestyle that will prolong the life of a loved one (Box 17.4).

▶ **HINT:** The grief process is very individualized. Not all people go through all of the stages of grief.

Box 17.4 Stages of Grief

Denial
Anger
Bargaining
Depression
Acceptance

Questions

1. Mr. Jones is being treated after a motor vehicle/pedestrian trauma. The patient is lethargic, pale, and has a blood pressure of 90/62 mmHg. Intravenous fluids were initiated and the physician was notified. The patient's daughter provides a do not resuscitate (DNR) form. The patient's hemoglobin comes back and the result is 6.2 mg/dL. What does the nurse do next?

   A. The nurse understands that the patient has DNR status and provides comfort care only.
   B. The nurse notifies the physician of the critical lab result and obtains an order for 2 units of blood to be transfused.
   C. The nurse talks to the patient and tells the patient that he needs a blood transfusion but that she is not going to transfuse him because of the DNR status.
   D. The nurse transfuses 2 units of packed red blood cells, but tells the patient that he will not need any further procedures because of the DNR status.

2. Providing physical comfort measures to the patient at the end of life is an important part of palliative care. Which of the following would not be an appropriate intervention for the patient at the end of life?

   A. Providing supplemental oxygen via nasal cannula
   B. Placing the patient in a lateral position
   C. Applying lip balm to the lips
   D. Leaving the patient uncovered and shivering because the patient is febrile

3. Mr. Kelly is in the intensive care unit, intubated and sedated. During the "sedation vacation," he remains unresponsive. The physician spoke to the family regarding the patient's poor prognosis. The spouse is clearly upset and states, "I wish I could talk to him just one more time, I need to tell him so many things." Which of the following responses would be the most appropriate in this situation?

   A. Encourage the spouse to talk to the patient even though the patient is unresponsive and sedated.
   B. The nurse encourages the spouse to talk to the patient, but informs her that he most likely will not comprehend what she is saying.
   C. "You are right, he won't be able to hear what you are saying. I'm terribly sorry for this poor prognosis."
   D. "It is highly unlikely that he can hear you, he doesn't even follow commands or even react to pain off sedation, there is no evidence to support that he will understand what you are saying to him, but you can try."

4. All of the following individuals can consent to allow organ donation if the wishes of the patient are not known except for the:

   A. Child of the patient younger than 18 years of age
   B. Spouse of the patient
   C. Sibling of the patient
   D. Legal guardian of the patient

5. Which of the following tests is required at the bedside to determine brain death before organ procurement can occur?

   A. Cerebral blood flow scan
   B. Meningeal testing
   C. Apnea test
   D. Babinski reflex

6. Which of the following should be corrected before brain death determination can occur?

   A. Metabolic alkalosis
   B. Tachycardia
   C. Hypothermia
   D. Apnea

7. Which of the following statements is *most* accurate regarding brain death?

   A. Brain-dead patients can continue to exhibit pupillary reaction to light.
   B. Spontaneous motor movement can occur in patients who are brain dead.
   C. The nurse should initiate the conversation of organ procurement with the family.
   D. An EEG can be obtained to determine brain death instead of a bedside evaluation.

8. Which of the following is a common complication of brain-dead patients?

   A. Syndrome of inappropriate antidiuretic hormone (SIADH)
   B. Cerebral salt-wasting syndrome (CSWS)
   C. Diabetes insipidus (DI)
   D. Cushing's syndrome

9. Which of the following would not be indicated in patients at the end of life?

   A. Oxygen therapy
   B. Elevating the head of bed
   C. Intubation
   D. Administering opioids and anxiolytics

Part VI

Professional Issues

Trauma Quality Management

■ *What is a database of information regarding traumatically injured persons and hospitals receiving injured persons called?*

■ **Trauma registry**

A trauma registry is a database in which information regarding the person involved in a traumatic injury and hospitals that care for the trauma patient are collected; the data are used to evaluate and improve the quality of patient management. The trauma registry can also be used to improve trauma prevention, education, research, and outcomes.

> ▶ **HINT:** When participating with a trauma registry, data are submitted regarding all admissions, readmissions, interfacility transfers, and deaths involving trauma.

■ *What are programs in the hospital that monitor services and initiate measurable changes in care to improve outcomes?*

■ **Quality improvement (QI) or performance improvement (PI) programs**

QI programs monitor and detect problems, effectively initiate change in trauma care services, and offer sustainable means to implement improvement initiatives. QI or PI programs focus on creating systems to prevent errors from happening. There is less focus on blame and reactive stances (Box 18.1).

> ▶ **HINT:** PI shifts the focus more on human performance, whereas QI focuses on the interaction of the system and the human component.

Box 18.1 Example of Error Types

Rule-based mistakes	Deviation from accepted guidelines or protocols
Knowledge-based mistakes	Errors made from lack of knowledge by the provider, either from inexperience or a new situation
Errors of execution	Correct decision is made, but the actual execution is incorrect
Diagnostic errors	Incorrect identification of an injury so management is incorrect

■ *When analyzing the trauma program, it is noted that there are delays in obtaining chest radiographs. The trauma coordinator reviewed the times at which x-rays were taken and compared them to the hospital's set goals. What is this is called?*

■ **Gap analysis**

Gap analysis is a part of the assessment process; it is the comparison of the actual outcome to a predetermined or identified goal. Gap analysis is used to determine whether the care provided is what the institute wants to deliver (Box 18.2).

Box 18.2 Process of QI or PI

Consider desired outcomes or performance
Identify gaps between desired and actual performance
Identify root causes
Select interventions to close the gap
Measure changes in performance

PI, performance improvement; QI, quality improvement.

- ■ *Who should be involved in QI for trauma patients?*
- ■ **Multiple disciplines**

Trauma care is multidisciplinary, extending across multiple departments and involving a wide range of hospital staff as well as various physical locations within the hospital. Everyone involved with the trauma patient may be a part of the QI or PI process. There should be a dedicated leader of the QI team who has the authority to recommend and make improvements.

> ▶ HINT: Multiple disciplines are necessary for the achievement of optimal patient outcomes and all should participate in QI.

- ■ *What is essential for a PI to be successful?*
- ■ **Action**

Following analysis, a corrective strategy or action plan is essential to effectively change a suboptimal performance or process. Just analyzing a situation and discussing the issues will not make the change occur; only implementation of an action plan can change the situation.

> ▶ HINT: Program improvement should be continuous. The trauma program should continually perform analyses and institute action plans to improve patient care (Box 18.3).

Box 18.3 Examples of Action Plans

Guidelines, pathways, and protocols	Development of new practices Implementation
Targeted education	In-services Posters Seminars Rounds
Peer review	Morbidity and mortality conference
Action targeted on specific providers	Further education Disciplinary action Restriction of privileges
Enhancement of resources	Additional personnel Communication Facility improvement

■ *What does the term closing the loop mean in QI programs?*

■ **Measuring corrective actions**

The program should measure what is achieved by the corrective strategies to confirm that they have the intended effects. Confirmation of the impact of the action plan is the closure needed to ensure an improvement was made.

> ▶ **HINT:** Documentation of the gap analysis, action plan, and loop closure is the final step in PI.

■ *What is the formal peer-review process for reviewing deaths and complications on a regular basis?*

■ **Mortality and morbidity (M & M) conference**

M & M conferences are held to review all trauma deaths and complications. This is a formal peer-review process that has been used as a foundation for medical quality-improvement programs. These conferences should be seen as not just a discussion of deaths and adverse events, but also as an opportunity to improve (Box 18.4).

> ▶ **HINT:** Deaths are typically determined to be nonpreventable, potentially preventable, and preventable.

Box 18.4 Examples of PI

Morbidity and mortality conferences
Trauma PI committee
Preventable death panel review
Case review
Rounds

PI, performance improvement.

■ *A trauma patient with a face mask for supplemental oxygen is brought into the emergency room with a Glasgow Coma Scale (GCS) of 6. The patient continues to deteriorate and goes into respiratory arrest. The physician is unable to obtain an airway and the patient expires. How would this death be classified?*

■ **Preventable**

A standard of care is to obtain an airway on a patient with a significantly depressed level of consciousness. This patient was admitted with a GCS of 6. An airway was not obtained until after the respiratory arrest.

> ▶ **HINT:** An example of a preventable death is one resulting from airway obstruction or isolated splenic injuries (Box 18.5).

> ▶ **HINT:** Even if a death is considered nonpreventable, the process should still be reviewed for potential improvement.

Box 18.5 Definitions

Preventable death	Injuries considered survivable; typically involves obvious deviation from standards of care
Potentially preventable death	Injuries severe, but survivable; death could potentially have been prevented if certain steps had been taken; some deviations from standards of care
Nonpreventable death	Injuries are not survivable even with optimal management

■ *What are preidentified variables that are routinely tracked to identify whether acceptable standards of care are being met?*

■ **Audit filters**

Audit filters can identify issues that may lead to adverse events, complications, and death. These frequently are used to identify "near misses" even if no complication occurred and the patient had a good outcome (Box 18.6).

▶ **HINT:** The trauma QI committee should review cases found by the audit filters (Boxes 18.7 and 18.8).

Box 18.6 Key Time Variables in Trauma

Estimated time of injury
Time until arrival at the scene by prehospital personnel
Time of arrival at the hospital
Time until transfusion
Time of general surgical evaluation
Time until disposition to operating room, ICU, or floor

ICU, intensive care unit.

Box 18.7 Examples of Prehospital Trauma Audit Filters

Field scene time more than 20 minutes
Missing EMS report or significant information
Appropriateness of triage and facility selection
Airway management

EMS, emergency medical services.

Box 18.8 Examples of Emergency Room Trauma Audit Filters

Abdominal injury with hypotension without laparotomy within 1 hour of arrival
Subdural hematoma without a craniotomy within 4 hours of arrival
Open fracture without debridement within 8 hours of arrival
Absence of hourly vital sign checks or neurological assessment on multisystem trauma patients
GCS less than 12 without a head CT scan within 2 hours
Unplanned return to OR within 48 hours

GCS, Glasgow Coma Scale; OR, operating room.

■ *What is an injury called that is caused by medical management rather than the underlying disease and that prolongs hospitalization, produces a disability at discharge, or both?*

■ **Adverse event**

The terms *complication* and *adverse event* are sometimes used interchangeably, but a complication can occur even without suboptimal care because of an underlying disease. An error can be considered a failure to follow an acceptable standard of care. An error that does not result in a bad outcome is considered a "near miss." A sentinel event is a severe adverse event with bad outcomes that prompts an immediate review and action plan. Complications should be tracked for rates that are considered higher than normal (Box 18.9).

> ▶ **HINT:** An adverse event does result in a complication, but not all complications result from an adverse event. Not all adverse events are sentinel events.

Box 18.9 Potential Complications to Track

Urinary catheter infections
Central-line infections
Wound dehiscence
Aspiration pneumonia
Sepsis
Surgical site infections
Skin breakdown
Compartment syndrome

■ *What is the investigation called when a sentinel event occurs?*

■ **Root cause analysis (RCA)**

When a particularly bad outcome occurs with an adverse event, a separate QI process called an RCA must occur. An RCA is a process used for identifying the etiology of an unanticipated outcome. The individuals involved in the RCA should come from multiple disciplines. RCA is a one-time investigation into the particular event.

> ▶ **HINT:** An RCA is not an ongoing collection and analysis, but rather a one-time event in which a particular case is investigated.

Questions

1. Which of the following is the emphasis of quality management in trauma?
   A. Reviews only the mortality
   B. Involves multidisciplinary teams
   C. Focuses on individual errors
   D. Involves reviewing cases without any corrective action

2. Which of the following is considered the *most* significant barrier to a quality-improvement program?
   A. Identify the problem, but fail to correct it
   B. Difficulty in determining preventable from nonpreventable deaths
   C. Inability to identify the problem
   D. Lack of adherence to protocols

3. Which of the following is the primary goal of morbidity and mortality conferences?
   A. Determine whether the trauma surgeon is meeting acceptable statistics
   B. Identify opportunities for improvement
   C. Identify all of the non-preventable deaths
   D. Track sentinel events

4. Which of the following is considered the step that is used to "close the loop" of a problem identified in the care of patients in the trauma facility?
   A. Identify the problem
   B. Develop reasonable corrective action plans
   C. Implement the plans
   D. Evaluate whether the action had the intended consequences

5. An identified variable that is routinely tracked to identify whether predetermined standards are being met is called:
   A. Scorecards
   B. Outcome scores
   C. Audit filters
   D. Closed loop

Staff Safety and Critical Incident Stress Management

■ *What is the key to preventing violence in a hospital setting?*

■ **Recognizing potential violence**

The key to preventing violence in the hospital setting includes early recognition of potentially violent patients or situations. Other interventions that may reduce the risk of violence include controlling environmental factors that provoke violent behaviors; a show of force; and in some situations, chemical or physical restraints.

> ▶ **HINT:** Situations that may induce patient violence include stress of the unknown regarding a diagnosis and pain (Box 19.1).

Box 19.1 Potential Situations That Trigger Violence in the ER

Small space
Long waiting times
Limited visitation
Patients in pain
ER accessible 24 hours a day
Continuation of trauma

ER, emergency room.

■ *What is the best position the nurse should take when confronting an angry person who may become violent?*

■ **Do not face the person directly**

When interacting with an angry person who is likely to escalate to violence, stand at a slight angle. Never stand directly facing the person and do not turn your back to the person. Stand close enough to have a conversation, but not too close so you remain out of reach.

> ▶ **HINT:** This stance is less provocative and intimidating to the person and provides a narrower target, which reduces exposure.

■ *What is the best response of the nurse when a family member begins to vent about the long wait for admission?*

■ **Allow a degree of venting**

Sometimes venting is a way to express one's frustration and concerns. Allowing some degree of expression of emotion can diffuse the situation. Avoid arguing or defending the actions of the health care providers or yourself. Remain calm and maintain control of your emotions.

> ▶ HINT: Following a degree of venting, calmly and firmly set limitations.

■ *What would be an appropriate response of an emergency room (ER) nurse if a patient in the ER suddenly pulls out a gun?*
■ **Protect yourself**

Apply the concepts of time, distance, and shielding. Avoid exposure to threat, put distance between yourself and the threat, and put protective barriers or equipment between yourself and the threat.

> ▶ HINT: In most situations, it is best not to fight back or attempt to remove the patient's weapon.

■ *What is the risk to ER personnel when caring for patients exposed to chemical or biological agents?*
■ **Secondary contamination**

Secondary contamination to the health care providers can occur with improper or incomplete decontamination of exposed patients, exposure of the toxic substance carried on the person's clothing or hair, and risk of exposure of the exhalation fumes of the chemical toxins in closed spaces. Ensure appropriate procedures are being followed during decontamination to limit the exposure to health care providers.

> ▶ HINT: Health care providers can become contaminated themselves as well as becoming spreaders of disease.

■ *What is the best way for health care providers to protect themselves from exposure to chemical or biological agents during the decontamination process?*
■ **Wearing appropriate personal protective equipment (PPE)**

PPE should be specific to the potential exposure, and appropriate gowning and use of these PPE devices can lower the risk of exposure. Staff training for disasters should include correct donning and removal of PPE following exposure.

> ▶ HINT: Different biologics and chemicals may require different PPE. If the substance is unknown, the staff should wear the maximal protective devices until the substance is determined (Box 19.2).

Box 19.2 Personal Protective Equipment for Unknown Substances

Powered air-purifying respirator
Chemical-resistant protective garment
Head covering
Double-layered protective gloves
Chemical-resistant protective boots

■ *Who has the priority for prophylactic antibiotics or chemical antidotes during mass exposures or contaminations?*

■ **First responders and health care providers**

First responders and health care providers place themselves at high risk when responding or treating patients who have been exposed to infectious disease, chemicals, or biological warfare. Health care providers should be trained to protect themselves from exposure, and should be the highest priority for receiving prophylactic antibiotics or chemical antidotes, if available.

> ▶ **HINT:** Safety for self should always be the highest priority for health care providers.

■ *What is a physical or psychological event or a threat to the well-being and safety of an individual or community called?*

■ **Critical incident**

A critical incident can be any event (e.g., shootings, deaths, or natural disasters) that causes a distressing or emotional response to a physical or psychological event. This response can cause the person to be unable to function during or after the event. It overwhelms his or her usual coping mechanism. The critical incident can cause a profound change in the person's psychological functioning.

> ▶ **HINT:** Those affected may include any emergency or public safety personnel (responders) involved in the traumatic event.

■ *When a person experiences a significant traumatic event or disaster, what is the most common initial reaction?*

■ **Shock**

Shock and denial are the two most common initial reactions when someone experiences a significant traumatic event or disaster. This shock phase can last days to weeks, and is characterized by confusion; disorganization; and an inability to perform simple, daily tasks. Denial takes the form of the person refusing to believe the event is happening.

> ▶ **HINT:** Not everyone experiences the shock phase. People trained as first responders frequently skip this phase initially.

■ *Following the initial phase of shock, what is a common emotional response a person may feel?*

■ **Anger**

The phase following the initial shock is commonly called the *impact phase*. It involves strong emotions such as anger, anxiety, crying, and outrage. The experience of helplessness and depression may also follow the shock phase.

> ▶ **HINT:** Self-doubt and self-blame may also contribute to some of the strong emotions experienced following a traumatic event.

■ *Does everyone move through these stages to the recovery phase following a critical event?*

■ **No**

Without proper counseling and being able to work through the traumatic event, people may get stuck in the impact stage. They commonly cycle from depression to anger. These people experience high levels of tension and stress.

> ▶ **HINT:** Posttraumatic stress disorder (PTSD) and drug or alcohol addictions are a complication that can occur without proper recovery.

■ *What is the purpose of a critical incident stress management (CISM)?*

■ **To lower the impact of trauma on the person**

A CISM should be initiated in any situation that could potentially create distress for those involved. The purpose is to mitigate the impact of the trauma on the people involved. It is a structured group that uses story-telling combined with sharing practical information to normalize the group's reaction (Box 19.3).

> ▶ **HINT:** Professionally trained counselors in CISM should lead the intervention of CISM.

Box 19.3 Goals of CISM

Mitigation of the impact of the traumatic event
Facilitation of normal recovery process
Restore adaptive functions in psychologically healthy people
Identify group members who may benefit from additional support

CISM, critical incident stress management.

■ *What is the immediate intervention following a critical or traumatic event called?*

■ **Defusing**

Defusing occurs immediately after the event and is a formal three-step process. This is typically the first intervention that occurs immediately after the event and provides one-to-one support. So soon after a traumatic event, most people are not ready for a debriefing. Defusing can be run by anyone experienced in counseling or support groups. Another name for this intervention is *immediate small-group support (ISGS)*.

> ▶ **HINT:** If defusing cannot occur within 12 hours, then a debriefing should be used instead.

■ *What is the supportive intervention technique that is a formal process initiated after the critical incident?*

■ **Debriefing**

Critical Incident Stress Debriefing (CISD) is the formal 8-step process that is recommended within days to 2 weeks after a critical event. This method becomes less effective the longer the time after the event. This intervention is intended for a small group of people who have encountered the same powerful traumatic event. It is a supportive, crisis-focused discussion of the critical event.

▶ **HINT:** This is not a substitute for psychotherapy for people in need of follow-up counseling and is not a stand-alone intervention.

■ *When should a CISD occur?*
■ **When a group shows signs of distress**

Typically, the CISD is used when the personnel from a particular homogenous group are demonstrating signs of distress caused by strong emotional reactions to the event. It aims at restoring group cohesion and performance.

▶ **HINT:** The distress may impair the ability of the personnel to function.

■ *What is the primary factor that makes up the group involved in the debriefing?*
■ **Homogeneity**

The group should be small enough for participation in discussions and should be homogenous. Group members should have about the same level of exposure to the event. An example is emergency room personnel who witnessed a hostage situation in the emergency department (Box 19.4). Even though other nurses in another area may have experienced fear and psychological trauma, it was at a different level than those in the emergency department.

Box 19.4 Common Situations Requiring Debriefing

Death in the line of duty
Emergency workers or peer suicide
Tragic deaths of children
Disasters (natural and man-made)
Bombings
Terrorist attacks
Shootings

▶ **HINT:** There may be several groups participating in the debriefing following a critical incident. These group members are paired according to their role and level of involvement (Box 19.5).

Box 19.5 Group Requirements

Homogenous mixture
Involvement in the event is complete
Members should have the same level of exposure to the event
All should be psychologically ready
Members should not be overly fatigued or distraught

■ *Is a debriefing designed to involve the cognitive or affective response of the group members?*
■ **Both**

The process of debriefing is designed to take a person from the cognitive aspect to the affective aspect and then back to the cognitive. The participants are encouraged to participate in the group, but participation is voluntary.

▶ **HINT:** Emotional content can occur anywhere within the process.

■ *During a CISD, following the introduction, what is the first phase during the debriefing?*
■ **Facts phase**

The group members are asked to talk very briefly about what happened in the critical event. All are given the opportunity to speak if they wish. This format is used to get the members talking. It is easier to talk about the actual traumatic event then to discuss with others the impact the event had on one's own life.

▶ **HINT:** This is the beginning, but it is not the real focus; it should remain very short.

■ *Which phase is the transition from the cognitive to the affective aspect?*
■ **Thoughts phase**

When the members are asked about their thoughts of the critical event, this moves the participants from the fact phase or cognitive domain into the beginning of the affective domain. The facilitator starts with inquiring about their thoughts, as these are easier to deal with than the deeper pain they may be experiencing.

▶ **HINT:** The questioned asked around the room is: "What was your first thought when you began thinking?"

■ *Which phase is considered to be the most crucial phase in the CISD intervention?*
■ **Reaction phase**

The reaction phase is the most crucial phase because it focuses on the impact of the event on the group members. This change of focus may become difficult for the group members. Different emotions may be exhibited including anger, sadness, fear, or confusion. Members are allowed to talk about the impact until the group no longer brings up new issues or concerns.

▶ **HINT:** The question at this phase is: "What is the very worst thing about this event for you personally?"

■ *What phase begins to move the group back to the cognitive domain?*
■ **Symptoms**

The symptoms phase begins to delve into what symptoms or changes the members have been experiencing since the traumatic event. This opens the way for the leaders to begin to teach.

▶ **HINT:** The question asked at this phase is: "What behavioral, cognitive, or emotional symptoms have you been experiencing since the event?"

■ *Following a mass shooting, the emergency room nurse tells you she has been experiencing excessive fatigue and an inability to sleep. What could these symptoms represent?*

■ **Distress from the critical incident**

Critical incidences produce common symptoms in people involved in a traumatic event (Box 19.6). Symptoms of distress are also commonly experienced by first responders and health care professionals involved in the traumatic event.

▶ **HINT:** Health care providers have been found to be at risk of developing PTSD.

Box 19.6 Symptoms of Critical Incidents

Restlessness
Irritability
Excessive fatigue
Sleep disturbances
Anxiety
Startle reactions
Depression
Moodiness
Muscle tremors
Difficulty concentrating
Nightmares
Vomiting
Diarrhea
Suspicion

■ *What phase of CISD allows the group members to begin to realize their symptoms are normal for the situation they have experienced?*

■ **Teaching phase**

The teaching phase is used to provide explanations for why the members are experiencing certain symptoms of after effects from the traumatic event. It is also a phase used to introduce stress management and interventions that may be used to allow the person to cope with his or her emotions. The final phases include summarizing the discussions and some social interaction to assist in anchoring the group members together (Box 19.7).

▶ **HINT:** Specific topics, which may be pertinent to the members of the group, may also be discussed at this time. If they were involved in a plane crash, for example future travel may be discussed.

Box 19.7 Phases of CISD

Introduction
Facts
Thoughts
Reactions
Symptoms
Teaching
Reentry
Follow-up

CISD, Critical Incident Stress Debriefing.

■ *What is the primary rule when people are sharing their thoughts or feelings about the critical event?*

■ **Do not criticize others**

The sharing of thoughts and feelings about the critical event or disaster should always remain positive and supportive. No one should criticize someone else during this sharing process; group members should use active listening. Everyone's feelings should be shared and accepted. Everyone should also know what is said is absolutely confidential.

> ▶ HINT: Everyone in the group needs to feel he or she can contribute to the group discussion and be accepted.

■ *How does CISM assist with the prevention of PTSD?*

■ **Allows person to work through the crisis**

Not all people who have been through a major trauma develop PTSD. It has been shown that when a person is able to work through the crisis about the event, the incidence of PTSD is significantly lower.

Questions

1. When the trauma nurse meets the family of a patient for the first time, the nurse introduces the health care team and each individual member. The nurse also describes what the patient looks like and the current situation in a calm manner allowing the family to process the information, encouraging them to express their feelings, ask questions, and visit the patient. This nurse is best exemplifying which of the following?

   A. Therapeutic communication
   B. Crisis intervention strategies
   C. Stress intervention strategies
   D. Concepts of psychosocial needs

2. Crisis intervention is frequently part of nursing care for the trauma patient. Denial is an important part of the grieving process. The nurse should handle denial by:

   A. Redirecting this defense
   B. Confronting the feelings
   C. Shying away from being honest
   D. Using reflection to confront thoughts

3. A critical incident stress management (CISM) team functions by providing all of the following except:

   A. Using debriefing techniques
   B. Leading debriefings
   C. Leading defusings
   D. Using critiquing techniques

4. Which of the following is the *best* definition of workplace violence?

   A. Does not include verbal abuse
   B. An act of physical violence only
   C. An act of aggression directed toward persons at work or on duty
   D. An act of theft only

5. When a trauma patient is brought into the emergency room in police custody, which of the following is the best nursing action when caring for the patient?

   A. The patient can be allowed to go to the restroom alone as long as a health care worker remains outside the restroom
   B. For safety purposes, do not allow the patient to be handcuffed or restrained in any manner
   C. Ask the police officers to leave the room during assessment for the patient's privacy
   D. Do not allow the patient to distract the nurse during assessment or while performing interventions

6. Which of the following is the best management of workplace violence?

   A. Crisis management classes for health care providers
   B. Prevention
   C. Perform deescalating techniques when violence occurs
   D. Provide force to restrain the violent patient

7. Which of the following interventions is *not* recommended in a violent patient to de-escalate the situation?
   A. Gently touch the angry patient's arm
   B. Speak in a slow calm voice
   C. Use continuous talking to distract the violent patient
   D. Avoid punitive or judgmental statements

8. Which of the following is *not* an appropriate stabilization technique used by health care personnel?
   A. Chest restraint
   B. Physical restraints
   C. Chemical restraint
   D. Sedation

20

Disaster Management

- *What is a low-probability but high-impact event that causes a large number of people to become ill or injured?*
- **Disaster**

Disasters are low-probability events, but if they do occur can have a high impact on the hospital and the community. These events cause a significant, short-term increase in demand of emergency services.

> ▶ **HINT:** During the time of disaster, hospitals frequently have to initiate a plan to free up resources and physical space.

- *Disasters can be grouped into two main categories: natural and man-made. How would a major train crash be classified?*
- **Man-made**

Man-made disasters include transportation incidents, terrorist bombings, and biological and chemical attacks (Box 20.1). Natural disasters include weather-related events (hurricanes, tornados, and earthquakes) and disease outbreaks (Box 20.2).

Box 20.1 Examples of Man-Made Disasters

Terrorism
Riots
Strikes
Bombs
Hostage situations
Transportation incidents
Structural collapses
Explosions
Fires
Chemical (toxic wastes)
Biological (sanitation)

Box 20.2 Examples of Natural Disasters

Hurricanes
Tornados
Earthquakes
Landslides
Tsunamis
Blizzards
Dust storms
Floods
Volcanic eruptions
Communicable disease epidemics

▶ **HINT:** Chemical emergencies can be unintentional such as a spill, or intentional as in a terrorist attack (Box 20.3).

Box 20.3 Categories of Terrorist Threats

Chemical
Biological
Radiological
Nuclear
Explosive

■ *What do hospitals need to have in place in case of enough warning of an impending disaster?*

■ **Evacuation plan**

All hospitals need to develop an evacuation plan, and staff need to be in service and aware of the plan. If there is a warning of an impending disaster (i.e., hurricane) and the patients would be safer in a different facility, then evacuation needs to occur in an orderly and timely fashion.

▶ **HINT:** If the hospital is able to evacuate the majority of the patients, then fewer patients are in harm's way and fewer casualties occur.

■ *What is a step in preventing a disaster in your hospital?*

■ **Recognize the hazard**

Disasters can happen at any time, and awareness of surroundings and people can assist with identifying potential hazards such as unusual behavior, unexplained liquids or smells, and suspicious packages. Know to whom to report this suspicious activity or behavior within your facility.

▶ **HINT:** An example of an unusual behavior that should be flagged as suspicious and reported is a visitor found in a restricted area.

■ *What is the first step in disaster management when preparing for a disaster?*

■ **Mitigation**

In preparing for disasters, the hospitals, counties, and regions perform a hazards vulnerability analysis. This step involves determining the hazards for which a hospital is at risk so that actions can be taken ahead of time to minimize the risks. This is performed annually. Hospitals need to focus their preparation on the most likely or potentially serious hazard, and it is not recommended that a plan be developed for every potential disaster.

> ▶ **HINT:** When performing the analysis, hospitals need to review both natural disasters (such as hurricanes) and man-made disasters (such as a plane crash).

■ *What stage of disaster management is the hospital performing when in the process of stockpiling enough antibiotics for 5 days?*

■ **Preparation**

Preparation is the stage during which the hospital takes steps to prepare for the disaster (Box 20.4). These steps may include stockpiling certain medications for a defined number of days. This may occur in response to the potential lack of access of critical medications during a disaster. Another example includes developing mutual-aid agreements and contracts with other health care facilities to take patients during the time of a disaster.

> ▶ **HINT:** The development of a disaster plan and education of staff is a part of the preparation for disaster management.

Box 20.4 Common Insufficiencies Found in Disasters

Available beds
Ventilators
Isolation rooms
Medications
Staff

> ▶ **HINT:** Some staff may have a difficult time getting to the hospital because of the actual disaster.

■ *What does the National Incidence Management System (NIMS) establish in the hospitals?*

■ **Incident Command System (ICS)**

The NIMS outlines the ICS, which defines the organizational structure for response. The ICS contains five functional areas: command, operations, planning, finance or administration, and logistics.

> ▶ **HINT:** The hospital ICS may be used in any unusual situation and is not reserved for a disaster only.

- *If a disaster is called and a nurse of the hospital involved is off duty, what is the best action of the nurse?*
- **Do nothing until called**

If a critical incidence command is set up for a hospital emergency or disaster, if more staff are required to handle the disaster, the staff will be notified by a prearranged communication system. It is recommended that the off-duty staff wait for the call and not call in or just show up at the hospital.

> ▶ **HINT:** Some staff may be needed during the incident and immediately following the incident, and call sheets should be developed and maintained before any unseen disaster.

- *The command center structure in the hospital includes a person with the title "public information officer." What role does this person have during a disaster?*
- **Works with the media**

The command infrastructure needs to have a process in place or a person who is in charge of patient care, media, safety, logistics of critical supplies, and staff or family support. These roles and processes should be well defined before the incident.

> ▶ **HINT:** Only the designated person should be talking with the media during a critical incident or a disaster.

- *During a disaster, what is important to maintain with the community?*
- **Communication**

Hospitals may need to work closely with the police and fire departments, power companies, utilities, and water department during the disaster. Communication routes and alternative routes should be established during preparation to prevent a loss in obtaining or providing critical information regarding the disaster. Phone lines and cell towers may be out with a loss of the phones during an emergency. The alternative may be walkie talkies or radio (Box 20.5).

> ▶ **HINT:** Health care providers working in the hospital during the disaster require real-time and up-to-date information about what is happening.

Box 20.5 Issues That Occur With Poor Communication

Patients transported to inappropriate facilities
Hospital becomes overwhelmed with too many patients
Lack of sufficient alert before patients arrive
Inappropriate allocation of resources in the community

■ *During the disaster, a triage unit is set up in front of the hospital. If a patient is considered likely to be salvageable but requires immediate intervention, what color would be assigned to him or her?*

■ **Red**

During triage of patients in mass casualty events, colors are placed on each victim depending on the patient's level of acuity. Red is used for patient injuries that are considered to be life threatening, but salvageable. These patients require immediate intervention for survival and are the priority during mass casualty events (Box 20.6).

▶ **HINT:** Most victims end up in the nearest hospital despite the appropriate capabilities of the hospital. Do not assume the patient was triaged in the field or properly decontaminated.

Box 20.6 Disaster Triage

Black	Deceased or likely to die from injuries despite treatment
Red	Likely salvageable with immediate intervention
Yellow	Requires medical care, but unlikely to die without immediate interventions
Green	Walking wounded, but likely to survive even if medical treatment is not provided

■ *What is the most common route of arrival to hospitals following a mass casualty event?*

■ **Private transportation**

The most common route for patients to arrive at the emergency room following a disaster or mass casualty event is by private transportation. Mass casualty victims arrive by private car, taxis, buses, and police vehicles. If able, victims walk to the nearest emergency room. They are called the *walking wounded*.

▶ **HINT:** The most serious often arrive in the emergency room first followed by the walking wounded.

■ *When a hospital has reached the maximum number of patients who exceed the hospital's medical infrastructure, what is this is called?*

■ **Surge capacity**

Surge capacity is the ability to manage increased patient care volume that otherwise would severely challenge or exceed the existing medical infrastructure. Surge capacity may involve physical space, medical personnel, necessary equipment, or medications and supplies. Surge capability is the ability to manage patients requiring unusual or very specialized medical evaluation and intervention, often for uncommon medical conditions.

▶ **HINT:** A large number of people may present to the emergency room at the same time following a mass casualty event, causing an initial surge to maximum capacity to handle the wounded.

■ *After the disaster, the recovery stage occurs. What is a primary action required during this phase?*

■ **Evaluation**

During the recovery stage after a disaster, the primary action is to evaluate how the hospital and community are, and what needs to be done now to restore them to their previous status. Interventions include restoring the physical building if damaged during the disaster, replenishing stocks of supplies and medications, assessing bed status, and disposing of garbage and other waste.

▶ **HINT:** Recovery is basically restoring the institute back to its previous status.

■ *What is considered a standard of care that must be maintained even in circumstances of disaster and mass casualties?*

■ **Maintaining airway and breathing**

During periods of uncontrolled, increased volumes of patients that can occur during a disaster or a mass casualty event, certain standards of care may be abandoned, but a few are critical and should be present always. This includes maintaining airway, breathing, and circulation (ABCs), maximizing patient and staff safety, and maintaining or establishing infection-control measures. Elective procedures, routine care, and complete documentation may not always be upheld when responding to a disaster or mass casualty event.

▶ **HINT:** In an emergency, the goal is to save lives. This works on the principle of the greatest good for the greatest number. This is called *sufficiency-of-care mode.*

■ *What is the mechanism that may be used in a disaster to allow students in health care or health care volunteers to work under guidance in the hospital?*

■ **Emergency response competencies**

These are competencies that can be used during a disaster to credential a person to be able to work under guidance during a disaster when more staff is needed to care for the increased volumes of patients. Emergency medical services (EMS) are another good source of nurse and physician extenders. The National Disaster Medical System has teams of volunteers from around the country. Volunteers should not be self-assigned or self-directed, but should be working under direct guidance of employed health care providers.

▶ **HINT:** Delegation of some care may be given to technicians or support staff or involve family of the patients during these times of crisis.

■ *What is a primary method used in an emergency situation to free up beds for victims from the mass casualty?*

■ **Discharge noncritical patients**

Victims of the emergency situation or disaster may be a higher level of acuity than current patients. Depending on the number of victims and resources, hospitals typically expand beyond capacity and require more beds to care for the victims. Discharging patients who are noncritical is an important step in increasing the hospital's capacity to care for the influx of patients.

> ▶ **HINT:** Other options include cancelling elective surgeries, transferring patients to other hospitals that are not a part of the emergency, and using extra space to place more beds.

■ *What does The Joint Commission require hospitals to perform regarding disaster management?*

■ **Disaster drills**

The Joint Commission requires hospitals to have an emergency management plan and to test the plan with practice drills. Disaster drills are needed to evaluate the plan and make appropriate changes, but may not actually address the educational needs of the staff.

> ▶ **HINT:** Education and competency of emergency nurses in a disaster is a recommendation for each hospital.

■ *What do patients suspected of exposure to chemical or biological agents require before entry into the hospital's emergency room?*

■ **Decontamination**

Patients suspected of exposure to chemical or biological agents require decontamination before entry into the hospital. EMS may do field decontamination, but often some of the people exposed walk in to the emergency without field decontamination. If the patients are not decontaminated appropriately and enter the emergency room, it can be shut down for operations.

> ▶ **HINT:** Hospitals must be prepared to lock down to prevent contaminated people from entering the emergency room before decontamination in extreme cases.

Questions

1. A community-based disaster has just occurred. A tornado has caused mass destruction, resulting in 220 people being injured; 50 of these injuries are life threatening, and 100 are casualties. This situation can be best described as:

   A. Multiple patient incident
   B. Multiple casualty incident
   C. Mass casualty incident
   D. Single hospital response team

2. Which of the following are categorized as the most toxic of all chemical agents and have a mechanism of action of inhibiting acetylcholinesterase, spread through inhalation or contact?

   A. Nerve agents
   B. Vesicants
   C. Pulmonary agents
   D. Blood agents

3. A patient was exposed to Tabun, a type of nerve agent, and is now experiencing rhinorrhea, salivation, and seizures. What is the appropriate antidote for this patient?

   A. Dimercaprol
   B. Sodium nitrate
   C. Atropine
   D. There is no antidote

4. Decontamination is a routine necessity for all chemical agent exposures, but it is the only treatment for what two exposure types?

   A. Pulmonary agents and incapacitating agents
   B. Pulmonary agents and riot-control agents
   C. Incapacitating agents and riot-control agents
   D. Riot-control agents and blister agents

5. A patient comes into the emergency room, lethargic and hyperventilating. Emergency medical responders report that there is a probability the patient ingested pesticides. The nurse is attempting to perform a quick neurological examination by asking the patient his name and location, but the patient keeps repeating that he smells almonds. What is the suspected blood agent exposure?

   A. Cyanide
   B. Carbon monoxide
   C. Chlorine
   D. Mustard

6. Emerging pathogens that can be used for mass destruction and have the potential to have a high morbidity and mortality rate in the future are categorized by the Centers for Disease Control and Prevention as:

   A. Category A
   B. Category B
   C. Category C
   D. Category D

7. A patient has arrived in the emergency room with nausea, vomiting, coughing, burning in the throat and eyes, burning pain in the hands with visible lesions, and shortness of breath. This patient has been exposed to a pulmonary agent. Considering the pulmonary agents phosgene and chlorine, what is a feature of phosgene that chlorine does not possess?

   A. The ability to have delayed effects
   B. Pulmonary edema
   C. Burning sensation in the nose
   D. Chest tightness

8. An emergency room has seen five patients in the past week with fevers higher than 101°F, productive cough with associated chest pain, and purulent sputum. These patients all had evidence of bronchopneumonia on chest x-rays. Because of this pattern, the physician follows up with the previously collected sputum samples and reviews the gram-negative rods results. Why are these results so significant?

   A. They present symptom clusters
   B. They are indicative of infectious agent involvement
   C. These symptoms are indicative of the plague
   D. All of the above

9. When treating a patient with smallpox, the nurse should educate the patient about the disease process and transmission to orient the patient to the plan of care and reduce the anxiety of the patient. All of the following are true facts about smallpox except:

   A. Smallpox can be contracted by contact or airborne sources; so the patient will be placed in reverse isolation and all health care providers will be in a gown, gloves, and face mask.
   B. There is no cure for smallpox, but if the smallpox vaccine is administered 2 days after exposure to the virus, the patient will not contract the disease.
   C. The patient will experience small spots on the tongue and mouth, which spread to the face, torso, and the rest of the body.
   D. The rash is erythematous initially, then turns into maculopapular lesions, then progresses into vesicles, and eventually ends up as pustules.

10. A patient with smallpox will experience many progressions during the virus's life cycle. When is the patient no longer contagious?

    A. When the pustules begin to crust over and scab
    B. When the patient becomes afebrile
    C. When all of the scabs have fallen off
    D. Two weeks after the pustules have been scabbed over

11. This is the most lethal substance possible and occurs from improperly preserved food. It presents with descending flaccid paralysis, dilated pupils, dry mouth, and gastrointestinal hypoactivity.

    A. Ricin
    B. *Yersinia pestis*
    C. *Clostridium botulinum*
    D. *Variola*

12. Terrorists use various radiological devices for destruction. This type of explosive device scatters radioactive materials. A "dirty bomb" is an example of this. What is this radiological method of destruction called?

    A. Simple radiological device
    B. Radiological dispersal device
    C. Reactor
    D. Improvised nuclear device

13. A patient has been exposed to ionizing radiation. Within 2 hours of exposure, the patient starts vomiting violently. What is the importance of this sign after radiation exposure?

    A. Survival is probable and decontamination needs to be initiated
    B. Survival is possible and the nurse should assess the patient with a Geiger–Muller survey
    C. Survival is improbable and supportive care should be initiated
    D. Survival is imminent and the nurse should begin removing the patient's clothing

14. Which of the following provides hospitals with a chain of command, organizational charts and checklists, and facilitates communication among other facilities in disaster situations?

    A. Hospital Emergency Incident Command System
    B. Emergency Medical Treatment and Labor Association
    C. Emergency Disaster Command Station
    D. Hospital Emergency Medical Disaster System

15. It is imperative for health care providers to participate in utilizing the proper personal protective equipment (PPE) available. In reference to the levels of PPE, what level of protective gear is utilized for vapors, aerosols, solids, and liquids?

    A. Level A
    B. Level B
    C. Level C
    D. Level D

16. What is the priority of care for large numbers of contaminated people presenting to the emergency room with traumatic wounds?

    A. Obtain an airway and ventilation
    B. Apply pressure bandages on the bleeding extremities
    C. Perform decontamination strategies before care is provided
    D. Obtain two large-bore peripheral intravenous catheters

17. Which of the following *best* describes plans to care for high volumes of patients in an unexpected event?

    A. Crisis planning
    B. Disaster planning
    C. Community planning
    D. Hurricane relief center

18. Which of the following is the *most* accurate statement regarding a mass casualty event?

   A. People injured rapidly seek care at the nearest hospital and may not present to facilities designated for mass casualties.
   B. Identification and tracking of patients should occur after the disaster to prevent delay of care.
   C. The clinics are the typical point of entry following a disaster.
   D. The response of an emergency department during a disaster is the same regardless of the magnitude of the disaster.

19. Which of the following areas within the hospital are critical for clearing beds to allow room for survivors following a mass casualty event?

   A. Emergency department
   B. Medical–surgical floors
   C. Intensive care units
   D. Operating room

20. During disaster triage, a patient is determined to be salvageable but requires immediate intervention to survive. What color tag would be used with this person?

   A. Yellow
   B. Red
   C. Black
   D. Green

Regulations and Standards

- **What does HIPAA stand for?**
- **Health Insurance Portability and Accountability Act**

HIPAA was developed to provide standards to address the privacy of an individual's health information. This protected health information allows people to control who and how their health information is used. A major goal of HIPAA is to ensure that individuals' health information is properly protected, yet still allowing health information to provide and promote high-quality health care and to protect the public's health and well-being. HIPAA ensures patients receive information about the way their health data are used and disclosed.

> ▶ **HINT:** The standard developed by HIPAA is called the Privacy Rule.

- **What does the Privacy Rule call individually identifiable health information?**
- **Protected health information (PHI)**

Individually identifiable health information is information, such as demographics, that can identify the person and his or her health records or health payments. HIPAA defines and limits the situations in which the health information can be used.

> ▶ **HINT:** The key to HIPAA is determining whether the health information can be identified as belonging to a certain individual.

- **Can you use a picture of an x-ray without permission from the individual who was x-rayed in a presentation if there are no individual identifiers on the x-ray?**
- **Yes**

There are no restrictions to the use of health information if it has been de-identified. De-identified health information does not have any identifiers and does not provide a reasonable basis on which to identify an individual.

> ▶ **HINT:** The use of patient cases and x-rays for education does not require permission from the patient if there are no identifiers used during the educational event.

- **When can a hospital provide information about a patient to another person?**
- **When the patient gives permission**

Patients can determine to whom they want to have their individual health information disclosed. This needs to be in writing before the hospital or hospital personnel can disclose the health information to that identified person.

▶ **HINT:** The patient has the right to change or amend the list of people able to access his or her individual health information at any time.

■ *A physician is asked to consult on a trauma patient. Does the patient need to give written permission to the consulting physician to review his or her individual health care information?*

■ **No**

The hospital may disclose individual health care information for treatment activities to any other health care provider. This includes physicians, nurses, therapists, and so on, who are involved in the patient's health care. There are also situations involving the overall public interest in which the individual health information may be shared without permission from the individual (Box 21.1).

▶ **HINT:** This does not allow a health care provider to review a patient's chart if the provider does not have any direct or indirect professional involvement with the patient.

Box 21.1 Routine Disclosures

Treatment by health care providers
Payment activities of insurance companies
Health care operations (e.g., quality management)
Required by law

Public health activities:
   FDA
   CDC

Victims of abuse, neglect, or domestic violence
Health oversight activities: Hospital audits
Judicial and administrative proceedings
Law enforcement purposes

Decedents:
   Medical examiners
   Funeral directors

Cadaveric organ, eye, or tissue donation
Research
Serious threat to health or safety
Essential government functions
Worker's compensation

CDC, Centers for Disease Control and Prevention; FDA, Food and Drug Administration.

▶ **HINT:** Obtaining consent from the patient for health care operations and third-party payers is optional under the HIPAA Privacy Rule.

■ *What is the assurance HIPAA provides patients about their own medical records?*

■ **Access to the records**

A component of HIPAA is the assurance that patients can have access to their own medical records. Patients have the right to review and obtain a copy of their individual medical records.

> ▶ **HINT:** There are exceptions to this; patients are denied access to certain health care information (Box 21.2).

Box 21.2 Exceptions to Right of Access

Psychotherapy notes
Information compiled for legal proceedings
Laboratory results that CLIA prohibits
Information by certain research laboratories

CLIA, Clinical Laboratory Improvement Amendments.

Questions

1. Which of the following *best* represents the law requiring that a person seeking medical care be provided a medical screening by a qualified medical professional?
   A. Health Insurance Portability and Accountability Act (HIPAA)
   B. Consolidated Omnibus Budget Reconciliation Act (COBRA)/Emergency Medical Treatment and Labor Act (EMTALA)
   C. Simple triage and rapid treatment (START) triage
   D. Trauma designation

2. Which of the following is the *most* correct statement regarding the Trauma and Injury and Severity Score (TRISS)?
   A. The lower score predicts greater mortality.
   B. It is used to calculate the probability of survival.
   C. A death of a patient with a higher score requires a quality review.
   D. The score is used to determine the amount of organ injury involved.

3. Which of the following is required by the Consolidated Omnibus Budget Reconciliation Act (COBRA)?
   A. Medical screening examination by initial hospital
   B. Receiving trauma center must accept the patient
   C. Receiving trauma center documentation stating patient has received the risks and benefits of the transfer
   D. Sending hospital must send a nurse with the patient

4. Which of the following would be a violation of the Health Information Portability and Accountability Act (HIPAA)?
   A. Sharing patient information between health care providers
   B. Sharing patient information with the insurance company for reimbursement purposes
   C. A nurse accesses the records of a family member
   D. Access for quality-improvement reasons

5. Which of the following is the most accurate statement regarding the transfer of a trauma patient from a nontrauma hospital to a trauma center?
   A. The transferring hospital should have all radiographic workups completed on the patient before transfer.
   B. The receiving trauma center must have an accepting physician.
   C. The receiving trauma center is responsible for determining the type and level of transportation.
   D. The receiving trauma center is responsible for complications of the patient during the transfer.

Ethical Issues

- ■ *What is the situation called when two or more unattractive courses of action are possible but neither has an overwhelming rational choice?*
- ■ **Ethical dilemma**

Ethical dilemmas exist when two or more unattractive courses of action are possible but neither is the overwhelming rational choice. Equally compelling alternatives and a moral argument can be made for and against each alternative.

> ▶ **HINT:** Ethical dilemmas are increasing in number and intensity in hospitals.

- ■ *What type of crisis does acting against one's consciousness cause?*
- ■ **Moral distress**

To act against one's own conscience causes feelings of shame or guilt, and violates one's sense of wholeness and integrity. Moral distress is caused when the ethically appropriate action is known but cannot be acted upon.

> ▶ **HINT:** Nurses frequently resort to their own personal values and receive guidance from other nursing peers when formulating their ethical beliefs (Box 22.1).

Box 22.1 Development of an Ethical Belief System

Parent's values and influence
Family's values and influence
Religious beliefs
Cultural traditions
Past experiences

- ■ *What is the ethical dilemma of withholding intravenous (IV) fluids from a patient at the end of life called?*
- ■ **Removal of life-sustaining therapies**

End-of-life issues and removal of life-sustaining therapies (nutrition, hydration, and ventilation) frequently can become ethical issues in the hospital (Box 22.2).

> ▶ **HINT:** Frequently, ethical dilemmas are a result of contradictory beliefs, competing duties, conflicting principles, and a lack of clear clinical or legal guidelines.

Box 22.2 Ethical Issues in the Hospital

Futility issues
DNR issues
"Slow codes"
Removal of life-sustaining therapies
Euthanasia
Physician-assisted suicides
Scarce resources
Organ donor/recipients
Protection of children's rights

DNR, do not resuscitate.

■ *What role do emotions play in making ethical decisions?*

■ **None**

Many decisions made in the intensive care unit (ICU) have an ethical component. Decisions need to be made based on a learned skill, not just an emotional response. Ethical decision making should use a systematic process and ethical principles provide direction. Without this guidance, decisions are made based on emotions, intuitions, or fixed policies.

> ▶ **HINT:** Everyone is unique and influenced by his or her own personal, cultural, and religious values.

■ *When an ethical dilemma is presented to the ethical committee, what is the first step in the process?*

■ **Data collection**

Data collection includes the gathering of medical facts, including the prognosis, alternatives, and assessment of patient/family knowledge. Social facts are also collected, including the living environment, family and significant others, economic concerns, current or previously stated wishes (Box 22.3).

> ▶ **HINT:** The ethical committee uses a process similar to the nursing process, which begins with the assessment.

Box 22.3 Steps in Making Ethical Decisions

Data collection	The gathering of medical facts, including the prognosis, alternatives, and assessment of patient/family knowledge; social facts are also collected, including the living environment, family and significant others, economic concerns, current or previously stated wishes

(continued)

Box 22.3 Steps in Making Ethical Decisions *(continued)*

Identify the conflict	Look at the values and determine where they conflict or agree, determine who is involved in the conflict; state the ethical position of the families, patients, and health care providers
Define the goals of therapy	Is the goal prolongation of life, relief of pain, or maximum recovery?
Identify the ethical principles	List the ethical principles that may be used in the situation and rank them to identify the primary principle; principles may conflict
Review alternative courses of action	Compare the alternatives to the goals; predict possible consequences of the alternatives and prioritize acceptable alternatives
Choose the course of action	This is the action that confronts the fewest ethical principles
Develop and implement plan of action	Requires the input of the health care providers and decision makers
Evaluate the plan	After the action is implemented, evaluate whether the plan effectively met the ethical principles and initial goals

■ *What is the ethical principle that is based on the greatest good for the greatest number of people called?*

■ **Utilitarianism**

Utilitarianism is also called *situation ethics*. This principle defines good as happiness or pleasure. It is based on two principles: the greatest good for the greatest number and the end justifies the means. When using this principle, the situation determines whether the act is right or wrong.

▶ **HINT:** Believers in utilitarianism do not believe in absolute rules, but believe that rules can change according to the situation.

■ *What is the ethical principle that is based on moral rules and unchanging principles called?*

■ **Deontology**

Deontology, in its purest form, focuses on the act, rather than the consequences of the act. Morality is defined by the act, not its outcome. The principles are human life has value, one is to always tell the truth, and—above all—do no harm.

▶ **HINT:** The standards used to make ethical decisions do not change no matter the situation, location, time, or people involved.

■ *When a hospital or country is experiencing scarcity of a resource, what ethical principle is used to determine the allocation of the resource?*

■ **Justice**

Justice incorporates ideas of fairness and equality. Most of the decisions on the allocation of scarce resources involve the use of this principle. Although every patient needs to be treated similarly, avoiding discrimination on the basis of age, gender, perceived social worth, financial ability, or cultural/ethnic background.

> ▶ **HINT:** The determination of which person on an organ transplant list will receive a donor organ is based on the principle of justice.

■ *Which ethical principle is commonly utilized when justifying the removal of life support on a patient in the intensive care unit (ICU)?*

■ **Beneficence**

Beneficence refers to health care's responsibility to benefit the patient, usually through acts of kindness, compassion, and mercy. This principle weighs the balance between benefit and harm and asks which action maximizes the benefit and minimizes the harm. The principle of beneficence is used to analyze futile care and withdrawal of life support.

> ▶ **HINT:** Although the principle of nonmaleficence is "to do no harm," the definition of harm becomes crucial when applying this principle.

■ *Who is the decision maker in the ethical principle of autonomy?*

■ **The patient**

Autonomy is the right of self-government (Box 22.4). This is the freedom to make choices that affect one's life. In the hospital setting, this is the belief that a competent patient has the right to make his or her own decisions about care and should be able to refuse therapy. This justifies our duty to obtain informed consent, to be truthful, and encourages the use of advance directives. Conflict occurs when the decision is in conflict with the health care providers or even family members. *Veracity* is the requirement to provide patients and decision makers with all the information needed to make an autonomous decision.

> ▶ **HINT:** Autonomy is used to justify the use of a family member as a primary decision maker if the patient is unable to make decisions at that time; the right of autonomy is recognized by the legal system.

Box 22.4 Components of Autonomy

The autonomous person is respected
The autonomous person must be able to determine personal goals
The autonomous person has the capacity to decide on a plan of action
The autonomous person has the freedom to act on those choices

■ *What is it called when health care professionals have the duty to benefit the patient, which outweighs the right of personal choice?*

■ **Paternalism**

The principle of paternalism maintains that the benefits provided outweigh the consideration of autonomy, the patient's condition severely limits his or her ability to choose autonomously, and the intended action may be universally justified in similarly relevant circumstances. Physicians may implement this belief by providing only partial information to the patient based on their own beliefs and personal preferences.

> ▶ **HINT:** When parents withhold the care of a child but the physicians believe that the intervention is in the child's best interests, then the hospital may take on the decision making for the child. When this occurs, the decision is based on the ethical principle of paternalism.

■ *At the end of life, terminal sedation is based on which ethical principle?*

■ **Principle of double effect (PDE)**

The principle of double effect states that the act must be morally good or indifferent and the bad effect must not be the means by which one achieves the good effect. The intention must be to achieve the good effect, with the bad effect as an unintended side effect only. The good effect must be at least equal to the bad effect.

> ▶ **HINT:** PDE is used to justify the administration of medication to relieve pain even though this may lead to the unintended, although foreseen, consequence of hastening death by causing respiratory depression.

■ *What is the ethical dilemma in which physicians and their consultants, consistent with the available medical literature, conclude that further treatment cannot, within a reasonable probability, cure, ameliorate, improve, or restore the quality of life that would be satisfactory to the patient?*

■ **Futile care**

In each situation, futile care may be hard to define. The survival rates or mortality rate of a certain disease process or situation is commonly used to assist with the definition of futility of care (Box 22.5).

> ▶ **HINT:** An example of futile care may be an emergency thoracotomy for a blunt chest trauma or an irreversible coma or vegetative state.

Box 22.5 Criteria Used to Assess Futility

Severity of illness
Chronic health conditions
Life expectancy
Quality of life
Expected long-term outcomes
Social support
Duration of therapy
Cost of treatment

■ *What is the document that identifies a person who will have the power to make medical decisions in the event that the patient is unable to do so?*

■ **Durable power of attorney for health care**

A durable power of attorney for health care is a legal document that identifies someone who will have the power to make medical treatment decisions in the event that the patient is unable. This power of attorney is initiated at a time when the patient loses the capacity to participate in the decision-making process (Box 22.6). This is part of one's advance directives, which may also include a living will.

> ▶ **HINT:** A dilemma may appear to exist when a patient has a living will that says he does not want to be intubated, but health care providers have already intubated him.

Box 22.6 Barriers to Initiating Advance Directives

Reluctance to talk about death
Belief that it is not needed at this time of life
Patient is waiting for physician to initiate the conversation
Completing the forms may be difficult
Ignorance of the option
Witness requirements may hinder or may make it more difficult to complete in the hospital setting
Health care professionals may not be knowledgeable about the process

■ *Which ethical principle is used to support physician-assisted suicides?*

■ **Autonomy**

Physician-assisted suicides involve a medical professional providing a patient the means to end his or her own life. The supporting ethical principle for this is autonomy, whereas the conflicting principle for this is nonmaleficence.

> ▶ **HINT:** It is well accepted that a patient may refuse treatment even if the health care professionals believe the treatment is in the patient's best interests. This is withholding treatment and is not considered assisted suicide.

Questions

1. Which of the following is the term used when a person acts against his or her own conscious or moral belief?

   A. Empathy
   B. Moral distress
   C. Beneficence
   D. Moral agent

2. An 84-year-old patient is in the intensive care unit (ICU) on a ventilator following a multisystem trauma. The physician has discussed a do not resuscitate (DNR) order with the family. The wife states the patient would not want to live like this but the son is adamant that everything should be done and would not discuss a DNR. Which of the following would be the *most* appropriate intervention by the nurse?

   A. Tell the wife that the son is right and she should support his decision.
   B. Ask the physician to make the decision for a DNR.
   C. Refer the situation to the ethical committee if it cannot be resolved.
   D. Continue treatment until the family can make a decision.

3. Which of the following ethical principles considers the balance between benefit and harm, in which an action maximizes the benefit and minimizes the harm?

   A. Paternalism
   B. Autonomy
   C. Nonmaleficience
   D. Beneficence

4. Which of the following ethical principles is commonly used for acts of kindness and mercy?

   A. Beneficence
   B. Nonmaleficience
   C. Veracity
   D. Fidelity

5. Which of the following is not an ethical dilemma commonly experienced with trauma patients?

   A. Accepting blood transfusions
   B. Emergency decision making for the patient by health care providers
   C. Futile care
   D. Inability to afford emergency treatment

Part VII

Questions, Answers, and Rationales

TCRN® Practice Test

1. A trauma patient in the intensive care unit is being monitored following repair of the liver. The central venous pressure (CVP) is found to be 2 mmHg. The nurse notifies the physician and anticipates the physician will order:

   A. Levophed
   B. Lasix
   C. Intravenous fluids
   D. Zosyn

2. A pregnant trauma patient comes into the emergency room and is required to be on a backboard until cervical and spinal clearance is obtained, the pregnant patient should be positioned:

   A. 15° to 20° in reverse Trendelenburg position
   B. 15 to 20° to the left side
   C. 10° to 15° to the left side
   D. 10° to 15° in Trendelenburg

3. Mr. Collins was in a motor cycle collision (MVC) and was not wearing a helmet. He arrives in the emergency room with obvious oral and facial injuries. A full trauma workup was completed, including CT scan of the head, spine, chest, abdomen, and pelvis. The patient is complaining of abdominal and back pain. A nasogastric tube is placed and connected to low-wall suction and salmon-colored fluid is noted in the gastric aspirate. Which of the following would be the most accurate statement by the trauma nurse?

   A. This is completely conclusive of a stomach injury
   B. This is indicative of blood from the oral facial trauma
   C. The patient needs immediate surgery for gastric bleeding
   D. This is why the patient is having stomach and back pain

4. A patient comes in to the emergency room with a blunt injury to the chest. The nurse knows that a blunt chest trauma injury is frequently associated with which of the following diaphragmatic injuries?

   A. Left-sided diaphragmatic rupture
   B. Right-sided diaphragmatic rupture
   C. Penetrated diaphragm
   D. Bilateral diaphragmatic rupture

5. A patient came into the emergency room after getting his hand caught in a rolling machine at work. The right hand has suffered a degloving injury. Which of the following best classifies the injury?

    A. Laceration
    B. Avulsion
    C. Contusion
    D. Abrasion

6. A patient was involved in a violent gang attack during which he was stabbed seven times in the abdomen. He is now returning to the emergency room with a possible overdose. What would be the *best* possible explanation of the cause of this patient's current state?

    A. Psychosis
    B. Manic-depressive state
    C. Posttraumatic stress disorder (PTSD)
    D. Addiction

7. A 19-year-old woman was diving into a pool when she hit her head on the bottom of the pool. After radiographic studies were performed, the x-ray revealed a cervical injury from C4 to C7 as a burst pattern of injury. What would be the suspected mechanism of injury for this patient?

    A. Rotational injury
    B. Hyperextension
    C. Hyperflexion
    D. Axial loading

8. A patient comes into the emergency room after an altercation in which he sustained a blow to the face. The patient's profile shows a compressed nose and the frontal view appears to be widened and flattened. What type of injury did this patient most likely sustain?

    A. Nasal fracture
    B. Ethmoid fracture
    C. Telecanthus injury
    D. Nasoorbitalethmoid (NOE) injury

9. A patient presented with a splenic injury and is now complaining of abdominal pain in the left upper quadrant and the pain is referring to the neck. What is this referred pain called?

    A. Positive Saegesser's sign
    B. Positive Kehr's sign
    C. Positive Cervicalgia sign
    D. Positive Kernig's sign

10. The nurse is performing a reflex assessment on a spinal cord–injured patient. A positive bulbocavernosus reflex would be:

    A. An anal contraction in response to squeezing the glans penis or clitoris, or tugging on an indwelling Foley catheter.
    B. Fanning out of toes and big toe dorsiflexion

C. Flexion of the knees when the neck is flexed

D. Plantar movement of the foot when the Achilles tendon is tapped

11. A patient who has been diagnosed with a grade III splenic injury after an automobile accident has started to deteriorate. The patient's blood pressure was 122/78 mmHg and it is now 100/54 mmHg, and the heart rate was 87 beats per minute but is now 105 beats per minute. The nurse notified the physician. What would the nurse expect the physician to order?

A. Embolization

B. CT

C. Laparotomy

D. Splenectomy

12. Which of the following is the 1986 federal law that requires anyone coming into an emergency department to be stabilized and treated, regardless of his or her insurance status or ability to pay?

A. Consolidated Origin of Budget Reconciliation Act

B. Emergency Medical Treatment and Labor Act (EMTALA)

C. Emergency Medical Treatment Act

D. Consolidated Omnibus Budget Reconciliation Act (COBRA)

13. A patient with a traumatic brain injury has come to the emergency department with hemorrhage into the posterior occiput with reports being on Coumadin. The patient is unresponsive, with blood pressure of 90/62 mmHg, heart rate of 112 beats per minute, and a respiratory rate of 12 breaths per minute. What should be the priority goals for adequate care of this patient?

A. Secure an airway, control the bleeding, and administer fluids

B. Secure an airway, blood transfusion, cerebral perfusion

C. Control the bleeding, secure an airway, vasopressor administration

D. Control the bleeding, blood transfusion, vasopressor administration

14. Mr. Francis experienced a crush injury following a motorcycle crash when the motorcycle landed on top of him. He was diagnosed with a colon injury and underwent a colon resection with primary anastomosis and a proximal colostomy. Mr. Francis is concerned with the duration of the colostomy and is worried about the maintenance after going home. The nurse informs the patient that the colostomy will most likely be:

A. Reversed in 6 to 8 weeks after surgery

B. Reversed in 4 to 5 days

C. Become permanent

D. Reversed in 6 to 8 months

15. The nurse is taking care of a newly diagnosed pelvic fracture. There is significant blood loss with the injury. Which of the following pelvic fractures most commonly result in significant blood loss?

A. Anterior fracture

B. Medial fracture

    C. Posterior fracture

    D. Posterior anterior fracture

16. Which of the following statements about burn shock is *most* correct?

    A. Burn shock is defined as hypotension and tachycardia that occurs rapidly after initial burn.

    B. Burn shock causes an increase in capillary permeability resulting in hypovolemia and cellular edema.

    C. Burn shock occurs within 48 hours and resolves spontaneously.

    D. Burn shock results in vasodilation and is the only shock that presents with bradycardia.

17. A patient's neurological assessment reveals bilateral nonreactive pupil dilation, decreased level of consciousness and a Cheyne–Stokes breathing pattern. The nurse is suspecting:

    A. Uncal herniation

    B. Subfalcine herniation

    C. Central herniation

    D. Tonsillar herniation

18. What intervention can be most helpful in preparing trauma staff to manage job-related stress effectively?

    A. Develop a stress support group

    B. Develop a critical incident stress management (CISM) team

    C. Consult a mental health professional

    D. Consult a peer for support

19. What is considered the "gold standard" diagnostic procedure for diagnosing facial fractures/injuries?

    A. Water's view x-rays

    B. Angiography

    C. CT

    D. Contrast studies

20. A nurse is transferring an injured patient to a level I trauma center. Which of the following should be the transferring hospital's responsibility?

    A. Ensure definitive airway control

    B. Perform all diagnostic studies before transfer

    C. Place a central line before transport

    D. Obtain consults of physicians in the patient's care

21. Which of the following is the preferred method for evaluating suspected pancreatic trauma?

    A. Endoscopic retrograde cholangiopancreatography (ERCP)

    B. Abdominal CT

    C. Abdominal ultrasound (US)

    D. Abdominal x-ray

22. A small fracture of the anterior vertebrae usually occurs with hyperflexion and axial compression injuries. This injury can also have associated posterior dislocation. This type of fracture is called:

    A. Simple fracture
    B. Compression fracture
    C. Teardrop fracture
    D. Burst fracture

23. The patient came to the emergency department with a cervical injury. The nurse is assisting by applying a halo vest to stabilize the injury. What is the important task that must be completed with halo utilization?

    A. Ensure the weights are hanging freely at all times
    B. Ensure the wrench is taped to the vest
    C. Cut hair that is around the pin sites
    D. Ensure that the liner is applied before the vest

24. Which of the following intracranial injuries is one of the leading causes of death in people with traumatic brain injury, who typically present to the emergency room as unresponsive or with a low Glasgow Coma Scale?

    A. Diffuse axonal injury
    B. Acquired brain injury
    C. Hypoxic brain injury
    D. Closed head injury

25. Paralysis is a late manifestation of compartment syndrome because it is typically a result of prolonged nerve compression and/or irreversible damage to muscle. Which of the following findings is a late sign in a patient who has compartment syndrome?

    A. Paralysis
    B. Pulselessness
    C. Paresthesia
    D. Pain

26. A patient has an odontoid type II fracture without cord involvement; the health care provider would anticipate treatment involving:

    A. Soft collar application
    B. C4–C5 surgical fusion
    C. Halo immobilization
    D. Traction with weights

27. Which of the following best describes trauma center designations?

    A. Federally mandated criteria for trauma centers
    B. Determined by the state and varying from state to state
    C. Designation is determined by the American College of Surgeons
    D. It is a self-subscribed designation by the hospital

28. A 34-week-pregnant patient comes in with bruising to the abdomen. She reports falling down the stairs this morning. After a complete examination and fetal heart tone

monitoring, no injuries were assessed besides the obvious bruising. Which of the following should the trauma nurse ask the patient about?

A. Current living situation
B. Self-mutilation
C. Safety features at home
D. Domestic violence

29. The nurse is caring for a patient with a compression injury to the thoracic cavity. The patient is intubated and sedated. On assessment, the patient has a heart rate of 119 beats per minute, the oxygen saturation reading is 91%, skin has a pallor, breathing is 18 breaths over the ventilator-setting rate of 12, the peak airway pressures are increasing, and crackles are auscultated throughout both lung fields. What diagnosis is most reflective of this patient's presentation?

A. Hemothorax
B. Myocardial contusion
C. Pulmonary contusion
D. Diaphragmatic injury

30. Which of the following *best* describes a focal brain injury frequently located on the frontal and temporal lobes in which the tissue is damaged and bruised?

A. Concussion
B. Subdural hematoma
C. Cerebral contusion
D. Diffuse axonal injury (DAI)

31. A facial trauma patient comes in with edematous swelling to the nose. Clear fluid is now coming from the nasal passages. The nurse suspects a cerebral spinal fluid (CSF) leak. This is typical of all fractures except:

A. Cribriform fracture
B. Ethmoid bone fracture:
C. Zygomatic fracture
D. Temporal bone fracture

32. A nursing colleague inquires as to why colloid solution, such as albumin, is not used more during aggressive fluid resuscitation in that it expands volume with less fluid. The *best* response would be:

A. Leaking proteins into interstitial spaces during increased capillary membrane permeable state may worsen lung injuries.
B. Leaking glucose into the vascular can cause hyperglycemia.
C. It increases platelet aggregation and results in clotting.
D. Colloids can cause metabolic alkalosis.

33. Stress is a state of mental or emotional strain or tension resulting from adverse or very demanding circumstances. This is the body's natural response to a perceived threat. The response to stress has been described biologically as a general adaptation syndrome that goes through three stages. Which is *not* considered a stage of stress?

A. Alarm reaction
B. Resistance

C. Exhaustion

D. Adaptation

34. Ms. Hall comes into the emergency trauma bay with a gunshot wound to the neck. The patient is short of breath and her oxygen saturation is decreasing from 98% to 92% with a nonrebreather mask. A chest x-ray is obtained immediately after emergently intubating the patient. The chest x-ray demonstrates correct placement of the endotracheal tube but also identifies an abnormality in the right mainstem bronchus. What would be the suspected injury in this patient?

A. Pneumothorax

B. Flail chest

C. Tracheal rupture

D. Tension pneumothorax

35. The nurse is assessing a patient with orbital ecchymosis and edema. The trauma nurse is having the patient follow the nurse's pen as she moves it across the full range of horizontal and vertical eye movements. The patient is having difficulty with extraocular movements. What type of fracture is *most* likely associated with this presentation?

A. Zygomatic fracture

B. Orbital blowout fracture

C. LeFort I fracture

D. Orbital rim fracture

36. A patient has a penetrating injury to the back. Upon assessment, it is discovered that there is a loss of pain and temperature below the level of injury on the contralateral side and a loss of motor function below the level of injury on the ipsilateral side. What type of injury is this patient presenting?

A. Central cord

B. Anterior cord

C. Posterior cord

D. Brown–Sequard syndrome

37. What type of chest injury is caused by lung parenchymal lacerations?

A. Open pneumothorax

B. Pneumothorax

C. Hemothroax

D. Tension pneumothorax

38. For which of the following traumatic eye injuries would the nurse avoid checking the eye motility and applying a pressure eye dressing?

A. Open-globe injury

B. Hyphema

C. Chemical burns to the eye

D. Orbital fracture

39. Which of the following mechanisms of injury would least represent risk of a diffuse axonal injury?

    A. Shaken baby syndrome
    B. Sports-related injuries
    C. Direct blow to the head
    D. Rollover vehicle crash

40. Mr. Minkins is a construction worker who was pouring hot tar and sustained a tar burn to the right hand. Which of the following would be the preferred treatment for a tar burn?

    A. Immerse the area in water
    B. Apply Neosporin cream to the site
    C. Dissolve the tar with neomycin cream
    D. Peel off as much tar as possible and apply antibiotic cream

41. A trauma patient comes into the hospital after a severe automobile collision in which he was ejected and dies after failed efforts of resuscitation. The patient is accompanied by six family members who are very hostile, angry, and upset. Which of the following would be the *most* appropriate approach to delivering the news to the family?

    A. Place the family in a private environment before going in to speak with them.
    B. Get security to accompany the nurse and the team members who are going to meet with the family.
    C. Use words like *expired* or *passed* instead of *died*.
    D. If a family member becomes aggressive have them escorted out of the room.

42. Mr. Fowler, a 22-year-old male trauma patient who had spent 10 days in the intensive care unit, has started becoming irritated with angry outbursts and is having trouble sleeping at night. Which of the following is the probable cause of these new symptoms?

    A. Posttraumatic stress disorder (PTSD)
    B. Bipolar disorder
    C. Delirium
    D. Psychosis

43. Radiographic studies found a bilateral pelvic ring fracture. What would this injury be classified as?

    A. Stable pelvic fracture
    B. Displaced pelvic fracture
    C. Unstable pelvic fracture
    D. Dislocated pelvic fracture

44. Orbital fractures can be associated with ocular injuries. Which of the following is not commonly associated with an orbital fracture?

    A. Vitreous hemorrhage
    B. Hyphema
    C. Optic nerve injury
    D. Opacification of the globe

45. A patient was driving and was struck on the left driver's side. The heart rate at the scene was 99 beats per minute, blood pressure was 140/90 mmHg, and respiratory rate was 24 breaths per minute with an oxygen saturation of 97% on room air. Upon admission to the emergency room, the patient's heart rate is 121 beats per minute, blood pressure is 98/60 mmHg, respiratory rate is 28 breaths per minute with an oxygen saturation of 91%. The patient is complaining of pelvic pain and chest pain. Upon assessment, the nurse notes petechiae to the chest and blood at the urinary meatus. What should the nurse suspect is occurring with the patient?

A. Fat emboli
B. Pulmonary emboli
C. Hypovolemic shock
D. Hemorrhagic shock

46. Documentation of events with trauma patients is crucial. All of the following are examples of improper forensic documentation techniques except:

A. The spouse is at bedside and seems to be feeling very guilty and remorseful by the way she is grieving over the patient.
B. The exit-wound bullet has been recovered and secured in a plastic bag.
C. Sheila Cohen, the patient's spouse, is at bedside and tells the patient that she is so "sorry that things got out of control."
D. None of the above

47. How would the nurse *best* explain the primary difference between occupational therapy (OT) and physical therapy (PT) to the family of a trauma patient?

A. "PT is more important during the rehabilitation process."
B. "OT and PT work as a team to improve the patient's outcomes."
C. "There is no a difference between OT and PT, clinically."
D. "PT primarily works with the legs, such as ambulation, and OT primarily works with arms for activities of daily living."

48. Hazardous materials, radiation contamination, significant hurricanes, major earthquakes, and structural failures all fall into which type of incident category?

A. Institutional-based mass casualty incident
B. Community-based mass casualty incident
C. Rural-based mass casualty incident
D. Institutional-based multiple casualty incident

49. Mr. Ross was diagnosed with of a traumatic aortic aneurysm. The trauma nurse knows that blood pressure management is a major priority in the delivery of care and can adversely affect outcomes for the patient. What would be a therapeutic goal for Mr. Ross's systolic blood pressure (SBP)?

A. Greater than 170 mmHg
B. Less than 130 mmHg
C. Between 150 and 170 mmHg
D. Between 130 and 150 mmHg

50. The nurse receives a trauma patient in the emergency room after a near-drowning incident. Despite all efforts of resuscitation, the medical team has exhausted all measures and the patient expires. The family is asking for all of the patient's belongings. Which of the following would be the most appropriate response by the trauma nurse?

    A. This was clearly an accidental drowning and all of the patient's belongings should be returned to the family.
    B. Do not give the family anything and instruct them that the belongings and valuables need to be kept at this time for evidence purposes.
    C. The nurse instructs the family that they can have the valuable items but all other belongings need to stay with the patient for evidence.
    D. Because the patient has expired, the family can have all of the personal items that were with the patient.

51. The "5 Ps" rule addresses the assessment of both the vascular and nerve supply of the extremity in compartment syndrome. Which of the following is *not* a part of the five Ps?

    A. Paresthesia
    B. Pallor
    C. Position
    D. Pressure

52. The nurse receives a patient with a traumatic amputation. The patient is bleeding profusely. The blood pressure is 100/62 mmHg, heart rate is 110 beats per minute, and breathing is 22 breaths per minute. The health care team's immediate priority would be to stop the bleeding. How would this best be executed?

    A. Place the tourniquet above the site
    B. Clamp the bleeding vessel
    C. Apply a pressure dressing
    D. Local digital nerve block

53. A patient experienced an extreme intravascular volume loss and now requires aggressive fluid resuscitation; what intravenous solution would be the best choice?

    A. Normal saline
    B. 0.45% saline
    C. Ringer's lactate
    D. 0.45% normal saline with dextrose

54. Which of the following scores is *not* used to evaluate the trauma patient for severity and predicted mortality?

    A. Subarachnoid hemorrhage score
    B. Revised trauma score
    C. Apache II score
    D. Emergency trauma score

55. The nurse received a patient post-reimplantation of the thumb. The digit begins to appear blue in color, is cool to the touch, and has brisk capillary refill. The nurse notifies the surgeon. What would the trauma nurse expect the trauma surgeon to order?

    A. Lower the extremity
    B. Leech therapy

C. Betadine scrub

D. Antiplatelet medication

56. Mr. Won has come into the emergency room severely beaten. The patient reports being robbed of his cell phone, thrown on the ground, and kicked multiple times in the abdomen. The primary assessment has been completed. Upon the nurse's abdominal assessment, hypoactive bowel sounds, right upper quadrant pain with rebound tenderness and involuntary guarding have been noted. What type of injury is highly suspected?

A. Splenic injury

B. Large bowel injury

C. Hepatic injury

D. Gastric injury

57. The receiving level 1 trauma center receives a patient from a lower level trauma center. When reviewing the transfer documentation and medical records, it is obvious that the benefits of transferring the patient have been misrepresented. This is a violating which of the following?

A. Certification of Transfer

B. Emergency Medical Treatment and Labor Act (EMTALA)

C. Trauma Transfer Guidelines

D. Consolidated Omnibus Budget Reconciliation Act (COBRA)

58. The once-stable spinal cord–injured patient is now becoming restless, flushed, and hypertensive. The nurse is concerned about autonomic dysreflexia (AD) and starts to assess for causative agents. Which of the following interventions would *not* be appropriate for the initial management of AD?

A. Assess the skin for pressure ulcers and reposition to relieve the pressure on the area

B. Catheterize the patient and send urine off for uranalysis and culture

C. Assess last bowel movement date for possible need for fecal disimpaction

D. Administer labetalol to address the hypertension

59. There are several causes of obstructive shock. Which of the following does not result in obstructive shock?

A. Cardiac tamponade

B. Spinal cord injury

C. Tension pneumothorax

D. Air emboli

60. A common error in the management of hypovolemic shock is failure to recognize it early. The diagnosis should be made by signs of decreased peripheral perfusion rather than reliance on alterations in blood pressure and heart rate. Which of the following is the best explanation for the preceding statement?

A. Elderly patients have less tolerance for hypovolemia

B. Patients taking beta-blockers may not have a tachycardic response to hypovolemia

C. Patients with pacemakers will not become hypotensive

D. Patients taking beta-blockers can be hypotensive without being hypovolemic

61. The goals of resuscitation for a burn patient are to stabilize vital signs, maintain urine output greater than 0.5 to 1 mL/kg/hr, and to have the patient maintain proper mentation. Intravenous fluids used for the fluid resuscitation should be:

    A. Warmed before administration
    B. Colloid solutions (in the initial treatment process)
    C. Administered in a central line
    D. Limited to prevent volume overload

62. A patient came into the emergency room with obvious severe facial trauma from a domestic abuse incident. Which of the following complications would be the highest priority?

    A. Cervical spine injuries
    B. Airway obstruction
    C. Assessing visual injury
    D. Brain injury

63. Mr. Wray is being treated in the emergency room after sustaining a blow to the head from a hammer while at work. He is bleeding from the site, but the amount of blood loss is unknown. His blood pressure is 100/60 mmHg, respiratory rate is 26, heart rate is 116 beats per minute, and his oxygen saturation is 93% on room air. The nurse places the patient on oxygen and administers 2 L of a crystalloid solution to fluid challenge the patient. How does the nurse know that the blood loss was probably less than 20%?

    A. His vital signs stabilize after the bolus but deteriorate when the fluids are stopped.
    B. His vital signs stabilize after administration of the fluids without further deterioration of status.
    C. His vital signs fail to stabilize with the fluid bolus.
    D. His vital signs stabilize after a second fluid challenge.

64. A trauma patient has been on multiple antibiotics during a 2-week hospital stay. The patient has begun to spike fevers again and has periods of diaphoresis and tachycardia. A fungal infection is suspected. Which of the following statements is the most accurate regarding fungal infections?

    A. There are more than 750,000 cases annually.
    B. Bacteremia has a higher mortality rate than fungemia.
    C. Fungal infections are more difficult to treat.
    D. Fungal infections are easier to diagnose than bacterial infections.

65. Which of the following *best* describes the primary goal of rehabilitation following a major trauma?

    A. To regain independence and to meet maximal recovery
    B. To return to the preinjury level of functioning
    C. To return to a productive life
    D. To increase the length of life

66. Which of the following is the *best* diagnostic study when evaluating for the presence of a suspected spinal cord injury without radiological abnormalities (SCIWORA)?

    A. Angiography
    B. Myelography

    C. MRI
    D. CT

67. A trauma patient came into the emergency room after being hit by a car. After receiving 8 units of packed red blood cells, he was transferred to the intensive care unit in stable condition. Two hours later, the patient spikes a fever of 102°F, is coughing and his oxygen saturation is 90% on 5-L via nasal cannula. The nurse calls the respiratory therapist and the intensivist to assess the patient and prepare for intubation. What is the most likely complication?

    A. Hemolytic blood transfusion reaction
    B. Exacerbation of chronic obstructive pulmonary disease (COPD)
    C. Pneumothorax
    D. Transfusion-related acute lung injury (TRALI)

68. Which of the following is *not* a description of a designated level 1 trauma center?

    A. Provides prevention through rehabilitation
    B. Involves research and formal teaching
    C. Comprehensive trauma center capable of providing total care for every aspect of trauma injury
    D. Prompt availability of a trauma surgeon

69. The presence of Grey–Turner's sign would indicate which of the following injuries?

    A. Retroperitoneal bleeding
    B. Esophageal tear
    C. Splenic injury
    D. Liver injury

70. Which statement is most correct with regard to hyperventilation in traumatic brain injury patients?

    A. Hyperventilation lowers intracranial pressure (ICP) and should be used.
    B. It induces hypocapnia leading to vasoconstriction, which will increase cerebral perfusion.
    C. It decreases cerebral blood flow, which results in brain ischemia and should not be used.
    D. Keeping a patient's CO_2 level at less than 35 is optimal.

71. Which area of the face requires assessment of the facial nerve and the parotid ducts if injured?

    A. Cheek
    B. Temporal area
    C. Eyebrow
    D. Forehead

72. A severely injured trauma patient is brought to the emergency room. The medical team cuts the clothing off to work on the patient. Which of the following are true statements regarding the handling of clothing?

    A. When cutting clothing, do not cut through defects on the clothing.
    B. Never shake the clothing and avoid throwing it on the floor for possibility of contamination of evidence.

    C. Place a white sheet on the floor before moving off gurney so that items can be better preserved.

    D. All of the above

73. An 80-year-old female patient missed a step while going down the stairs and dislocated her left knee. The patient is not complaining of pain to the left knee; in fact, she is reporting a decrease in sensation to the area. What injury should the nurse suspect that could explain this presentation?

    A. Peroneal nerve injury

    B. Popliteal vein involvement

    C. Popliteal artery involvement

    D. Avascular necrosis

74. After the nurse used the simple triage and rapid treatment (START) method and assigned a color to the patient, she should:

    A. Explain what the color means to the patient

    B. Group like colors together

    C. Move on to assess another patient

    D. Instruct the patient to go to the receiving area

75. A 32-year-old male was involved in a domestic dispute and received a single stab wound to the right side of his chest with a kitchen knife. On arrival, he has a pulse of 136 beats per minute, a blood pressure of 63/42 mmHg, a respiratory rate of 32 breaths per minute, and an oxygenation saturation level of 90% on a nonrebreather face mask. During intubation, the patient suffers a cardiac arrest with pulseless electrical activity (PEA). Which of the following emergency interventions would the nurse expect the physician to perform?

    A. Emergency thoracotomy

    B. Transfer to the operating room

    C. Chest tube placement

    D. Pericardial window

76. The nurse has a patient in septic shock in the intensive care unit. Vasopressors have been ordered to keep mean arterial pressure (MAP) greater than 65 mmHg for adequate perfusion. The nurse should keep in mind that administering vasopressors can cause further problems such as:

    A. Decreased organ perfusion

    B. Worsening cardiac output

    C. Renal insufficiency

    D. All of the above

77. The Centers for Disease Control and Prevention (CDC) revised the field trauma criteria and provided guidelines for field triage in trauma patients. There are four steps in this process. Which of the following steps are *not* included in these guidelines?

    A. Psychological criteria

    B. Anatomic criteria

    C. Mechanism of injury criteria

    D. Special considerations criteria

78. A patient who was involved in a house fire presents to the emergency room with hoarseness and singed nasal hairs. The patient is placed on a 100% nonrebreather face mask and an arterial blood gas (ABG) has been obtained. When the ABG results are obtained, the carboxyhemoglobin level is 26%. What do the results indicate?

A. Normal carboxyhemoglobin level
B. Elevated carboxyhemoglobin level
C. Toxic carboxyhemoglobin level
D. A lethal level of carboxyhemoglobin

79. A patient was admitted after being hit by a train. The patient has traumatic bilateral amputations and has suffered a large volume of blood loss. The patient is obtunded with a temperature of 96.2°F, oxygen saturation is 90% on a nonrebreather mask, blood pressure is 89/55 mmHg, and heart rate is 55 beats per minute. Which of the following is one component of the triad of complications in trauma?

A. Hyperthermia
B. Metabolic acidosis
C. Decreased hemoglobin level
D. Hypotension

80. Which of the following statements is the *most* accurate to explain the use of hypotensive resuscitation in a trauma patient?

A. Hypotensive resuscitation causes blood clots to dislodge from the site of injury.
B. Hypotensive resuscitation promotes tissue hyperperfusion.
C. Hypotensive resuscitation prevents development of compartment syndrome.
D. Hypotensive resuscitation increases blood viscosity.

81. A 19-year-old patient came in with a traumatic injury playing hockey without protective gear. He is complaining of pain upon inspiration. His chest x-ray reveals a facture to rib 2. What should be suggested as the next diagnostic test for this patient?

A. Chest x-ray
B. Arteriogram
C. Ultrasound of kidneys
D. Ultrasound of the carotids

82. A trauma patient who had an open fracture of the tibia after a motorcycle accident is 4 days postoperative. The patient is now spiking a temperature of 101°F and has a heart rate of 122 beats per minute. Which of the following would be the initial action after identifying these signs of sepsis?

A. Obtain blood cultures
B. Administer an antipyretic
C. Administer antibiotics
D. Obtain a central venous pressure reading

83. What law was passed that required all hospitals receiving Medicare and Medicaid funding to notify the nearest organ procurement organization of death or imminent death?

A. Uniform Anatomical Gift
B. Omnibus Budget Reconciliation Act

C. Routine Referral

D. Organ Donation and Recovery Improvement

84. The Parkland formula uses the formula: 4 mL of crystalloid solution multiplied by the patient's body weight in kilograms multiplied by the percentage of total body surface area burned. A 52-year-old male patient comes into the emergency room after a house fire. He weighs 176 pounds and 27% of his body surface area is burned. Which of the following would be the appropriate resuscitation?

A. 8,640 mL Ringer's lactate

B. 8,640 mL 5% dextrose normal saline

C. 37,840 mL normal saline

D. 37, 840 mL 5% dextrose normal saline

85. Mrs. Jones arrived at the hospital emergency room this morning with a placental abruption following a motor vehicle collision. She has just arrived to the postpartum unit following an emergency cesarean section. Her newborn baby is in the nursery. She is slightly lethargic and resting; her Foley catheter is still in place. The nurse takes the patient's blood pressure; it is 90/64 mmHg, but when the nurse removes the cuff, there is petechia where the cuff was. The nurse then goes to empty the catheter and notes pink-tinged urine. The nurse places a call to the physician and suspects the patient to possibly be experiencing:

A. Disseminated intravascular coagulation (DIC)

B. Hypovolemic shock

C. Antigen–antibody reaction

D. Amniotitis

86. A patient comes into the emergency department after gunshot wounds to the lower left lateral chest. A chest tube has been placed and the patient is transferred to the intensive care unit. While a handoff report is being conducted, the patient's heart rate increases to 134 beats per minute and the patient begins breathing at 43 breaths per minute. The nurse notes that the chest tube drainage system is beginning to rapidly fill with blood. The team begins to prepare for autotransfusion. Which of the following would be a contraindication to autotranfusion?

A. Suspected bowel injury

B. Bright-red chest tube drainage

C. Suspected tracheobronchial injury

D. Chest tube output greater than 500 mL

87. A patient suffers a skull fracture from a hammer injury and is diagnosed with an epidural hematoma (EDH). The family comes in and looks to you for an update on the injury and the status of the patient. You should communicate to the family that:

A. Because the patient is 23 years old, the mortality of the patient is increased and a poor outcome is expected.

B. This type of injury is usually a rapid bleed because it is frequently arterial in nature.

C. Because the patient is talking and conscious right now he should be okay.

D. All EDH injuries require immediate surgery and a neurosurgeon will be speaking with you shortly.

88. Which of the following presents with hypotension and bradycardia?

    A. Neurogenic shock
    B. Spinal shock
    C. Autonomic dysreflexia
    D. Hypovolemic shock

89. A 24-year-old patient was brought into the emergency department with a gunshot wound to the head. A family member was present during all resuscitation efforts. The patient unfortunately expired. Who is the best person to speak with the family about possible organ donation?

    A. The person who reports the death to the family
    B. The attending physician on the case
    C. The organ procurement personnel
    D. The nurse who is comforting the family

90. Following a motor vehicle collision, the patient and spouse come to the emergency room after suffering a brief loss of consciousness post airbag deployment. The CT of the head was unremarkable. The nurse provided discharge instructions to the patient and the patient's spouse. What symptom would *not* be considered a reason to return to the emergency room?

    A. Clear fluid leaking from the nose
    B. Nausea and vomiting
    C. The patient is harder to wake than normal
    D. Persistent headache

91. A trauma patient presents into the emergency room with blunt chest trauma. The patient is hypotensive, tachycardic, and is noted to have elevated jugular distension. Which of the following would the trauma nurse suspect the physician to perform on this patient?

    A. Thoracotomy
    B. Autotransfusion
    C. Pericardiocentesis
    D. Needle thoracentesis

92. A burn victim comes to the emergency department with a severe burn to the right arm after a grease fire from cooking. The burn involves most of the dermis and there are large areas of waxy white injury. What degree of burn does this *best* describe?

    A. Superficial
    B. Superficial partial thickness
    C. Deep partial thickness
    D. Deep full thickness

93. A small amount of blood loss in children can trigger compensatory mechanisms. Evidence of hypovolemic shock presents differently in children versus adults. What is the *best* indicator of shock in a pediatric patient?

    A. Hypotension
    B. Tachycardia

C. Tachypnea
D. Fever

94. After patients experience a major traumatic event, depression can frequently occur. When discussing depression with a patient all of the following should be mentioned to assist in ameliorating its effects except:

A. Allow yourself time to grieve, do not try to rush recovery
B. Volunteer your time or join a charity
C. Even if you do not want to do anything, keep your daily routine
D. Continue to make major life decisions

95. The trauma patient with multisystem injuries is now being managed by palliative care. The nurse is performing comfort measures to the patient at end of life. The patient has nausea and decreased appetite and the family is concerned about the patient's nutritional status. Which of the following is the *least* correct regarding a patient at the end of life?

A. Obtain an order for Zofran for the nausea.
B. Comfort the family by informing them that, at this stage, going without food and water is not painful.
C. Instruct the family to bring in the patient's favorite foods from home so that he can be forced to eat.
D. Comfort and educate the family that losing appetite is a common and normal finding in the dying process.

96. A physiatrist specializes in which of the following fields of trauma?

A. Care of feet
B. Psychology
C. Psychiatry
D. Rehabilitation

97. Using the simple triage and rapid treatment or START triage system, what color should the nurse tag a patient who is unable to follow simple commands?

A. Red
B. Green
C. Black
D. Yellow

98. Which of the following is associated with a high mortality rate in multisystem trauma patients?

A. Pelvic fractures
B. Cranial fractures
C. Hip fractures
D. Extremity fractures

99. Which of the following examination is strongly recommended to evaluate abdominal trauma patients in the emergency department who are hemodynamically unstable?

A. Focused assessment with sonography for trauma (FAST)
B. Computed tomography scan

C. Diagnostic peritoneal lavage (DPL)
D. Intravenous pyelogram (IVP)

100. The trauma nurse has received a patient who is in cardiopulmonary arrest. Cardiopulmonary resuscitation efforts have been exhausted and, unfortunately, the patient is pronounced dead. All of the patient's family live in another state. How should the nurse proceed in informing them of the patient's status?

A. Do not tell them that the patient has died over the telephone
B. Inform the family of the time of death
C. Wait for the physician to call the family
D. Tell the family that there has been a terrible accident and to come to the facility

101. Common organs injured in blunt mechanism abdominal trauma include all of the following except:

A. Spleen
B. Liver
C. Small bowel
D. Large bowel

102. Which of the following levels of trauma prevention actually prevents the traumatic event or injury from occurring?

A. Primary
B. Intermediate
C. Secondary
D. Tertiary

103. An 84-year-old man slipped in the kitchen and fell, hitting his head on the counter. He lay unconscious until found by his spouse. On arrival at the emergency room the spouse approximates that the man was down for about 30 minutes to an hour. The patient has a hip dislocation with decreased peripheral pulses and greater than 3 seconds capillary refill. What plan does the nurse anticipate for this patient?

A. Immediate angiography
B. Immediate reduction
C. Immediate traction
D. Immediate cast application

104. Ms. Swartz had a splenectomy following a motor vehicle collision. The nurse provides the patient with pneumovax before discharge. The patient understands that her immune system's effectiveness will be lowered now that she does not have a spleen, but asks which vaccines are absolutely necessary to have and which are not? Which of the following vaccine is *not* routinely suggested for this patient?

A. Pneumococcal vaccine
B. Influenza vaccine
C. Meningococcal vaccine
D. Polio vaccine

105. A patient is presenting with gross hematuria in the emergency room. An intravenous pyelogram (IVP) is ordered. The nurse prepares the patient for the IVP by informing the patient that:

    A. Contrast dye is injected intravenously and consecutive ultrasound images are obtained
    B. Contrast dye is injected intravenously and consecutive x-rays are obtained
    C. The test views the urethra and the bladder
    D. The test views the urethra and the ureters

106. What diagnostic study is recommended to be used cautiously and only if needed for the pregnant patient?

    A. Cardiotocography
    B. Peritoneal lavage
    C. Focused assessment with sonography for trauma (FAST)
    D. CT of the abdomen and pelvis

107. A traumatic head-injured patient in the intensive care unit deteriorates neurologically. The nurse takes the patient down for imaging and the results demonstrate a significant increase in edema and shift. The health care surrogate receives an update from the neurosurgeon that the patient has a poor prognosis and further treatment modalities are limited. The health care surrogate decides to assign the patient do not resuscitate status and withdraw life-sustaining support. The focus of care shifts to comfort measures. Which of the following would be an inappropriate order?

    A. Discontinue serial labs
    B. Discontinue the MRI of the head
    C. Discontinue the order for morphine sulfate
    D. Discontinue the order for hospice consult

108. Psychosocial needs of trauma patients and their families are commonly centered around three major issues. Which of the following is the *most* commonly identified need of a trauma patient and family soon after the incident?

    A. The need for sleep, trust, and hope
    B. The need for information, trust, and hope
    C. The need for nourishment, spirituality, and information
    D. The need for spirituality, compassion, and independent decision making

109. A trauma patient who was involved in a motor vehicle collision has been in intensive care on a ventilator for 3 days. The patient is exhibiting periods of oxygen desaturation, overbreathing the ventilator, tachycardia, and hypotension. The nurse should have a high suspicion that the patient is experiencing symptoms of:

    A. Pulmonary embolism
    B. Cardiogenic shock
    C. Hypovolemic shock
    D. Acute respiratory distress syndrome (ARDS)

110. Which of the following is the best time to initiate rehabilitation for a trauma patient?

    A. After the patient is hemodynamically stable
    B. When the patient can interact with a physical therapist

    C. Upon admission to the hospital

    D. Upon initiation of discharge planning

111. The circumstances surrounding the death of a child greatly affect how parents grieve. When a traumatic event causes the death of the child, the trauma nurse should:

    A. Ask the parents whether they want to see the body

    B. Allow the parents to stay with the deceased child

    C. Encourage the parents to leave because viewing the body will cause more emotional trauma

    D. Discourage the parents from seeing the body

112. A patient comes into the emergency department with an anterior chest wall stab wound. The patient is grimacing and moaning in pain. The pain is located in the epigastric area and is severe. The patient is short of breath and tachypneic. The nurse should assess the patient for:

    A. Hemothorax

    B. Diaphragm injuries

    C. Flail chest

    D. Pulmonary contusion

113. Which of the following is considered the "gold standard" in diagnosing an aortic injury or transection?

    A. Chest x-ray

    B. CT of the chest

    C. Angiography

    D. Focused assessment with sonography for trauma (FAST)

114. An occurrence causing widespread destruction places great strain on caregivers because it changes the paradigm of care to patients. Disaster relief care focuses on:

    A. Using optimum resources to achieve the best outcome for each patient

    B. Allocating resources to achieve the best outcome for the greatest number of patients

    C. Using optimum resources to achieve the best outcome for the greatest number of patients

    D. Allocating available resources to achieve the best outcome for each patient

115. The nurse is assessing a patient for rehabilitation services. Which assessment is not appropriate for a rehabilitation consult?

    A. Cognitive dysfunction

    B. Respiratory dysfunction

    C. Behavioral dysfunction

    D. Musculoskeletal dysfunction

116. Worldwide disasters happen yearly, but which type of natural disaster is the *most* common and has the greatest effect on public health?

    A. Tornados

    B. Hurricanes

C. Floods

D. Fires

117. What is the most frequent complication in the pregnant patient sustaining a trauma?

A. Abruptio placentae

B. Uterine rupture

C. Fetal demise

D. Premature labor

118. A hot zone should be defined as the area with the highest probability of contamination and in this scenario needs to be confined to the parking area only. There are patients who need to go through decontamination. Where should the decontamination process actually take place?

A. In the hot zone

B. In the warm zone

C. In the parking area only

D. In the emergency department

119. When a patient comes in with a burn of irregular size and depth, it is most effective to use which of the following methods to determine the extent of the burn's surface area?

A. Rule of nines

B. Lund and Browder chart

C. Rule of ones

D. Any of the above

120. Which of the following is *not* a goal of rehabilitation?

A. Compensation

B. Restoration

C. Recovery

D. Adaptation

121. A patient came into the emergency room after a recreational vehicle fire. The patient is obtunded and in respiratory distress with a respiratory rate of 44 breaths per minute and an oxygen saturation of 75% on a nonrebreather face mask. An advanced airway is placed, the patient is being hyper-oxygenated, and intravenous fluid resuscitation is being administered. Which of the following is the most likely cause of the respiratory failure?

A. Asphyxia

B. Hypermetabolism

C. Adult respiratory distress syndrome

D. Carbon monoxide poisoning

122. A patient has signs of sepsis accompanied by a low blood pressure of 90/60 mmHg and an $ScVO_2$ reading of 65% after fluid resuscitation and initiation of a vasopressor. Which of the following would the patient most likely be experiencing at this time?

A. Severe sepsis

B. Septic shock

C. Sepsis

D. Multiple organ dysfunction

123. A burn patient has arrived at the emergency department. After primary assessment, it is determined that the patient has third-degree burns over 45% body surface area and needs to be transferred to a specialized burn unit to receive adequate care. The patient has a heart rate of 110 beats per minute, a blood pressure of 98/64 mmHg, and an oxygen saturation of 94% on a nonrebreather mask. What should the nurse do in this situation?

    A. Place a hold on the transfer until the patient is hemodynamically stable

    B. Prepare to intubate the patient to secure the airway to keep the patient at the current facility

    C. Administer intravenous fluid resuscitation as ordered and prepare for transfer

    D. Call the receiving facility for direction on wound care

124. A patient presents to the emergency room with obvious facial trauma. What is the nurse's *first* priority in the care for this patient?

    A. Clearing the cervical spine of injury

    B. Assessing the level of consciousness

    C. Assessing for upper airway for hemorrhage

    D. Cleansing the facial lacerations

125. Which of the following is *not* a purpose of a trauma registry?

    A. Compile data to show trends in trauma injuries

    B. Identify individual physicians not practicing according to current guidelines

    C. Use the data obtained to develop preventive programs

    D. Perform outcome studies

126. Mr. Harrison sustained a crush injury to the right arm last night after a large rock fell on him while landscaping. He is experiencing pain rated 10/10 on a 1 to 10 severity scale, his blood pressure is 140/94 mmHg, heart rate is 110 beats per minute, pulse oximeter is reading 98% on room air, and his urine output is less than 30 mL/hr and is a reddish-brown color. The nurse should be suspicious that the patient might be experiencing:

    A. Hypovolemia

    B. Adverse reaction to antibiotics

    C. Rhabdomyolysis

    D. Urinary tract infection (UTI)

127. A nearly drowned patient presents to the emergency department. The patient is obtunded and the events leading up to the injury are unobtainable. In caring for the patient, the health care provider would suspect:

    A. Seizure activity

    B. Possible cord injury

    C. Hyperthermia

    D. Carbon monoxide poisoning

128. During a disaster, color-coded disaster triage categories should be used to better allocate benefits to the greatest number of patients in order to achieve optimal outcomes. When triaging during the disaster, the trauma nurse comes across a patient who is agonal breathing and unresponsive. What should the trauma nurse do at this time?

    A. Immediately begin resuscitation efforts
    B. Place a black tag on the patient
    C. Keep surveying the area for other treatable patients
    D. Place a red tag on the patient

129. Which of the following involves enhancing the quality of life in any stage and integrating physical, social, spiritual, and psychological aspects of care of patient/family who has been involved in a traumatic situation?

    A. Hospice
    B. Psychosocial centered care
    C. Palliative care
    D. Rehabilitation

130. Which of the following is *not* considered a correct statement about obtaining serum lactate levels?

    A. If obtaining a level by venipuncture, do not use a tourniquet.
    B. Arterial lactate levels are more conclusive than venous lactate levels.
    C. A lactate level needs to be obtained within 6 hours of onset of sepsis.
    D. Lactate levels should be obtained early to recognize occult hypoperfusion.

131. While treating a chemical burn patient, the nurse notices a powdery substance on the patient's skin. The nurse suspects that it is lime. What should the nurse do next to treat this injury?

    A. Identify a neutralizing agent
    B. Irrigate copiously
    C. Brush off the substance with a dry towel
    D. Apply a petroleum substance

132. The family of a trauma patient is requesting a transfer to another facility. The patient is unstable. Which of the following statements is *not* true regarding the transfer request?

    A. Risk and benefits of transfer must be clearly documented using the Certificate of Transfer.
    B. Responsibility for arranging transfer falls on the receiving institution.
    C. The receiving hospital must be notified before initiation of the transport and cannot refuse to accept the patient unless physically unable to care for the patient.
    D. The transferring facility must provide proper level of trained personnel to accompany the patient.

133. When does the rehabilitation start after the traumatic injury?

    A. During the acute in-house rehabilitation
    B. Immediately before discharge

C. At the time of transfer to a progressive care unit

D. At the time of admission to hospital

134. A nurse is preparing a trauma patient with multiple injuries who is being transferred to a level 1 trauma center in order to provide the level of care required. The nurse wants to ensure that adequate circulation is maintained during the transfer. Which of the following would be the most appropriate action by the nurse?

A. Provide extra intravenous fluids for the transport

B. Place extension tubing on the intravenous tubing

C. Ensure that the transport team has extra chest drainage systems

D. Place an uninflated shock garment under the patient

135. What is the overall goal of the Trauma Quality Improvement Program?

A. Collect accurate data from trauma facilities

B. Identify improvement processes

C. Improve the quality of trauma care

D. Establish benchmark comparisons of trauma centers

136. A speech therapy consultation is very beneficial to patients with dysarthria or dysphagia; however, there are many other reasons why speech therapy may be initiated for patients. All of the following are examples of when a speech therapist consultation is warranted except:

A. Recently extubated patients

B. Traumatic cases that involve aspiration

C. Psychiatric patients

D. All of the above

137. Mr. Miller, a pedestrian involved in a pedestrian versus motor vehicle collision, arrived in the emergency room 1 hour ago and has just returned from radiology. When reviewing the results, the nurse notes a positive pelvic fracture. Upon reassessment, the patient has difficulty breathing, a slightly distended abdomen, has not urinated yet, is complaining of abdominal pain, and is nauseous. The nurse is suspicious of possible complications, but what would be the primary concern?

A. Hypovolemia

B. Abdominal compartment syndrome (ACS)

C. Infection

D. Cholangitis

138. A trauma series is ordered for a genitourinary trauma patient. Which of the following examinations requires Foley catheter insertion and filling the bladder with contrast to evaluate for peritoneal extravasation following bladder rupture?

A. Cystogram

B. Retrograde urethrogram

C. Intravenous pyelogram

D. Voiding cystourethrogram

139. During crisis intervention, the trauma nurse demonstrated calmness, remained emotionally available, stayed neutral while maintaining eye contact, and used touch to calm the family member. Which of the following is *not* always a therapeutic way to respond during a crisis situation?

A. Using touch
B. Using eye contact
C. Staying neutral
D. Being emotionally in touch

140. A patient thrown from a moving vehicle presents with gross hematuria and severe flank pain. The nurse suspects a renal injury. Which kidney would be more likely to be affected by an injury?

A. Right kidney
B. Left kidney
C. Bilateral kidneys
D. Neither kidneys

141. Which of the following symptoms is significant in differentiating a septic patient from a severe sepsis patient?

A. Body temperature below 96.8°F
B. Heart rate greater than 90 beats per minute
C. Change in mental status
D. Respiratory rate greater than 20 breaths per minute

142. After a gunshot wound to the abdomen, the patient sustained a colon injury. A Hartmann's procedure was performed. Which of the following is the *best* explanation of this procedure?

A. A type of surgical resection with primary anastomosis
B. Double-barrel colostomy and complete diversion
C. A type of loop colostomy that is easily constructed and reversed
D. Hemicolectomy procedure

143. A patient is brought into the trauma bay. The patient was in a motor vehicle collision, was restrained, and airbags deployed. Upon examination, the nurse notices tenderness in the suprapubic area, and the patient is complaining of lower abdominal pain. The nurse suspects a possible pelvic fracture and obtains an order for CT scan of the pelvis. Because there is a chance that there could be further damage to the bladder, the nurse also obtains an order for:

A. Cystogram
B. Foley catheter placement
C. CT of the bladder
D. Sonography of the bladder

144. Where do the majority of aortic transections occur?

A. Ascending aorta
B. Level of the isthmus
C. Descending thoracic aorta
D. Infrarenal abdominal aorta

145. There are different levels of responders to disaster situations. At what level are hospitals and receiving facilities categorized?

    A. Level 1
    B. Level 2
    C. Level 3
    D. Level 4

146. The nurse assesses the patient and discovers that the patient has apraxia confabulation. Which consult order is most appropriate for this patient?

    A. Speech therapy
    B. Occupational therapy (OT)
    C. Physical therapy (PT)
    D. Psychologist

147. Ms. Carrington slipped and fell while at home. She attempted to brace herself for the fall and fractured the shaft of her radius. Which of the following injuries is *least* associated with radial fractures?

    A. Wrist fracture
    B. Clavicle fracture
    C. Elbow fracture
    D. Shoulder fracture

148. A 23-year-old male patient comes in after a nuclear explosion. He is unresponsive and agonal breathing. What would be the caregiver's *first* priority be in the care of this particular situation?

    A. Decontaminate the patient to limit exposure to others and then initiate resuscitation efforts.
    B. The health care provider should initiate resuscitation efforts.
    C. The health care provider should rapidly place all contaminated objects, including clothing, into a double bag and then initiate immediate resuscitation efforts.
    D. Place a waterproof drape over the patient and immediately begin resuscitation efforts.

149. A patient comes to the emergency room with burns to bilateral lower extremities, groin, and the anterior chest and abdominal walls. Using the rule of nines, what is the appropriate calculation of the percentage of total body surface area burned?

    A. 55% of the body
    B. 31% of the body
    C. 28% of the body
    D. 45% of the body

150. Proper medical management of a traumatic brain injury patient includes all except:

    A. Administering analgesics
    B. Administering 3% saline infusion
    C. Maintaining cerebral perfusion pressure (CPP) greater than 60
    D. Administering steroids

151. The nurse receives a patient with third-degree burns to the face. Which of the following is the priority nursing intervention for this patient?

    A. Obtain intravenous access to start fluid resuscitation
    B. Place a sterile dressing on the burn site
    C. Prepare for intubation
    D. Obtain a history of comorbidities and home medications

152. There are many complications from cardiac contusions. Which of the following is *not* considered one of them?

    A. Cardiogenic shock
    B. Congestive heart failure
    C. Hypovolemic shock
    D. Thrombus formation

153. What is the data-collection system that is composed of uniform data elements that describe the injury event, demographics, prehospital information, diagnosis, care and outcomes of injured patients?

    A. National Trauma Data Bank
    B. Trauma registry
    C. ACTION Registry
    D. IMPACT Registry

154. Which type of incomplete cord syndrome is the most common and usually occurs as a result of hyperextension injuries or interrupted blood supply to the cord?

    A. Central cord
    B. Anterior cord
    C. Posterior cord
    D. Brown–Sequard

155. Abdominal compartment syndrome (ACS) includes all of the following except:

    A. Metabolic acidosis
    B. Decreased cardiac output
    C. Metabolic alkalosis
    D. Decreased urinary output

156. A pregnant patient presents to the emergency room after being involved in a fender bender. Upon vaginal examination, the nurse notes umbilical cord prolapse. What is the *most* important intervention for this situation?

    A. Attempt to push the cord back in
    B. Position to relieve cord pressure
    C. Place the patient in Trendelenburg position
    D. Cover the cord in moist sterile gauze

157. The nurse is assessing a burn patient. After the nurses inspects and auscultates, the nurse moves onto a palpation assessment. Which of the following palpation assessments is abnormal for a burn patient?

    A. Palpation of the burned extremity detected decreased sensation
    B. Does not feel pain when palpated around the full thickness burn
    C. Burn tissue feels cold
    D. Peripheral pulse in circumferential burn is decreased

Chapter Review Answers and Rationales

CHAPTER 1. NEUROLOGICAL TRAUMA

1. **A**

   Increasing the head of bed (HOB) angle to 30 to 45 degrees facilitates venous drainage and lowers intracranial pressure (ICP). Decreasing the HOB does the opposite and increases the ICP by interfering with venous drainage. The fluid order is inappropriate because the goal is euvolemia, and dextrose is not indicated in neurologically impaired patients. Mannitol is frequently used in patients with a sustained increase in ICP greater than 20 mmHg, but the ICP was only 18 mmHg. Mannitol can increase cerebral perfusion, but this is not the first nursing intervention in this situation.

2. **D**

   This is a coup injury because the injury is on the same side of impact, accelerating the brain forward so it hits the side of the skull. A contre-coup injury is when the injury is on the opposite side of impact. An accelerated injury is when a moving object impacts a stationary object; an example of this would be a blow to the head. A subluxation is the displacement of the bone from the joint.

3. **C**

   Wrapping the eyes with gauze and nasal packing is inappropriate and contraindicated. Patients with basilar skull fractures frequently present with "raccoon eyes"; this is expected. Frequent level of consciousness (LOC) and pupillary assessments can reveal changes in pupil size and reactivity, and decreased LOC, which warrants suspicion for increased intracranial pressure (ICP), and indicates need to call the MD to notify of changes. If cerebral spinal fluid (CSF) leak is suspected, these patients are at increased risk for developing meningitis and should be placed on antibiotics. Placing nasal drainage on a gauze reveals a halo ring around the drainage, indicating a CSF leak.

4. **B**

   In an attempt to increase cerebral blood flow, cerebral perfusion pressure (CPP) may be maintained by raising the mean arterial pressure (MAP), or by lowering the intracranial pressure (ICP). Increasing systolic blood pressure (SBP) in turn increases MAP, thereby increasing cerebral blood flow. When CPP is maintained above 60 mmHg, the reduction in mortality is as much as 35% for those with severe brain injury. There is substantial evidence now that early hypotension is associated with increased morbidity and mortality following severe brain injury.

5. **C**

Ipsilateral pupil dilation and contralateral motor weakness occur because an uncal injury is below the midbrain; contralateral weakness is expected. This herniation compresses cranial nerves (CN) III leading to dilation of the pupil on the ipsilateral side. These patients usually have a severely decreased level of consciousness (LOC) and would not be awake or oriented. Having a Glasgow Coma Scale (GCS) of 12 would not reflect this injury because these patients often have a GCS of about 3 to 5, depending on the severity of injury.

6. **B**

Respiratory insufficiency is usually not seen in midbrain injuries. The midbrain lies just above the pons at the top of the brainstem. It plays a part in sensory functions, such as in helping to control eye movement, depth perception, other visual and auditory system functions, and helps to control body movements. Midbrain injuries present with loss of pupillary reaction, abnormally shaped pupils, resting tremors, rigidity, auditory changes, and even coma.

7. **C**

Trauma patients can go through stages of anxiety, fear, isolation, and grief, but a traumatic brain injury patient exhibits characteristic behavioral changes such as loss of control of emotions, combativeness, and abusiveness.

8. **A**

A cerebral concussion is a diffuse injury because of tearing or shearing of the axons. These injuries are caused by circumstances of rapid acceleration or deceleration or rotational injuries of the brain. CT of the brain is usually negative but the patient has a poor neurological status. CT of the head would reveal blood in the subdural space if a traumatic subdural hematoma. An epidural hematoma is a clot between the dura and the skull; the bleed expands rapidly and increases intracranial pressure (ICP), hemiparesis, and pupillary dilation. A patient with subdural hematoma acquired from bleeding in the subdural space would present with increased headache, declining level of consciousness (LOC), and motor deficits.

9. **B**

The Cushing's triad includes an increased systolic pressure, a widened pulse pressure, bradycardia, and respiratory insufficiency. This response is initiated in an attempt to increase cerebral blood flow. It occurs during herniation and is considered a very late sign of increased intracranial pressure (ICP).

10. **B**

In autonomic dysreflexia, 80% of patients with thoracic (T6) injury and above suffer from symptoms, including hypertension, sweating above the level of injury, piloerection, restlessness, anxiety, bradycardia, pounding headache, and a flushed face. In spinal shock all reflexes, sensation, and movement are lost below the level of injury, and usually there is no change in vital signs. Neurogenic shock is the impairment of sympathetic pathways, therefore, although the patient is bradycardic, a patient in neurogenic shock is usually not hypertensive after the acute phase and loses the ability to sweat for thermoregulatory control. Patients in distributive shock lose autonomic sympathetic function and vasodilation occurs.

11. **C**

Stimulating the rectum encourages regular bowel movements. A bowel program is needed with spinal cord injury (SCI) patients because they typically have a spastic or hyporeflexive bowel, and would benefit from bowel training. For immobilization, the Roto Rest bed is already implemented by the physician. The "quad cough" should be included in the pulmonary toileting order. The nurse should change the position of the patient *slowly* (not quickly) to avoid postural hypotension. Frequent positioning should also be implemented to decrease the risk of pressure ulcers.

12. **D**

Pregnancy and a normal delivery are still possible, there is no evidence that spinal cord–injured females cannot have normal pregnancies and deliveries, but autonomic dysreflexia should be monitored and managed closely during the pregnancy and delivery. The dysfunction of the autonomic nervous system (ANS) does not change the ability of female menses or ability to get pregnant. Indications for vaginal deliveries versus caesarian sections (C-sections) are essentially the same for women with spinal cord injury (SCI) as with able-bodied women. Research has shown, however, that C-sections are more frequently performed in women with SCI.

13. **A**

Bronchial constriction is a result of parasympathetic stimulation. This originates from nerves in the craniosacral region of the central nervous system (CNS) and regulates function under normal conditions. Increased respiratory rate, bronchial dilation, and pulmonary vascular constriction are a result of sympathetic stimulation. The sympathetic nervous system originates from the thoracolumbar region of the spinal cord, and increases during physiologic and psychological stress.

14. **B**

Spinal cord contusions occur because of bruising, swelling, and possible necrosis to the tissue caused by compression. Spinal cord concussion is a temporary loss of function caused by narrowing of the vertebral foramen. Spinal cord transection is disruption in the spinal tracts, including incomplete and complete injuries. Spinal cord ischemia occurs because of an interruption in vascular supply (not necessarily compression) to the spinal cord, resulting in ischemic injury, or even necrosis.

15. **A**

Vertebral fracture stability is defined as no potential for injury to the spinal cord, no potential for displacement during healing time, no displacement or angulation from normal loading after healing. The loss of ligamentous integrity is defined as an unstable spinal injury. All spinal injuries should be presumed unstable until further evaluation.

16. **A**

Spinal cord injury without radiologic abnormality (SCIWORA) accounts for up to 30% of severe cervical injuries in children aged 8 years and younger, and usually occurs in the cervical spine region. This occurs because elasticity in the pediatric cervical spine can allow severe spinal cord injury in the absence of radiographic findings. Compressed nerves, spinal lesions, and lumbar hematomas may cause some paresthesia, but considering the age of the patient and the severity of the presentation, SCIWORA is more likely.

17. **B**

Neurogenic shock is associated with spinal cord injuries level T6 or above. The impairment, if sympathetic, pathways to the spinal cord results in the loss of vasomotor tone and sympathetic innervation to the heart. This results in pulses being slow and strong in neurogenic shock, as opposed to hypovolemic shock, in which patients display rapid, weak pulses.

18. **A**

Skin presentation in neurogenic shock patients is warm and dry, and assumes the temperature of the surrounding environment. This is called *poikilothermia*. Hypovolemic shock patients' skin presentation is cool and moist because of the decrease in circulating blood volume.

19. **D**

The toe is innervated at the level of the fourth lumbar vertebrae. All of the other answers are correct in regards to level of innervation. Knowing these landmarks aid in localizing the level of injury to the affected dermatome site.

20. **A**

Tactile stimuli such as a pinprick or a light touch, should be used during assessment. The nurse should begin at the level of no sensation and proceed to the area of sensation. This aids in localizing the level of the injury.

21. **C**

Cervical spine images should be performed in order to visualize all seven cervical vertebrae and T1. If C7 to T1 cannot be accurately visualized, a CT of the cervical spine is recommended. Chest x-rays (CXR) visualize anterior ribs 5 to 7 at the midclavicular line and 9 to 10 posterior ribs. MRI is the most commonly used mechanism to evaluate cord injuries; CT scan is used more to evaluate bony injuries. An MRI may be used with caution because the patient could have metal devices in place.

22. **C**

Hypotension is a frequent symptom of patients in neurogenic shock because of hypovolemia from occult injuries. Hypotension and bradycardia occur when blood vessels below the level of injury vasodilate, and blood pools in the lower extremities. Intravenous fluids and vasopressor medication are frequently utilized for these patients. Orthostatic hypotension and autonomic dysreflexia are also long-term complications of spinal cord injuries, and result in significant blood pressure changes, which need to be monitored closely.

23. **B**

Administering an ordered sedative or short-acting paralytic aids in the maintenance of adequate immobilization in the patient who is agitated or restless. Education on the importance of immobility and proper alignment should be implemented to increase the understanding of the patient's safety. Administering methylprednisone does not aid in the agitated and restless state, and actually can cause agitation as a side effect.

High-dose steroids are no longer recommended in managing acute spinal cord–injured patients.

24. B

A patient who sustains an initial concussion may develop cerebral edema, loss of consciousness, memory impairment, disorientation, dizziness, and headache. The brain's autoregulatory mechanisms compensate for the injury and protect against massive swelling but when the patient sustains a "second impact," the brain loses its ability to autoregulate. In severe cases, this may lead to rapid cerebral edema followed by brain herniation. Death has been reported to occur in a matter of minutes. Cardiac arrest did occur but was not the primary injury. The patient did suffer from a traumatic brain injury when he injured his head with the initial concussion, but second-impact syndrome is more descriptive and fits the injury presentation. Double-impact injury is not a recognized injury.

25. C

The nonbleeding head injury patient can take ibuprofen for pain and swelling, which can cause stomach bleeding and renal complications in certain people, but is not contraindicated for this injury. The patient can also take acetaminophen. Utilizing ice packs for pain at the site is appropriate, just ensure that patient is aware of the length of time ice is recommended. Waking in intervals of 3 to 4 hours is recommended in the first 24 to 48 hours to be on alert for amnesia, postconcussion syndrome symptoms, or changes in mentation. A return to contact sports is not recommended until patient is completely back to normal.

26. D

Hypercalcemia is a common complication of spinal cord–injured patients. Hypercalcemia is caused by immobility and, if left untreated, patients may develop dehydration, personality changes, calcium oxalate nephrolithiasis, and renal failure. Treatment is aimed at early mobilization, hydration, and restoration of balance between calcium excretion and resorption. Misdiagnosis of an acute abdomen is a common complication of these patients because they are plagued with gastroparesis, paralytic ileus, constipation, and colitis, which can mimic the signs and symptoms of acute abdomen. The degree of pain perception below the level of injury in patients with spinal cord injury (SCI) is highly variable and unpredictable, depending on the level and completeness of the injury. Placing a urinary catheter would be incorrect because patients with SCI are at an increased risk for urinary tract infection (UTI), placing an indwelling urinary catheter increases that risk. It is more beneficial to first begin a bladder program with intermittent catheterization and utilization of bladder scanning.

27. C

After a spinal cord injury (SCI) above the T6 level, the autonomic nervous system (ANS) can be disrupted, which affects those automatic responses that we do not have any control over such as blood pressure, stuffy nose, headache, and flushing. The ANS does include digestion, but the other nervous systems have a greater effect on gastrointestinal (GI) processes. The CNS provides extrinsic neural inputs that regulate, modulate, and control GI functions. The peripheral nervous system (PNS) exerts both excitatory and inhibitory control over gastric and intestinal tone and motility. The enteric nervous system (ENS) functions to control the GI system by controlling mobility and secretions.

28. A

Dantrolene is an antispasmolytic agent that prevents muscle stiffness and spams. Steroids, like methylprednisolone, are given to reduce damage to nerve cells and decrease inflammation near the site of injury. Lexapro and other serotonin-norepinephrine reuptake inhibitors used for depression, block or delay the reuptake of the neurotransmitters serotonin and norepinephrine by the presynaptic nerves. This increases the levels of these two neurotransmitters in the synapse and tends to elevate mood. Lyrica and other medications for neuropathic pain interact with descending noradrenergic and serotonergic pathways originating from the brainstem, and reduce neuropathic pain transmission from the spinal cord.

29. B

Diuresis (not oliguria) and shivering are known complications of therapeutic hypothermia. Coagulopathy (not hypercoagulable state) and arrhythmias are also complications experienced with therapeutic hypothermia.

30. D

Mild brain injury patients can present with headache, dizziness, irritability, fatigue, or poor concentration. A patient with continual confusion, unconsciousness, or seizure activity may have a more severe injury. Infants with an increased intracranial pressure (ICP) may experience irritability, lethargy, and vomiting. The pattern of unconsciousness, consciousness, followed again by unconsciousness is typically seen with an epidural hematoma and is a severe brain injury.

31. C

Neuropsychological assessment by evaluation of the symptoms a person reports after sustaining the injury is typically the best method used to assess for a mild brain injury. There are newer, more sophisticated imaging technologies that show promise in more effectively capturing damage in a mild brain injury such as single-photon emission CT, but these are expensive and typically not readily available. CT scan or MRI show no evidence of injury because damage to white matter of the brain is harder to detect on scans.

32. B

The patient is experiencing some of the later symptoms of the injury and it is disrupting the patient's life by affecting performance at work. Rehabilitation evaluation can be very beneficial to this patient and performing exercises for the brain may be recommended to restore useful function. Making an appointment with a psychiatrist or neurologist for medication management does not have the benefit value that rehabilitation services can provide to this patient. If the patient feels like a neurological reevaluation is needed, encourage the patient to seek aid here, but the symptoms experienced are expected of a mild brain injury.

33. B

It is always important to obtain the smoking status of a patient during any history obtainment; however, it is not as relevant as the other questions when assessing a suspected brain-injured patient. Drug and alcohol use can explain a decreased level of consciousness (LOC), and need to be ruled out or addressed. If the patient has a history of seizure activity, the patient could have a decreased LOC because of the postictal state. If a loss of consciousness occurred after the injury, this could indicate a possible concussion or severe brain injury.

34. **A**

A patient with linear, depressed, or basilar skull fracture is expected to experience a headache and a change in level of consciousness. The possibility of an open fracture and palpation of a depression of the skull over the fracture site are associated with depressed skull fractures. Periorbital ecchymosis, also known as "raccoon eyes," is seen in basilar skull fractures only.

35. **B**

This patient gets 2 for best eye opening because the eyes opened to painful stimuli. The patient receives a 1 for no verbal response; gasping does not count as an incomprehensible or inappropriate verbal sound. The best motor response would be a 4 for the withdrawal from painful stimuli, take great care not to misinterpret grasp reflex or postural adjustments as a response to a command. The total Glasgow Coma Scale score (GCS) for this patient is 7.

36. **D**

The patient is currently stable with oxygenation; a nonrebreather mask is the recommended method of oxygenation for this patient because many patients with brain injuries are hypoxic and need to be hyperoxygenated initially. Because this airway is secure at this time, intubation is not warranted, but airway assessment and securement should always come first in any assessment. Usually, the nurse's priority after airway has been assessed is to stop any bleeding, but because this patient is presenting with a depressed skull fracture, applying direct pressure to the site can cause further damage. Therefore, the next step should be establishing two large-bore IV (intravenous) sites to initiate fluid resuscitation and possible blood transfusion. Assessing the patient's pupils is important because it is a component of the neurological assessment, and can indicate an increased intracranial pressure; however, circulation is the priority of care.

37. **A**

These injuries describe a hyperflexion injury involving the posterior ligament and anterior vertebral body fracture. Hyperextension injuries involve the anterior ligament and compression fracture of posterior vertebrae. Vertical compression fractures usually are burst fractures caused by forceful blows to the top of the head. Odontoid fractures involve fracture of the odontoid (dens) bone, which is a small bony protrusion from the anterior ring of C2.

38. **A**

A fracture of the anterior and posterior arch of C1 without cord damage is usually a burst fracture, frequently without displacement of the cord. This is called *Jefferson's fracture*. A displacement fracture at this level is fatal. A bilateral fracture through arch C2 would be a hangman's fracture, and is frequently seen in deceleration motor vehicle collisions or falls. An atlanto-occipital fracture is the avulsion of C1 from the occipital bone; death is usually imminent. The odontoid fracture is known as a "dens" fracture. This is the body extension of C2 into the anterior portion of C1, allowing C1 to rotate C2.

39. B

Complete cord injury is correct because there is no preservation of motor or sensory below the level of the injury. Central cord syndrome is the most common incomplete cord injury; it involves a loss of motor and sensory function, but the loss is usually greater in the arms than in the legs, and there is a gradual return of function. A posterior cord injury is an incomplete cord injury that usually presents with a loss of proprioception, vibration, fine touch, and fine pressure below the level of injury, but motor, pain, and temperature remain intact. Necrosis of the spinal cord postinjury is a secondary ischemic injury because impaired blood supply causes necrosis of the spinal cord after injury.

40. C

Vibration, position sense, deep pressure, two-point discrimination, and light touch are all expected because anterior cord syndrome allows posterior column preservation. Although this injury has a poor prognosis, with about 10% to 20% of patients regaining motor function, to tell a patient he or she can never move his or her legs again is not a therapeutic response, but offering false hope is also inappropriate. With anterior cord syndrome, progression would be to regain motor, pain, and temperature sensory function. Usually people with central cord syndrome have a recovery rate of about 50%; anterior cord syndrome has a worse prognosis. Stating that patients always regain motor movement with this type of injury is inaccurate.

41. D

The patient has an absence of vasoconstriction and loses the ability to conserve heat with shivering and the ability to dissipate heat by sweating. Poikliothermia occurs in injuries above thoracolumbar outflow of the sympathetic nervous system, and the patient lacks internal regulation of body temperature with an absence of vasoconstriction.

42. D

Memory notebooks assist in improving the patient's memory by reinforcing events and plan of care. This provides a written reference to aid the patient in recalling events and emphasizing the plan of care.

43. D

Patients with mild brain injury often present with headache, dizziness, irritability, fatigue, or poor concentration following the injury. This is called postconcussion syndrome. The return to normal may take several weeks to months following injury. Infants presenting with irritability, lethargy, or vomiting following a brain injury indicate the presence of increased intracranial pressure (ICP); this is considered a severe traumatic brain injury.

44. A

A diffuse axonal injury causes brain cells to die, which causes intracranial swelling. This increased pressure in the brain decreases cerebral blood perfusion, causing additional injury. About 90% of survivors with severe diffuse axonal injury remain unconscious. The 10% who regain consciousness are usually severely neurologically impaired. Acquired brain injuries result from damage to the brain caused by strokes, tumors, anoxia, hypoxia, toxins, degenerative diseases, near drowning, or other conditions not necessarily caused by an external force. Hypoxic brain injuries are caused by oxygen deprivation and prolongation of this state leads to cell death. Encephalopathy is altered mentation caused by multiple different underlying etiologies. Some encephalopathies are reversible by managing the underlying etiology.

45. **C**

Diffuse axonal injury is not the result of a penetrating trauma to the brain. This injury results from the brain moving back and forth in the skull as a result of an acceleration–deceleration mechanism of injury, or rotation forces in the brain. Automobile collisions, sports-related injuries, falls, and shaken baby syndrome are common causes of diffuse axonal injury. Acceleration, deceleration, and rotation movement causes the brain to move within the skull, tearing or shearing the axons. The shearing is caused by tissues sliding over tissue.

46. **B**

When a patient has an altered level of consciousness (LOC), agitation is most likely a sign of hypoxia, and if hypoxia persists the patient progresses to being obtunded because of hypoventilation and hypercapnia. Hypoglycemia can cause patients to be shaky but not necessarily agitated, but there is no hint in the question about the patient being a diabetic. People who are intoxicated can be agitated but typically don't progress to being obtunded, this would be seen more in an overdose situation. Hypotension alter mentation because of decrease in blood flow and perfusion to the brain does not necessarily lead to hypoxia.

47. **C**

The neck is shorter in children, which makes evaluation of the trachea more difficult, but does not increase the risk of traumatic brain injury. The head is larger and heavier in relation to the rest of the body, and the occiput area is more prominent in pediatric patients making it a larger area for probable injury. White matter is not well myelinated yet, which increases risk of cranial shearing injuries.

CHAPTER 2. MAXILLOFACIAL TRAUMA

1. **C**

The chin-lift maneuver is utilized in cervical patients to avoid hyperextending or flexing the neck in order to open the airway, not actually to inspect the airway. Vocalization; the presence of secretions, blood, vomit; noting loose teeth, foreign objects, edema, or tongue obstruction are all part of assessing for a clear airway.

2. **C**

Discoloration or bruising, loss of function such as opening the mouth, loss of tissue, bone exposure, sources of bleeding or lacerations, and deformities of the face are all other signs of facial trauma and potential fracture. Cranial nerves are commonly injured in facial trauma and should be assessed, but a loss of a corneal reflex is more likely associated with a brain injury.

3. **A**

   Clear fluid from the laceration site indicates a posterior table fracture with a dural injury. The dural injury causes cerebrospinal fluid (CSF) leaks. Pneumocephalus is the presence of air or gas within the cranial cavity and is not associated with leaking fluid. It is usually associated with disruption of the skull such as a depressed skull fracture. Maxillary and mandible fractures alone do not cause a CSF leak.

4. **D**

   Skin adhesives would not be appropriate in a bleeding scalp wound. Holding direct pressure or applying a pressure dressing to the site helps control the bleeding. Sutures and staples are ways to control blood loss in scalp lacerations.

5. **C**

   Hydrogen peroxide would not be an appropriate medication to use when cleansing a deep facial laceration because of potential damage to healthy tissue. The use of hydrogen peroxide is also contraindicated in wounds with possible sinus involvement. Cleansing the wound with normal saline and irrigating it with an antibiotic solution are recommended. Lidocaine is utilized as local anesthesia for suturing facial lacerations.

6. **D**

   A razor would be inappropriate because the eyebrows should not be shaved. Eyebrows should not ever be shaved because they serve as landmarks and for approximation of wound edges. All of the other supplies are appropriate for cleansing and treating the facial wound.

7. **C**

   A cold compress should be applied to minimize edema, not a warm compress. Placing the patient in High Fowler's position may decrease facial edema and assists with maintenance of the airway. Inserting an orogastric tube is recommended. Nasogastric tubes are contraindicated in basilar skull fractures and severe midface fractures. Direct pressure should be applied to the facial site if bleeding is present.

8. **D**

   Control epistaxis with direct pinch pressure for up to 30 minutes; if that is ineffective, cauterization may be utilized. If this fails, nasal packing can be used with ribbon gauze impregnated with petroleum jelly. Posterior epistaxis requires posterior packing or balloon tamponade. Surgical reduction is not recommended as early management of nasal fractures.

9. **D**

   A cerebrospinal fluid (CSF) leak is not specifically caused by a hematoma of the septum. Nasal passage obstruction by a hematoma can result in severe deformity of the septum, an abscess within the nasal passage, and a central nervous system (CNS) infection. Careful examination and cleaning of the nares are required to prevent hematomas and epistaxis.

10. **C**

   Cranial nerve I, the olfactory nerve, is located in the nasoorbitalethmoid (NOE) region. Damage of the medial orbital wall can injure the ethmoid bone, which is connected to the cribriform plate. All of these can result in injury to the olfactory cranial nerve, resulting in the loss of smell. Frontal lobe injuries can also result in the loss of smell and are a common complication of traumatic brain injuries. Maxillary fracture can present with rhinorrhea, and the injury can extend through the tooth-bearing region, or through the nasal or sinus mucosa, but does not usually cause injury to the olfactory cranial nerve.

11. A

This is an indirect injury to the optic nerve. An indirect injury occurs with a blunt trauma in which the forces are transmitted through the optic canal to the optic nerve. This is a delayed presentation of the injury. A direct injury to the optic nerve resulting in visual changes occurs when the injury is a penetrating injury, or when bony fragments directly damage the optic nerve fibers. There is no object that directly entered the eye; therefore, labeling this a penetrating wound would not be accurate. It was a blunt force injury, but not directly to the optic nerve.

12. D

Signs of a globe injury with fracture include visual impairment, extrusion of intraocular contents, hyphema or subconjunctival hemorrhage, restricted extraocular movements, and decreased intraocular pressure. Severe orbital fractures may communicate with the anterior cranial fossa, involving a direct brain injury, internal carotid injury, or a cerebrospinal fluid (CSF) leak; the signs provided in the scenario were of the actual orbital fracture with entrapment of the extraocular muscles.

13. B

When a patient comes in with an ocular trauma, the nurse should obtain an accurate history and ask the important questions asked of all trauma patients during the primary survey. Blepharospasm is prolonged uncontrolled blinking and may be misinterpreted as an ocular injury. Knowing whether the patient has had prior eye surgery is important because the eye may have compromised vessels or abnormal structures. If the patient was wearing eyeglasses or contacts at the time of the injury, then the eyeglass may have shattered, or the contacts may still be in place. The patient with dysphonia would present with a neck trauma, not an ocular trauma, and have difficulty with speech.

14. D

The nurse should assess for the presence of enophthalmos. This occurs when the globe recedes posteriorly and may result in the loss of function of the orbitalis muscle, or a blowout fracture. The nurse should also assess the lid appearance but not necessarily invert the eyelid. Applying pressure is contraindicated in blowout fractures and open orbital injuries. There is no indication in this scenario of the need to perform a halo test to determine the presence of cerebrospinal fluid (CSF) drainage.

15. C

Rounded medial palpebral fissure is a sign of a nasoorbitalethmoid (NOE) injury, not a zygomatic fracture. The palpebral fissure is located between the medial and lateral canthi of the two open eyelids. A zygomatic fracture has pain with opening the mouth or limited motion of the jaw, the frontal view appears to be "flattened." Other symptoms include upward gaze, facial edema, periorbital ecchymosis, and endophthalmus.

16. A

Airway obstruction can occur in mandibular fractures because the tongue is secured to muscle attached to the mandible, and a fracture with damage to those securing muscles results in a loss of tongue control. The tongue can fall backwards and obstruct the airway. Assuring patency of the airway is the primary goal of treatment in mandibular fractures. Zygomatic fractures may involve the mandible, but the tongue is not usually involved. Oral cavity injuries can cause airway issues involving the tongue when there are lacerations to the tongue; this is not as common as mandibular fractures. Nasoorbitalethmoid (NOE) injuries have more sinus involvement and are not associated with tongue injuries.

17. C

The patient's airway is always the first thing considered, therefore securing the airway with intubation is the first intervention. Then, controlling the pharyngeal bleeding by packing the throat to limit blood loss should be the second intervention. The third step is to transport the patient to radiology because the patient may require an emergency angiography to determine the extent and location of the injury and to guide interventions.

18. D

Patients who sustain an oral cavity injury can have many complications, such as massive hemorrhage, because of arterial injury, aneurysm formation, basilar skull fractures with cerebrospinal fluid (CSF) leaks, thrombosis, expanding hematomas, and cranial nerve (CN) defects. The most commonly involved cranial nerves are V (trigeminal), VII (facial), VIII (acoustic), IX (glossopharyngeal), XI (accessory), and XII (hypoglossal). CN III (oculomotor) is typically not involved with oral trauma.

19. A

Patients with soft tissue injuries and lacerations to the lateral side of the face can result in injury to the parotid gland and the parotid duct, which are responsible for producing saliva. Therefore, the clear fluid leaking from the wound in this scenario is saliva. The sublingual glands usually are not affected because they are the smallest of the salivary glands. The submandibular gland is located below the floor of the mouth and is not affected by this injury. The Stensen's duct is involved in the route that saliva travels from the major salivary glands to the parotid gland into the mouth. The most common injury is actually to the parotid gland itself.

20. B

The face is divided into three main regions and traumatic fractures can be identified based on the region injured. The middle-third region of the face includes the zygoma, maxilla, and the nasal bones. The upper third involves the frontal bones and orbits, and the lower third contains the mandible.

21. C

Assessment for a LeFort type I fracture is performed by gently holding the maxilla with the thumb and forefinger, and carefully attempt to rock the maxilla forward and back. If the maxilla moves independently of the face, then a LeFort type I fracture is present. If there is separation of the midface in a pyramid shape (appearing like an oxygen facemask) then it is a LeFort II fracture. A LeFort III fracture appears as a complete separation of the face from the cranium. This is also called *craniofacial dysfunction*. Placing two fingers in the lower jaw to assess for movement is not a correct technique to assess for LeFort I fractures.

22. C

The LeFort II fracture is a LeFort I fracture with an extension through the orbital rim, medial orbital wall (not lateral orbital wall), ethmoid sinus, and the nasal bone. The term *zygomaticomaxillary complex* refers to fractures of the frontal, maxillary, temporal, and sphenoid bones, and is not a part of the LeFort II fracture. LeFort II fractures do not include mandible fractures.

23. A

Lefort II and III fractures are at risk for a cerebrospinal fluid (CSF) leak and upper airway obstruction. They both involve some degree of orbital fractures. These patients are more likely to get intubated or have a cricothyroidotomy. The LeFort III patient has a higher associated loss of consciousness with brain injury and increased blood loss, leading to hypovolemia and altered cerebral perfusion.

24. B

This describes the Water's view. Caldwell's view is when the patient's forehead and nose are against the x-ray plate; it is used to identify similar structures as Water's but with a different view. Lateral view is used to identify nasal bones, frontal sinus, and multiple small maxillofacial floors fractures. The mandibles view shows anterior–posterior, right, and left lateral views of the mandible.

25. C

The loss of hearing is an unlikely complication of facial trauma unless a temporal bone fracture or brain injury are involved in the trauma. Complications of facial trauma are aspiration pneumonia because of the increased risk for aspiration of blood. Optic nerve injury, both direct and indirect, as well as entrapment of extraocular muscles places the patient at risk for visual loss following injury. Hemorrhage because of injury of major arteries can occur with facial trauma. Other complications may include upper airway obstruction; loss of vision and the inability to close eyes; hemorrhage; lacrimal duct injury; parotid duct injury; facial nerve injury; cosmetic issues; and associated injuries to the brain, neck, spine, and eye injuries.

26. D

Facial, sensory, and motor losses may occur and it may take up to 24 months to recover function, so they are not always permanent. Routinely use artificial tears to lubricate the eyes to aid in moistening. The patient may tape the eyes shut at night to prevent corneal desiccation.

27. A

A dacryocystorhinostomy is a silastic tube used to cannulate and repair a lacrimal duct injury. It typically remains in place for 3 to 6 months after injury. Disruption of the lacrimal duct leads to epiphora, or tear overflow, and usually requires repair. Removal of the duct is not recommended. Bypass is not a procedure used for parotid ductal repair.

28. B

All of these are appropriate assessments and interventions, but securing an airway takes priority over a diagnostic study. The patient is drooling, lethargic, and has stridor, there clearly is an upper airway problem. Assessing for a cerebrospinal fluid (CSF) leak is important because it places the patient at high risk for central nervous system (CNS) infection, but is not more important than securing the airway. Assessing for a subconjunctival hemorrhage should be done in suspected facial fractures, but again, it's not as important as checking the airway.

29. A

The primary treatment for facial fractures is open reduction with internal fixation. The procedure may be delayed for up to a week depending on the patient's status, other injuries, and swelling or edema of the face. Wiring is used more in maxillomandibular fixation, but a complication of wiring is temporomandibular joint (TMJ) and masticatory wasting, which occur with prolonged immobility. Titanium is the choice of metal for craniofacial plates because it doesn't interfere with MRI machines and because of its "pseudobiological" activity in bonding with the host tissue.

30. B

Common mechanisms of injury for ocular trauma include thermal burns, foreign bodies, blunt trauma, and chemical burns. Less common mechanisms of ocular injury include machinery accidents, motor vehicle collisions, and firearms.

31. B

Corneal abrasion is a type of ocular injury that can be associated with a coup traumatic brain injury. Symptoms include ocular pain, a feeling that there is something in the eye, tearing, redness, sensitivity to light, blurred vision or a loss of vision, and a headache. Subconjunctival hemorrhage is a broken blood vessel in the eye, causing the area to appear bloody. This was not in this patient's presenting symptoms. Choroidal hemorrhage is bleeding into the suprachoroidal space or within the choroid, and is caused by the rupture of choroidal vessels. Choroidal hemorrhage and retinal necrosis present with a red, bloody eye, periorbital pain, decreased vision or color vision, and reports of the appearance of "floaters."

32. D

An ocular injury that can occur following a traumatic brain injury with a direct force of impact to the skull is a corneal abrasion. Retinal necrosis is most commonly caused by viral infection. Commotio retinae and choroidal hemorrhage are usually a result of a direct blunt impact to the eye itself.

33. D

Burns to the eyelids and skin can cause scarring and contraction of the eyelids. Exposure of the cornea and ocular surfaces occurs because of the eyelid scarring and contraction. This exposure can then lead to corneal abrasions and to prevent this, frequent eye care is required. Hyphema can occur with ocular trauma, but is not a result of eyelid burns and scars.

34. A

Pure orbital floor fracture involves the fracture of the orbital floor only, without an associated orbital rim fracture, and typically occurs because of low-impact trauma. Impure orbital floor fracture involves both the orbital floor and the orbital rim. It is usually a result of high-impact trauma to the face. A blowout fracture typically involves the floor of the orbit, but it also includes multiple orbital fractures. A LeFort I fracture does not involve orbital fractures.

35. D

Forced duction tests may be used to evaluate the presence of ocular muscle entrapment. This is done to distinguish between a muscle paralysis and a mechanical restriction. The procedural steps include instilling a local anesthetic, using forceps to grab the inferior rectus muscle, then rotating the globe in all directions to assess motion. Oral antibiotics and nasal decongestants are frequently administered following orbital fracture reconstruction. Orbital fractures typically require reconstruction of the orbital floor and medial wall with titanium mesh, synthetic orbital plate constructs, or bony grafting. Neither of these answers the question about what is used to evaluate the entrapment. Needle decompression of the ocular muscle is not a correct assessment or treatment of this injury.

36. B

Oculocardiac reflex presents with bradycardia, heart blocks, nausea, vomiting, and syncope following an orbital injury. Immediate evaluation for surgery is required to repair the ocular fracture in patients presenting with oculocardiac reflex. Entrapment of eye muscles and retrobulbar hemorrhage may also require immediate evaluation and management, but the patient does not present with these signs. Brain injuries can be associated with facial trauma but this patient is awake and light-headed. These are not common symptoms of a severe traumatic brain injury.

37. D

Risk factors of a patient developing a retrobulbar hemorrhage following an orbital fracture are increased when associated with the Valsalva maneuver postoperatively. The administration of stool softeners and antiemetic medications decreases the chance of Valsalva and increased intraocular pressures. In addition, hypertension has been shown to be a risk factor for retrobulbar hemorrhage in postoperative patients; therefore, the administration of beta-blockers to manage the blood pressure may be indicated. Administering anticoagulation medication to postoperative trauma patients has been shown to increase the risk for developing retrobulbar hemorrhage and should be avoided.

38. A

Patients with corneal abrasions should have a light, semipressure dressing applied. The dressing should not compress the eye too firmly, just enough to keep the eyelid from blinking. Too much pressure on the eye causes central retinal artery occlusion. The dressing should be taped from the forehead to the cheeks. Some abrasions require instillation of antibiotic eye drops to prevent infection of the epithelium, but treatment does not typically involve oral antibiotics for 14 days.

39. B

Corneal infection is a complication of corneal injury or abrasions. Symptoms are increased eye pain and an enlargement of the gray area on the corneal surface. If a foreign body is left in the eye and not removed, it becomes a nidus of infection. Conjunctivitis and conjunctival infection are bacterial or viral infections in the eye, usually presenting with symptoms of pink eye. Corneal abrasion is most likely involved with this injury, and the patient is complaining of pain, which is a symptom of a corneal abrasion, but the question is reflective of infection symptoms of the gray area.

40. C

The physical examination for an ocular injury includes the external inspection, pupillary assessment, visual acuity measurement of each eye, photo documentation, and extraocular movement assessment. The slit-lamp examination and the fundus dilation are also key parts of diagnosing an ocular injury, but these examinations should be done by an ophthalmologist and not the trauma nurse.

41. D

An order for an MRI should be questioned when attempting to detect a foreign body in the eye because the material in the eye could be metal. The MRI can cause movement of the metal, resulting in further ocular damage. Ultrasound can evaluate the eye from the cornea to the optic nerve. CT scan and x-ray are both appropriate tests to detect foreign bodies that may be present in an ocular injury, depending on the type of material.

42. C

Fluvoxamine is a selective serotonin reuptake inhibitor used to treat depression, it also has an anticholinergic effect that may cause pupil dilation and is not used in patients with increased intraocular pressure. Diamox is an oral carbonic anhydrase inhibitor, Timolol is a topical beta-blocker; glycerin is a hyperosmotic agent. All are used to decrease intraocular hypertension and would be indicated in this patient. Normal intraocular pressure is less than 21 mmHg.

43. A

Irrigate 1 L of fluid with Morgan lens, test pH afterward; this process may be repeated until the pH is neutral. If the pH does not neutralize, sweep the fornices with a cotton swab to remove crystalized particles. The pH of the ocular surface is checked using litmus paper.

44. B

This is true of an ocular injury from bases (alkali). Acids can cause denaturation and precipitation of proteins within the cornea and sclera. This type of injury rarely penetrates into the anterior chamber. Neutrals shouldn't cause injury like acids and bases do to the eye, and corrosives are not recognized as a type of chemical burn.

45. A

The Fox eye shield, also known as the *Fox screen*, is a malleable and light-weight perforated metal screen that is frequently placed over an injured or postoperative eye. The Tungsten eye shield provides adequate protection of the ocular structure from ortho-voltage x-rays up to 9 mEV. A suction shield is a disposable shield used for Yankauer devices. The Uvex shield is a face shield used for heavy-duty work protection, such as welding.

CHAPTER 3. NECK TRAUMA

1. A

Starting the intravenous bolus with normal saline is the first line of treatment for the hypotensive patient in neurogenic shock. Levophed may be the next line of treatment if the patient is not responding to fluid resuscitation, but should not be used until fluid resuscitation occurs. Checking the airway is always the first assessment, but this patient is not in respiratory distress and her airway is secure, therefore, we need to address the hypotension. This patient is hypotensive and bradycardic because of the neurogenic shock; bradycardia is only treated when symptomatic. Cardizem would be inappropriate for the treatment of this patient, as it is commonly used to slow the heart rate and can lower blood pressure.

2. **A**

The C4 and C6 levels of injury patients require ventilatory support. C4 level innervates the diaphragm and C6 level with edema up the cord may need intubation in the acute phase. The C8 and below injury should be closely monitored, but most likely do not need ventilatory support.

3. **A**

The patient does not need to stay on cervical spine (C-spine) precautions if he or she is awake, alert, oriented, and experiencing no pain. X-ray images are not always a requirement to clear C-spine. An altered level of consciousness (LOC) or tenderness on palpation warrants x-rays, and for the patient to remain on C-spine precautions. A CT or MRI scan would not be indicated in this patient

CHAPTER 4. THORACIC TRAUMA

1. **A**

Flail chest is defined as three or more fractures occurring in two or more places, resulting in a freely moving chest wall. Flail chest displays paradoxical movements, tachypnea, and frequently requires intubation with positive pressure ventilation. Fracture of the sternum is associated with myocardial contusions and intrathoracic injuries. Rib fractures 4 to 12 may cause a bowing effect in the chest, resulting in midshaft fracture. A clavicle fracture is not considered a serious injury and would not contribute to respiratory distress.

2. **B**

The nurse should pinch or temporarily clamp the tubing at the insertion site and assess for bubbling in the water-seal chamber. If the bubbling stops, the leak is in the lung and the physician should be notified. If the bubbling continues, the air leak is in the system, which will need to be replaced. Chest tube drainage systems should always be positioned below the chest and not used to assess for an air leak. If the leak is found to be in the patient, the system would not have to be replaced. A chest x-ray does not determine whether the air leak is in the system and does not need to be ordered immediately.

3. **C**

Sternal fractures are usually associated with heart or great vessel injury because of the location and force of impact. The angle of Louis is the most common fracture site of the sternum; it is adjacent to the second intercostal space. Left lower rib fractures may be associated with splenic injuries and rupture, and not the right side. Right lower rib fractures may be associated with hepatic lacerations, and not the left side.

4. **A**

Damage to the tracheobronchial tree can occur with aspiration of liquids or objects. The aspiration causes an obstruction in the airway, resulting in respiratory insufficiency.

A bronchoscopy is the most *definitive* study to diagnose a true tracheal rupture. A chest x-ray is the most *standard* radiographic study but does not definitively identify a tracheal rupture. CT scan of the chest is the most *preferred* study because endoscopic reconstructions can be more easily clarified with it and tracheal tears can be highly suggested, but it still results with questionable findings. Ultrasound is not utilized with this type of suspected injury.

5. **A**

Aortic injuries are usually the result of blunt force trauma. The more common site of damage is the descending aorta at the level of the isthmus immediately below the arch. Pericardial tamponade will present with hypotension but will have distended neck veins and muffled heart sounds. Blunt cardiac injury patients will have a suspected injury to the heart, but will not have the poor circulation to the lower extremities or the systolic murmur. Ascending aortic injury is not as common and will typically result in death.

6. **A**

This patient has both aortic injury and abdominal involvement with intraabdominal hemorrhage. This patient may be hemodynamically unstable from the liver injury, and hemorrhage control remains the primary priority. If the aorta is injured, but is not the source of active hemorrhage, it can wait for bleeding or neurologic stabilization to be corrected. A pericardial window is utilized for patients with pericardial tamponade. This patient has evidence of aortic injury and not pericardial tamponade. Blood pressure control is necessary in order to stabilize the patient appropriately, but control of the hemorrhage is the priority of care.

7. **D**

The presence of an expanding aortic transection or aneurysm is a criterion for immediate surgery to repair the aorta. If the facility in which the patient is currently located does not have the capability of repairing the aorta, then the surgery has to be delayed until transfer occurs. A severe head injury, such as an epidural hematoma, may take precedence over aortic repairs as the priority for surgical management. An aneurysm that is less than 5 cm in size and not expanding may be stable and managed with observation.

8. **C**

Mr. Carson is exhibiting pericardial tamponade. An open thoracotomy in the emergency room is the most appropriate intervention for a hemodynamically unstable patient with a penetrating injury to the chest. Pericardiocentesis and surgical repair are acceptable treatments for a patient with pericardial tamponade, but an open thoracotomy would be more appropriate in this case because of the patient's declining status. An arteriogram of the aorta is not indicated in this situation. A cardiac injury should be suspected over an aortic transection based on mechanism of injury.

9. **B**

Pulmonary contusions can be life-threatening because of hypoxemia, intrapulmonary shunting, and reduced lung compliance. Inflammation and edema occur after injury. The combination of atelectasis, interstitial edema, and the presence of blood and fluid produce a decrease in pulmonary compliance and an increase in airway pressure. Hypercarbia does not increase airway pressure.

10. **C**

The diagnosis of pulmonary embolism (PE) is confirmed by a pulmonary angiogram, which is considered the most definitive diagnosis. A ventilation perfusion scan can recognize a high-probability ventilation/perfusion (V/Q) defect suspicious of a PE. A CT arteriogram (CTA) scan can demonstrate one or more filling defects or obstructions in the pulmonary artery or pulmonary artery branches. Chest x-ray (CXR) changes may be found but are nonspecific for a PE.

11. **C**

Lower respiratory rates would not be beneficial to the pulmonary contusion patient. If tidal volumes are decreased or the patient is placed on pressure control ventilation, the respiratory rate should actually be increased to maintain normal minute ventilation. The use of smaller tidal volumes to lower the peak and plateau pressures limits the trauma to the lungs. Positive end-expiratory pressure (PEEP) is favorable to improve oxygenation because it allows pressure to remain in the alveoli at end-expiration, recruits collapsed alveoli, and improves oxygenation. Pressure control ventilation limits barotrauma to the lungs, which occurs when ventilating with high tidal volumes and pressures.

12. **A**

Histologically, myocardial contusions are similar to myocardial infarctions because they both share myocardial cell necrosis, infiltration of leukocytes, absorption of hemorrhage, and healing by scar formation. Myocardial contusion is hemorrhage within the myocardium, marked by cellular injury. Hemorrhagic contusion is not recognized as a disease process. Pulmonary contusions and liver lacerations do not have these described properties.

13. **B**

There is no ischemic zone in myocardial contusions, there is only the necrotic zone followed by healthy tissue. Myocardial infarctions have a necrotic zone, followed by an ischemic zone, and end with healthy myocardial tissue.

14. **D**

Echocardiography, radionuclide angiography, transesophageal echocardiogram (TEE), 12-lead EKG, cardiac enzymes, and technetium scanning are all appropriate diagnostic studies to evaluate patients with suspected cardiac contusions.

15. **A**

Without adequate treatment, 40% of the patients with an aortic dissection die within hours of coming into the hospital, 75% within 3 weeks, and 90% by 10 weeks after injury. With operative intervention, the mortality rate is 15% to 25%.

16. **B**

The patient is exhibiting symptoms of a traumatic aortic aneurysm and the most common mechanism of injury is from sudden deceleration such as a fall or motor vehicle collision. The nurse should assess pulses of the upper and lower extremity because the patient could be presenting with pseudocoarctation syndrome. Pseudocoarctation presents with bounding pulses in the upper extremity with diminished pulses in the lower extremity. Traumatic aortic aneurysms patients do not typically experience symptoms that would require a papillary assessment, bowel sounds, or skin-color assessment to be completed before pulse checks.

17. C

Sonography is not typically used as a diagnostic test for a traumatic aortic aneurysm. A CT arteriography (CTA) of the chest is frequently used to diagnose the aortic injury. Aortography reveals the presence of aortic aneurysm and great vessel injuries, and is considered the "gold standard" for diagnosing a traumatic aortic aneurysm. Chest x-rays are used as a screening tool and would reveal a widened mediastinum, obliteration of the aortic knob, and obvious double-lumen contour of the aorta.

18. C

During cross-clamping of the aorta to repair the aortic transection, the organs that are usually perfused distal to the site of the cross-clamp may become hypoperfused, resulting in multiple organ failure. Partial left heart bypass is commonly used to move blood around the cross-clamped area to perfuse organs distal to the cross-clamp. A clamped aorta without distal canalization can be performed but the procedure has to be very quick to prevent hypoperfusion. Autologous grafts are not typically used and autotransfusion from chest tubes is not indicated in this surgical repair.

19. B

Myocardial infarction can occur because of the increased resistance to the heart with the cross-clamped aorta. Organ dysfunction can also occur during this procedure because of the risk of hypoperfusion below the clamp. All the other answers are potential complications of the surgical repair of an aorta but are not specifically the result of the cross-clamping of the aorta.

CHAPTER 5. ABDOMINAL TRAUMA

1. A

The abdominal cavity is actually divided into the peritoneal cavity and the retroperitoneal space. These organs are present in the peritoneal cavity of the abdomen. The retroperitoneal space contains the duodenum, ascending colon, descending colon, kidneys, part of the bladder, pancreas, and major vessels. The pleural space is the thin, fluid-filled space between the visceral and parietal areas of each lung, and does not contain any of these organs. The splenic flexor is not a compartment of the abdomen to contain organs.

2. B

A sudden increase in uniform pressure causes blunt abdominal trauma. Blunt abdominal trauma causes entrapment of organs between the vertebral column and the impacting forces. Solid organs commonly involved are the spleen, liver, and pancreas. The hollow organs, such as the stomach, tend to collapse with the increased pressure on the abdominal cavity. Kidney avulsion from the vascular supply is commonly a result of changes in organ position. Rib fractures may cause traumatic injuries to underlying organs in the abdomen, causing lacerations to the spleen, kidney, and liver.

3. **A**

When assessing the abdomen after a traumatic injury, percussion of the abdomen identifies the presence of dullness or hyperresonance. Hyperresonance indicates the presence of air and may reveal the type of injury present. If dullness is heard, this is indicative of fluid accumulation.

4. **D**

Liver injuries are scaled from grades I to VI. Lacerations that are 1 to 3 cm in length are categorized as grade II. Grades I to III are often successfully managed non-operatively and through close observation. Lacerations less than 1 cm are categorized as a grade I, lacerations greater than 3 cm and deep into the parenchyma are categorized as a grade III. Grades IV to VI typically result in surgical management of the liver.

5. **B**

CT is the most appropriate diagnostic study for the hemodynamically stable patient. CT of the abdomen with intravenous contrast aids in the diagnosis of active abdominal bleeding if the patient's presentation displays suspected abdominal bleeding. A plain CT of the abdomen would not show the vascular structures. Oral contrast CT scans reveal no significant benefit in the initial diagnosis and delays the treatment. Diagnostic peritoneal lavage (DPL) is a method used to detect intraabdominal bleeding and is best utilized in the hemodynamically unstable patient.

6. **B**

The insertion of a gastric tube decompresses the stomach, prevents aspiration, minimizes gastric leakage, and subsequently contaminates the abdominal cavity. A nasogastric tube allows for observation of blood in the aspirate, prevents (not increases) vagal stimulation and the resultant bradycardia.

7. **C**

Repeat or serial CT scans are usually ordered in patients with abdominal bleeding in order to evaluate the progression or stabilization of the bleeding, and to ensure a pseudoaneurysm does not develop. If a patient has abdominal distention, a CT scan may be warranted to evaluate the cause of the distention, but that is not a reason for serial or repeated CT scans in a patient with abdominal bleeding.

8. **B**

The nurse should never attempt to push abdominal contents back into the abdominal cavity; this increases the risk of infection. The care of the wound should be to place a sterile dressing over both the site and the intestines. Leaving it open to air causes drying and increases the risk of infection from exposure. Vaseline gauze is not recommended for the treatment of eviscerated intestines.

9. **D**

Abdominal distention, pain with palpation, and dullness to percussion would indicate further intraabdominal bleeding, which is the number one complication of a liver laceration. The liver is extremely vascular, hemorrhage and hemorrhagic shock are the most common complications in abdominal trauma, especially to the liver. Although the nurse should assess distal and proximal pulses for presence and quality, the correct answer should be looking for signs of hemorrhage following liver laceration. Localized pain to palpation and bony crepitus sites is seen in areas of a long bone fracture and splinting is required, but not with abdominal trauma. Loss of breath sounds indicate pneumothorax. A hemothorax is dullness on percussion of the chest cavity and is found when blood is present. This is an important part of the assessment when the nurse suspects bleeding into the pleural space, but the primary focus of the abdominal assessment is looking for signs of further bleeding from the liver laceration.

10. B

Solid organs are commonly associated with blunt abdominal trauma. Penetrating injuries commonly affect both solid and hollow organs, but most commonly affect the larger organs. Gunshot wounds are associated with a higher percentage of intraabdominal injuries and typically require surgery. Stab wounds to the abdomen require diagnostic studies to determine the need for surgical intervention.

11. C

Assessing the pain level is the most important missed assessment. Abdominal pain present following a trauma may indicate abdominal injuries. A negative examination does not preclude an injury. A change in bowel sounds is nonspecific to abdominal injuries. Auscultation of an abdominal bruit would be indicative of an arteriovenous fistula, atherosclerotic plaques within the arteries, or turbulent flow, but nonspecific for trauma. A rectal examination is extremely important and informative because it can elicit tenderness from an inflamed and swollen appendix, but lack of rectal tone is not indicative of abdominal injury.

12. A

The abdomen may sequester large amounts of fluid without marked abdominal distention. Patient manifestations of abdominal trauma are sometimes subtle. Abdominal injuries present with abdominal pain, tenderness, board-like abdomen, and absent bowel sounds.

13. A

A CT of the spine helps to diagnose or rule out spinal column damage in injured patients, but is not used to evaluate the abdomen. A CT of the abdomen allows the ability to view the retroperitoneal cavity as well as intraabdominal injuries, identify the organs involved, and grade the severity of the injuries. A chest x-ray (CXR) can identify free air in the upper abdomen, especially in a ruptured hollow organ, and can detect the presence of foreign bodies. An abdominal x-ray can identify retroperitoneal free air, gross organ injury, presence of blood in the abdominal cavity, and foreign objects.

14. C

Morbidly obese patients are not eligible for a laparoscopy, neither are patients in advanced pregnancy, those with pelvic injuries, previous abdominal surgeries, advanced cirrhosis, and coagulopathy because the risk of a conversion to a laparotomy is higher. A focused assessment with sonography for trauma (FAST) examination can estimate the amount of blood in the abdomen preventing unnecessary laparotomies, and can be performed in obese patients. Peritoneal lavage diagnoses occult intraabdominal bleeding in abdominal trauma patients but can result in false findings in obese patients. CT scanners have weight limits and might not be able to be used in morbidly obese patients.

15. **A**

Focused assessment with sonography for trauma (FAST) is indicated in trauma patients with suspected abdominal trauma. It allows evaluation in the emergency room without having to transport patients to radiology when hemodynamically unstable. FAST is used to evaluate the chest, abdomen, and pelvis, but is not used to evaluate the brain. It is used to detect the presence of perisplenic fluid, perihepatic and hepatorenal space fluid, pericardial tamponade, and fluid that may be present in the pelvis.

16. **C**

The neck is not an area where the focused assessment with sonography for trauma (FAST) examination would be beneficial. Neck diagnostic studies include plain radiographic studies, CT, MRI, and angiography. FAST is recommended in areas such as the chest, pelvis, peritoneum, flanks, and abdomen.

17. **D**

A delayed presentation of peritonitis is common with a duodenal tear because it spills alkaline fluid into the abdomen. As the fluid is alkaline, unlike acidic gastric fluid, the alkaline fluid causes less of an immediate irritation and delayed presentation of symptoms. Although patients in liver failure have an increased bilirubin level and jaundice, this typically does not occur within 2 days of the trauma. Gallstones are unlikely with this presentation of a trauma patient. The patient is febrile and has sepsis, but the source is more likely to be from peritonitis.

18. **D**

This would describe a grade IV splenic laceration. Grade I splenic injury includes a capsular tear less than 1 cm of parenchymal depth. Grade II is a 1- to 3-cm parenchymal injury without vessel involvement. Grade III is greater than 3-cm parenchymal depth or involvement of trabecular vessels. Grade V is a completely shattered spleen with devascularization. Grades I to III are less severe and are frequently managed with observation, not surgery.

19. **D**

Current evidence reveals that routine follow-up CT scans can be omitted in stable patients with blunt splenic trauma because they do not change the course of management. All of the others are proper interventions for this patient.

20. **C**

Always insert an indwelling bladder catheter using sterile technique. The transducer is leveled at the symphysis pubis. The patient should be in a supine position during measurement in order to reproduce and compare readings. Sterilely instill 35 to 50 mL of normal saline before obtaining the reading. Too much water causes bladder distention and an inaccurate reading. A normal bladder pressure reading is between 12 to 15 mmHg and a reading greater than 20 mmHg may require decompression of the abdomen.

21. D

A drain is usually placed for 8 to 10 days until the patient can tolerate feeding without an increase in pancreatic fluid. Pancreatectomies are hardly ever performed. It is possible to survive without a pancreas, but then patients are insulin dependent and require digestive enzymes. Debridement is avoided unless infected necrosis is present because it can potentially induce hemorrhage. Vaccinations are important for splenectomy patients but not for pancreatic injuries.

22. A

Following a splenectomy, the platelet count is typically elevated and can cause a thrombotic event such as a myocardial infarction or deep vein thrombosis. Postsplenectomy patients should be placed on a venous thromboembolism (VTE) prophylaxis medication such as Lovenox. Aspirin is considered an antiplatelet but is not a therapeutic anticoagulant. Neulasta is a medication that would increase the number of white blood cells (WBCs). This would be inappropriate because postsplenectomy patients typically have leukocytosis. For treatment of anemia, a daily dose of folic acid is generally used, but this patient is not anemic.

23. D

If the patient has had a splenectomy, a minor infection can potentially develop into a life-threatening infection. Postsplenectomy sepsis patients (overwhelming postsplenectomy sepsis [OPSS]) may occur within 1-year postsplenectomy, but also can occur several years later. The patient should be instructed to seek medical attention if experiencing fever, chills, nausea, vomiting, petechia, and palpitations. All of these are signs of possible sepsis and need immediate medical attention.

24. C

Pancreatic trauma is difficult to recognize because of coexisting injuries to other intraabdominal organs and pancreas's the retroperitoneal location, which makes signs and symptoms less obvious. The triad symptoms of pancreatic injury include midepigastric abdominal pain, leukocytosis, and elevated serum amylase levels. Lactate levels would not be routinely elevated, but are elevated in liver injury or septic patients.

25. A

Amylase levels are nonspecific to trauma injuries of the spleen and are not useful in diagnosing injuries. Hepatic injuries and duodenal injuries also have elevated amylase levels. Traumatic injuries to the face can have salivary gland involvement and present with an elevated amylase level. A raised amylase level after blunt pancreatic trauma is time dependent, and a persistently elevated or a rising amylase level is a more reliable indicator of pancreatic trauma, but it does not indicate the severity of the injury.

26. B

This laceration would be considered a grade II pancreatic laceration. Grade I laceration would be a superficial laceration without ductal injury. A grade III laceration would have distal transection or pancreatic parenchymal injury with ductal injury. A grade IV laceration would present with proximal transection or pancreatic parenchymal injury involving the ampulla. Lastly, a grade V laceration is a massive disruption of the pancreatic head.

27. **B**

Seat belt syndrome refers to the spectrum of injuries associated with lap belt restraints, particularly flexion–extension injuries to the spine. The child had a lap belt on, which created ecchymosis to the lower abdomen and potentially a cord injury. Pelvic fractures and cervical fractures are unlikely with this mechanism of injury. To avoid these injuries, a child should have a shoulder strap along with a lap belt on even in the backseat of a car.

28. **B**

A forceful injury may still result in injury to underlying organs without any evidence of rib fracture because in children the chest wall is more pliable, and the liver lays more anterior with less protection by the ribcage. Cardiac injury and renal injury are unlikely according to where the child was struck. However, renal injuries in children are common because of the lack of fat protection around the organs. A lung contusion is possible, but the liver is more likely to be damaged in this particular situation.

29. **B**

The focused assessment with sonography for trauma (FAST) examination would be the test of choice in pediatric patients with suspected intraabdominal trauma because it is a rapid evaluation of the abdomen for presence of fluid. Abdominal distention in a pediatric patient may not always be accurate, especially in a crying patient because children tend to swallow large amounts of air when crying. CT remains the imaging device of choice to evaluate suspected injuries in pediatric patients, but the FAST examination should be used first to evaluate whether further imaging may be warranted. Peritoneal lavage is not commonly performed in children, and a kidneys, ureter, and bladder (KUB) x-ray could be useful, but a CT is preferred if further diagnostic testing should occur.

CHAPTER 6. GENITOURINARY TRAUMA

1. **A**

The mechanism of injury is usually a crush injury of air-filled organs, such as the bowel, and fluid-filled organs, such as the bladder. These are the most commonly injured organs from the use of a seat belt. The stomach is located higher in the abdominal cavity and injury is less likely caused by a seat belt injury.

2. **B**

Bowel obstruction increases intraluminal pressure, which makes the bowel edematous, and in turn compromises arterial blood flow, leading to bowel ischemia. Bowel ischemia increases the risk of perforation, infection, and increases a patient's mortality rate. Nutrition is important and is addressed after a bowel obstruction is corrected. Decompressing the stomach with a nasogastric tube is significant, but tissue death because of ischemia is more important. An air or barium enema is used to enhance imaging of the colon that may be warranted for certain suspected causes of obstruction, but a soapsuds enema is not the most important.

3. B

The three classifications of bladder injuries are partial-thickness wall contusions, extra-peritoneal rupture, and intraperitoneal rupture. The classification is made based on a retrograde cystography or CT cystography. A pelvic x-ray is used to recognize pelvis fractures, but cannot identify bladder injuries. Bladder ultrasound and a kidneys, ureter, and bladder (KUB) x-ray will not identify bladder injuries.

4. D

Deceleration forces usually result in vascular damage to the renal artery. As there is minimal collateral circulation to the kidney, any type of ischemic injury could lead to tubular necrosis, but would not be the immediate injury for this patient. Bleeding injuries would be more likely if there has been a deep penetrating injury to the site. Rupture of the kidney presents in a hemorrhagic shock state.

5. B

The presentation of the patient can be mistaken for peritonitis; but the correct answer is ureteral injury. The clue would be the hematuria, elevated creatinine, and taking into account the mechanism of injury. Ureteral injures are only present with hematuria about 40% of the time, but are most common with penetrating-injury trauma patients. Kidney injury is possible but unlikely because there is no complaint of flank pain and the mechanism of injury would not match. Renal injuries are usually caused by deceleration, not penetration. Sepsis is inconclusive because of the incomplete workup, lack of white blood cell (WBC) count, and lactic acid level.

6. C

Straddle injuries occur when the bulbous urethra is compromised against the symphysis pubis, and usually result in a posterior urethral injury. Posterior injuries present with blood at the meatus, inability to void, bladder distention, butterfly bruising, and a high prostate with rectal examination for male patients. Anterior urethral injuries present with perianal pain, blood at the meatus, perianal edema, scrotal swelling in male patients, cellulitis, and ecchymosis. Buck's fascia surrounds the anterior urethra, corporal bodies, and penile skin. A medial urethral injury is not medically recognized.

7. D

Intravenous antibiotics are routinely administered for prophylaxis and should cover common urinary tract pathogens. Urethral catheters can remain for 2 to 3 weeks after primary repair. Suprapubic catheters can be maintained for 2 to 3 weeks for a straddle injury and 3 to 6 months for prostatomembranous injuries. Alpha-adrenergic blockers, such as tamsulosin (Flomax), are used for benign prostatic hyperplasia but not as a treatment for urethral tear.

CHAPTER 7. OBSTETRICAL TRAUMA

1. B

Pregnant women are at an increased risk for falls because they experience increased fatigue, relaxation of the pelvic girdle ligaments, altered balance, and gait disturbances. These cause balance issues, and an enlarged uterus with a growing belly shifts the body's center of gravity forward, making it even harder to stay upright. Syncopal episodes, bradycardia, and transient ischemic attacks (TIA) are not common reasons for falling and may be a complication.

2. **D**

Falls are the second leading cause of injury during pregnancy, not the second leading cause of mortality. Motor vehicle collision is the number one cause of death in pregnant women. Penetrating injuries cause trauma to the pregnant patient, with gunshot wounds having a higher mortality rate than stab wounds.

3. **B**

Estimation of gestational age and the presence of fetal heart tones should be done rapidly, emergency cesarean section (C-section) needs to be initiated within 5 minutes to improve survival of both the mother and fetus, and resuscitation measures need to be continued throughout the C-section. It is optimal for a neonate resuscitation team to be in the operating room when the baby is delivered. A vaginal or uterine examination would take too much time, would interfere with resuscitation efforts, and is meaningless because a C-section is going to occur.

4. **D**

Positioning the patient on the left lateral side increases circulation because it keeps the uterus off the vena cava, and allows for improved blood return and cardiac output, as well as flow to the fetus, uterus, and kidneys. The nurse may repeat the blood pressure, but it would be more effective if the nurse positioned the patient, and then repeated the blood pressure. Placing the patient in reverse Trendelenburg position increases the blood pressure, but placing on the left side promotes increased circulation to the fetus. Even if the patient is not symptomatic of hypotension, left-side positioning increases needed circulation and perfusion.

5. **A**

There are landmarks on the abdomen that helps to determine gestational age. The fundus measure for about 20-weeks gestation is the level of the umbilicus. If the fundus is located at the pubic symphysis, the patient is about 12-weeks pregnant, and about 36-weeks when at the xiphoid process of sternum.

6. **A**

The Kleihauer–Betke (KB) test is important for this particular patient because the patient is Rh negative. The KB test detects fetal red blood cells in maternal circulation, indicating fetal hemorrhage; the need for Rh immune globin therapy is imperative. A beta human chorionic gonadotropin (HCG) test is not very important because the trauma team already knows that the patient is 32-weeks pregnant. A prothrombin time (PT) and partial thromboplastin time (PTT), and hemoglobin and hematocrit (H & H) are significant to know in a bleeding patient and should be drawn as well, but because the patient is Rh negative the KB test is indicated for accurate treatment.

7. **A**

Preeclampsia is a pregnancy complication usually beginning after 20-weeks gestation and characterized by high blood pressure in a woman whose blood pressure had been previously normal. Patients commonly complain of headache, blurred vision, and epistaxis. Usually, organ dysfunction is involved, frequently the kidneys, therefore testing for protein in the urine is recommended. Eclampsia is the onset of seizures in a woman with preeclampsia. Pregnant women are usually hypervolemic because blood volumes increase by week 10 of pregnancy. This does not account for the symptoms this patient developed. Status preeclampsius is not a real complication.

8. **B**

Pregnant women frequently have cardiovascular changes during pregnancy. Blood volumes increase by 50% at week 34. Heart rates can increase by 15 beats per minute (bpm) to 20 bpm by the second trimester, therefore a heart rate of 65 bpm in the third trimester is considered bradycardic and is abnormal. EKG changes include inverted T waves, elevated ST segments, and Q waves because of the pressure of the diaphragm on the heart, which causes the heart to push upward and rotate.

9. **A**

Hematocrit may be lower in pregnant patients (30% to 40%). Anemia can occur because erythrocyte production cannot be maintained during pregnancy, and leukocyte level is usually slightly elevated, but not usually as high as 24,000. Glycosuria is common and considered normal in the pregnant patient. Calcium, phosphate, and magnesium levels may decrease while pregnant. Pregnant women have additional requirements, such as calcium, phosphate, and magnesium, because they are needed for the fetus's growing and developing body.

10. **D**

When a pregnant patient is in cardiac arrest, she is managed as if she were not pregnant. No cardiac arrest drugs such as epinephrine, amiodarone, or sodium bicarbonate are contraindicated and the code should be running normally as if the patient was not pregnant. The main difference is the need to assess viability of the fetus and perform an emergency cesarean section (C-section) during the resuscitation attempt.

11. **B**

These are normal arterial blood gas (ABG) readings for a pregnant patient. Normal parameters for pregnant women are: Ph of 7.35 to 7.45, PaO_2 of 101 mmHg to 104 mmHg, SaO_2 greater than 95%, $PaCO_2$ of 25 mmHg to 35 mmHg.

12. **A**

Fluid shifts along with uterus compression on the vena cava interrupting venous return tend to cause a fluid volume deficit leading to tissue hypoperfusion. Alteration in tissue perfusion for the pregnant patient can occur because of increased metabolism or hypovolemia (decrease in delivery and increase in demand). Premature labor can be a result of hypoperfusion, but is not typically a cause of it.

CHAPTER 8. MUSCULOSKELETAL TRAUMA

1. **B**

Stabilization of pelvic fractures is commonly performed by wrapping the pelvis in a folded sheet knotted or clamped at the front. The application of a pneumatic antishock garment to splint the unstable or open pelvic fracture may be used. Considerable blood loss requires immediate stabilization by external fixation. An air splint is filled with air and used to temporarily immobilize an injured extremity, not a pelvic fracture.

2. C

The forces that result in pelvic injuries include external rotation by anteroposterior rotation or abduction, shear, and lateral compression. Paying attention to both anatomic and biomechanical features is important in assessing pelvic fractures. Internal rotation is not considered a force that would cause a pelvic fracture.

3. B

Motor status assessment, neurovascular status assessment, stabilization of the extremity, immobilization of the extremity, and application of a sterile dressing to the open wound all take priority in an open femur fracture injury. Infection and osteomyelitis are complications of an open femur fracture but are not an early finding, and do not need to be assessed with the initial presentation of an open fracture.

4. B

The nurse should inspect for ecchymosis, muscle spasms, edema, nail-bed color, and capillary refill. The nurse should palpate for crepitus, pain, or muscle spasm, the presence of a pulse, and interruption in bone integrity.

5. D

Proper immobilization includes immobilization above and below the level of injury. This technique provides the best stabilization of the extremity. Immobilization devices should be checked frequently for effectiveness, the extremity monitored for swelling, and to ensure splints are padded appropriately to prevent further injury. Immobilizing the actual injury can cause further damage to the site.

6. B

The nurse should notify the physician of the need for pain management so that proper irrigation and cleansing can be performed with the patient as comfortable as possible. The initial wound care includes removal of gross contaminates from the wound and covering exposed bone or tissue with a sterile saline dressing. The patient should be informed of the importance of cleaning the debris and the significance of treatment and infection prevention; however, pain is the fifth vital sign and should be addressed. A significant complication of fractures is infection, therefore antibiotics are indicated, but the wound still requires appropriate cleansing.

7. A

If there is vascular or nerve involvement associated with a humeral fracture, it usually is caused by the axillary nerve or axillary artery. Rarely, the brachial artery, brachial plexus, or radial artery are involved with a shoulder injury. Identification of an anterior or posterior bulge may suggest a dislocation. Tenderness and swelling often are diffuse, making it difficult to detect clear point tenderness. Neurologic and vascular examinations of the upper extremity should be performed completely.

8. **B**

Anterior dislocation is almost always traumatic and is usually from falls. It is the most common shoulder dislocation experienced after a traumatic event. A fracture of the humeral head, neck, or greater tuberosity can occur at the same time. Posterior dislocation is less common and is generally caused by forces applied, although the shoulder is held in internal rotation and adduction positions. This injury may be seen in violent seizure activity. Inferior, superior, and intrathoracic shoulder dislocations can also occur but are extremely rare.

9. **D**

Distal pulses may still be present because of the extensive collateral flow of the arm. The arm would be cool to the touch and have absent axillary pulses. There is usually a hematoma present in the axillary region. Although this complication is very rare, consider it if a brachial plexus injury is identified, especially in patients older than 50 years of age.

10. **C**

Altered sensation, altered mobility, vascular compromise, and pain are early complications of an open fracture. Late complications are associated complications frequently with issues of prolonged immobilization such as contractures.

11. **A**

Considering the mechanism of injury, thoracolumbar vertebral compression fractures should be suspected. The upward force of the impact when the patient jumped compressed the vertebral bodies causing burst fractures. Sacral, pelvic, and femur fractures are all possibilities, but vertebral fracture should have the highest suspicion.

12. **D**

The impact of the injury to the patella may also cause an associated posterior hip fracture or dislocation, popliteal artery injury, and a femur fracture in the affected leg.

13. **D**

Neurovascular injury should be suspected with any injury to a bony extremity, especially with dislocation. Nerves, arteries, veins, and soft tissue injuries may be compromised when an extremity fracture occurs and need to be evaluated. Cranial and vertebral injury can be present with extremity trauma, but this depends on the mechanism of injury. However, this is not likely the answer here because no mechanism of injury was given in this scenario.

14. **B**

A traction splint would be most appropriate for tibial and femur fractures. Rigid splints are made of plastic, metal, or cardboard and are used for extremities such as an injured forearm. Soft splints are devices like air splints and slings used to treat an injured arm, wrist, or hand. Contraction splint is not a recognized splint type.

15. **B**

It is important to avoid excessive movement of the fractured bone fragments because this can increase the risk of bleeding, fat emboli, and movement can also convert a closed fracture to an open fracture. An open fracture is already a displaced fracture.

16. **B**

Open fractures can be irrigated with normal saline and a sterile dry dressing applied to the site. However, frequent dressing changes are contraindicated because they increase the risk of bacterial contamination with each wound exposure. Monitoring the site for bleeding is standard and a marked increase in bleeding should prompt the nurse to notify the physician of the change. To decrease the risk of infection, antibiotics and a tetanus shot are frequently ordered with open fracture.

17. **A**

An alteration in tissue perfusion can be related to vessel compression, interruption of circulatory flow, and hypovolemia. The nursing interventions described are indicated to achieve expected outcomes of adequate capillary refill, normal skin assessment, strong pulses, and the absence of pain and motor paralysis. Impaired physical mobility interventions would be the actual splinting, positioning, and pain management. Nursing interventions for impaired skin integrity would include the actual application of the splint, assessing skin integrity, and maintaining aseptic technique. Fluid volume deficits require interventions, such as the administration of intravenous fluids and blood products, but would not include correction of the constricting devices that impair adequate circulation.

18. **A**

During the initial injury, fluid shifts into the tissue surrounding the injury, causing edema, which compromises surrounding structures. This is part of the injury, not the repair. The body's physiological mechanisms that aid in minimizing damage include the initiation of the clotting system, restoration of cellular membranes to improve fluid reabsorption, and collateral circulation to improve blood flow and promote healing.

19. **B**

Femur fractures can result in a collection of 1,000 mL to1,500 mL of blood in the thigh. Femur fractures present with pain, shortening of the affected leg, external or internal rotation, edema or deformity of the thigh, and possible neurovascular compromise. Tibial fractures lose up to approximately 750 mL of blood. Hip dislocation and vertebral fractures cause minimal blood loss.

20. **D**

An impacted fracture has distal and proximal fracture sites wedged into each other. A displaced fracture has proximal and distal fracture edges out of alignment, a greenstick fracture occurs when the bone buckles or bends, and a complete fracture is when there is total interruption in bony continuity.

21. **B**

This patient's injury is a grade II. Grade II involves an open fracture with a wound greater than 2 cm with the presence of a slight crush injury. Grade I open fracture has minimal tissue damage, and grade III open fractures has an extensive soft tissue damage and a high risk of severe contamination such as osteomyelitis, sepsis, and poor wound healing. There is no grade IV open fracture category.

22. B

Ischemic pain is described as burning and throbbing in the injured extremity. Compartment syndrome pain is a type of ischemic pain, and is usually out of proportion to the injury and present on passive range of motion to the affected side. Patients with nerve compression usually report decreased pain and sensation. Crush injury patients usually report intense pain and a tingling sensation in the area. Muscle spasm is frequently described as sharp or cramping.

23. A

To provide adequate stabilization of the pelvic binder, it should be placed at the level of the greater trochanters. The binder should not be placed over the iliac crest or the abdomen. Application of a pelvic binder above the level of the greater trochanters is an inadequate method of reducing pelvic fractures and is likely to delay cardiovascular recovery.

24. D

Subtrochanteric fracture is a fracture of the proximal femur, categorized as a hip fracture, not a pelvis fracture. A straddle injury is an injury to the bilateral pubic rami that occurs when a person falls while straddling an object. It is associated with urethral and bladder injuries. Open-book pelvic injury occurs when the front of the pelvis opens like a book, this injury results in damage to pelvic ligaments that hold the pelvic bones together as well as major arteries. Vertical shear pelvis injury occurs when one half of the pelvis shifts upward.

25. B

Destot's sign is the presence of a hematoma above the inguinal ligament, over the scrotum, or in the upper thigh and is associated with pelvic fractures. Murphy's sign refers to a maneuver used during an abdominal examination. It is useful for differentiating pain in the right upper quadrant, especially in cholecystitis. Earle's sign is a bony prominence or large hematoma noted on rectal examination. Roux's sign is a decrease in the distance from the greater trochanter to the pubic spine on the affected side in a lateral compression fracture.

26. D

Fat emboli occur when fat globules are filtered out of the pulmonary system and obstruct at the pulmonary capillary level. This causes release of oxygen free radicals, increased capillary permeability, vasodilation, and pulmonary interstitial edema, which results in acute respiratory distress syndrome (ARDS). ARDS is inflammation that occurs throughout the lungs. In the lung tissue, tiny blood vessels leak fluid, and alveoli collapse or fill with fluid, which prevents adequate oxygen exchange. The development of pneumonia would require an infectious source, such as bacteria. Chronic obstructive pulmonary disorder (COPD) is a progressive respiratory disease that makes it harder to breathe over time. Sepsis would also need a source of infection and by itself does not result in pulmonary edema.

27. A

A patient with a fat embolus presents with a productive cough and coarse crackles because of the inflammation and the fluid leakage into the alveoli, which cause the alveoli to fill with fluid. A dry cough with scattered rhonchi would indicate a patient with asthma, bronchitis, or pneumonia. Productive cough with diminished breath sounds could belong to multiple diagnoses, including pneumonia. Dry cough with inspiratory wheezes is usually identified in asthma patients.

28. D

Right bundle branch block, depressed ST segments, and inverted T waves are all changes that would be seen on EKG when a patient has a fat embolus because the embolus causes right heart strain and increased pulmonary resistance. Because of this, dysrhythmias, S waves in lead I, and Q waves in lead III may also be present.

29. B

Appearance of petechiae usually occurs on the upper trunk, axilla, chest, conjunctiva, and mucous membranes. This is because the embolization of small dermal capillaries leads to extravasation of erythrocytes, which produces a petechial rash in these areas. Petechiae do not commonly appear on the upper extremities with fat emboli.

30. A

Pain is the most sensitive indicator of compartment syndrome because it is known to be reported as out of proportion to the injury, and is not relieved with analgesic medication administration. Paresthesia would be the second most sensitive sign, followed by pulselessness and paralysis together, which are strong indications for compartment syndrome.

31. C

Pressure readings less than 20 mmHg are considered normal, although pressures greater than 30 mmHg require immediate surgical evaluation. Even though this patient's compartmental pressure is only 28 mmHg, the patient is hypotensive, which indicates a greater perfusion deficit even with lower compartmental pressures. The intervention would be a surgical evaluation for potential fasciotomy. Close observation, frequent assessment, and pain management should be performed, but the surgical evaluation is needed because of the hypotension and the higher compartmental pressure reading.

32. D

Serum creatine phosphokinase (CPK) and urinary myoglobin measurements are frequently inappropriately ordered in patients with compartment syndrome. These tests are specific to muscle injury, but not to compartment syndrome. There is no definitive lab test that would diagnose compartment syndrome, only symptoms and compartmental pressure readings.

33. A

Elevating the extremity would decrease perfusion and would not promote adequate circulation to the extremity with compartment syndrome. Maintain the extremity in a neutral position and remove constricting clothing, casts, or dressings that may be present to correct management of an extremity with suspected compartment syndrome.

34. B

Infection is not a complication of untreated compartment syndrome patients. Infection would be a complication of having a fasciotomy because of compartment syndrome. Volkmann contracture occurs when there is ischemia to the forearm from the increased pressure and ischemia from compartment syndrome. Swelling presses on blood vessels and can decrease blood flow to the arm. A prolonged decrease in blood flow injures the nerves and muscles, causing them to become scarred, and leads to gross muscle necrosis. Amputation would be a complication from untreated compartment syndrome, because of the lack of circulation to the area and severe muscle necrosis.

35. B

Reperfusion injuries to muscle occur when there is an increased blood flow to the muscle following a period of ischemia, resulting in the washout of lipid-soluble intracellular metabolites. These metabolites can cause further injury called *reperfusion injury*. Inadequate decompression is a complication of a fasciotomy. Volkmann contracture is a complication of untreated compartment syndrome. Hypoperfusion occurs during compartment syndrome but is not associated with an increased blood flow.

36. B

An avulsive injury is a result of a forceful stretching, twisting, or tearing away of tissue and bone, resulting in an amputation. A cut or guillotine type of amputation has well-defined edges. A crush amputation involves more soft tissue damage of the amputated part.

37. B

Initial emergency care for an amputated body part in the emergency room includes rinsing with isotonic solution, wrapping in sterile gauze or moistening with aqueous penicillin, wrapping in a moist sterile towel, placing in a plastic bag, and then placing on crushed ice. Do not freeze the part by directly placing it in ice or adding coolants like dry ice. Never float a part in a bag of solution and do not use antiseptics, hydrogen peroxide, iodine, or other solutions.

38. C

Partial amputation occurs when bone, muscle, or ligament remain attached to the body. Partial amputations should be treated as if fully intact and eligible for reimplantation. Partial amputations are managed by splinting the attached part, applying a saline-moistened sterile dressing, applying pressure to control bleeding, and placing oximetry on a distal part to monitor oxygen saturation.

39. B

Choices between amputation and reimplantation are usually based on clinical presentation and the limb involved. Fingers have less muscle and more tendon, which is less susceptible to ischemia and results in better reimplantation outcomes. Fingers are good candidates for reimplantation and are more commonly reimplanted than hands. Clinical variables include the extent of tissue damage, duration of limb ischemia, hypotension, age (older victims tend to not do well), preservation of protective sensation, of potential of limb length discrepancy and vascular injury.

40. B

When the continuity of major vessels is damaged, such as the sciatic or posterior tibial artery, reimplantation becomes less of an option. Lower extremities are not usual candidates for reimplantation because of the risk of two different lengths of legs, which would adversely affect the ability to ambulate. The loss of sensation to the sole of the foot because of nerve injury can make the reimplanted foot unable to be used for ambulation.

41. C

Toes are rarely reimplanted unless multiple toes or the big toe are lost. The scalp, penis, nose, extremity, hand, and foot can be potential candidates for reimplantation.

42. B

The occupational and functional value of the digit or extremity is a part of the decision making for reimplantation. The occupational and functional value of the extremity or digit is evaluated when determining the need to attempt reimplantation of the extremity. Bilateral hands, thumb, multiple digits, dominate hand, amputation proximal to the most distal interphalangeal are associated with a high occupational value, and should be considered for reimplantation.

43. C

Prophylactic antibiotics are usually ordered for 2 to 5 days postoperatively, 14 days would be out of the norm. Postoperative care for the reimplantation patient should include frequent Doppler tones, pulse oximetry, neurovascular checks, antiplatelet or anticoagulation therapy such as heparin or aspirin, heat lamps, and heating pads. Leech therapy is sometimes utilized to vasodilate and anticoagulate to improve venous outflow.

44. A

The proper method for leech therapy is to puncture the site to initiate bleeding, attach the leech and wrap with gauze to prevent migration. The leech is allowed to feed until it detaches on its own, which is usually 10 to 20 minutes. Remove the leech, place in an alcohol-filled container, and dispose with other waste material. Never reuse the leech because of risk of infection. Do not forcefully detach the leech because it can regurgitate and cause a wound infection.

45. B

Systemic complications occur after the release of the compressive forces, causing blood flow to reperfuse the injured area, releasing chemical mediators. Hypovolemia can occur because of the shift of fluid from the vascular to the interstitial space. Compartment syndrome can occur because of the increased pressure within the damaged compartments of the extremity. Rhabdomyolysis is the breakdown of muscle following the crush mechanism. This releases myoglobin into the blood, which is then filtered by the kidneys, resulting in acute renal failure. Coagulopathy can occur following a trauma, but not necessarily a hypercoagulable state.

46. C

Administration of calcium following a crush syndrome can be harmful to the patient's kidneys because there is a greater concentration of calcium intracellularly. Infusions of mannitol cause osmotic diuresis and may be used to flush the myoglobin through the kidneys. Diamox is a diuretic usually administered in conjunction with mannitol to prevent serum alkalosis. Sodium bicarbonate may also be administered to alkalinize the urine and decrease the renal toxicity of myoglobin.

47. D

The description and mechanism of injury here is of an abrasion. Abrasions are no deeper than the dermis and occur with rubbing or friction against hard objects or surfaces. Traumatic tattooing is also an abrasion, but debris gets trapped under the dermis or epidermis and causes discoloration that sometimes requires surgical intervention. An avulsion is a full-thickness injury, and a contusion is a closed wound that results from ruptured blood vessels.

48. A

A complex laceration is a type of compression energy injury that causes potential complications of infection, scarring, devitalized tissue, and compartment syndrome. Complications from avulsions include tissue ischemia, moderate scarring, infection, and vascular disruption. Punctures and abrasions are types of shearing injury and involve minimal scarring and minimal risk of compartment syndrome.

49. C

Human saliva can cause both gram-positive and gram-negative organisms, therefore, antibiotic coverage should be for both. Puncture wounds such as bites are grossly contaminated and require both wound care and antibiotics.

50. B

Wound irrigation is the most important step in initial wound care because it is effective in reducing bacterial contamination and decreases the risk of infection. Copious irrigation with normal saline is recommended to thoroughly clean a wound. Wound cleansing may only remove visible contaminants and some antiseptics can cause delayed wound healing. Hair clipping facilitates wound cleansing but is not as important as irrigation. Antibiotic administration is controversial because it is only prophylactic until cultures are obtained.

51. D

Aftercare treatment is the last of the four steps and includes all of the wound care described in addition to educating the patient on signs of infection, proper wound care, dressing changes, and follow-up wound assessments. Hemostasis is the first step and involves controlling the bleeding. Wound preparation comes next and this includes irrigation, cleansing, hair clipping, anesthetics, antibiotics, culture, and possible debridement or exploration. Wound closure, if indicated, is next and there are many methods that may be utilized to achieve the least-invasive method of closure.

52. B

Ulcerations, punctures, full- or partial-thickness abrasions, and some human bite wounds are best healed by secondary intention because of the high risk of wound contamination. Lacerations are usually treated by primary intention or delayed primary intention in which cleaning, irrigation, debridement, and antibiotics are administered for 3 to 5 days before closure is conducted.

CHAPTER 9. SURFACE AND BURN TRAUMA

1. A

Cigarette-smoking accidents are the number one cause of fatal fires. This is typically because a person carelessly discards or abandons the smoking materials and end up igniting trash, bedding or upholstered furniture. Cooking equipment is the leading cause of home fires and of injuries in home fires. Candle fires are not very common, but one out of three fatal candle fires in the home occurred when the candles were used for light because the power was out. Incidence of arson has decreased over the past 30 years, but remains the leading cause of property damage in the United States.

2. D

The upper extremity of the body is the most commonly burned area of the body, followed by the head-and-neck regions. This may be the result of using the arms in an attempt to shield the face or body or in carrying flammable material/explosives. Lower extremities tend to be the least commonly burned body part.

3. B

This accurately describes the zone of stasis. If resuscitation is promptly initiated following a burn injury, it may restore blood flow to the zone of stasis, allowing tissue to survive. The zone of hyperemia involves the most peripheral and superficial areas of the burn; it is erythema of a first-degree burn. The zone of coagulation is the area that contains irreversible cell death and involves the most severe burn area, which had the most intimate contact with the heat source.

4. C

Full-thickness burns are as also called third- and fourth-degree burns. These burns may have charring, dark brown, or white skin and will be hard to the touch. Pain is usually only present at the periphery of the burn. Superficial burns (first-degree) have red skin and pain at the site. Partial-thickness (second-degree) burns have blisters, intense pain, white, or red skin and is moist or mottled but does not involve muscle or bone.

5. B

The resuscitative phase begins with the hemodynamic response and lasts until capillary integrity is restored and the plasma volume is replaced. The acute phase starts with the onset of diuresis of edematous fluid mobilized from the interstitial space and continues until the closure of the burn wound. The last phase, the rehabilitation phase, includes prevention and correction of functional deficits, contracture releases, psychological support, and job retraining. The recovery phase is not a recognized phase of the three phases of burn shock.

6. D

The greatest amount of fluid loss for partial-thickness burns occurs on the first day of injury (within 24 hours). Full-thickness burns have the greatest fluid loss at 4 days postburn.

7. **C**

The intravascular fluid shifts actually cause a fluid deficit and a decrease in cardiac output. Hemoconcentration, not hemodilution, is a result of the fluid shifts occurring with burn shock. Hypercoagulopathy with platelet aggregation occurs with burn shock, resulting in decreased organ perfusion. Compensatory response begins with increasing peripheral resistance and the release of catecholamines.

8. **B**

The hypermetabolic response following a burn results in hyperglycemia, negative nitrogen balance, catabolism, and increased oxygen consumption. During the hypermetabolic state, burn patients frequently experience hypoproteinemia not hyperproteinemia.

9. **C**

Glomerular filtration rate is frequently decreased in burn patients. Red blood cells (RBCs) are destroyed from the heat, so RBCs will be lower than normal. There will be a decrease in platelet count, not an increased platelet count. Fibrinogen level will also be decreased following a major burn.

10. **C**

Peritonitis is not a systemic response to burn injuries because it is usually caused by a bacterial or fungal infection that occurs in the peritoneum. Sepsis is a systemic complication resulting in multisystem organ failure (acute respiratory distress syndrome [ARDS] and acute kidney injury).

11. **B**

The patient with a second-degree burn should be medicated for pain. This patient is hemodynamically stable with an uncompromised airway and adequate evidence of perfusion. A dressing is already applied and the intravenous fluids may be continued with the management of pain.

12. **A**

A patient with carbon monoxide poisoning should be immediately placed on 100% FiO_2 (fraction of inspired oxygen). This will accelerate the clearance of the carbon monoxide and promote oxygenation, oxygen carrying by hemoglobin, and tissue perfusion.

13. **B**

The least important information would be whether any others were involved. The cause of the burn will aid in treatment modality and assessing for complications such as inhalation injury. The time of the injury is important to determine the fluid resuscitation. Noxious chemical involvement is important because it will also change the treatment modality and give possible indication of inhalation injury.

14. **A**

The Parkland formula is: $4 \times$ weight (kg) $\times$ body surface area. In this patient: 4×70 kg $\times 40 = 11,200$ mL. Hint: The 154 pounds needs to be converted to kilograms by dividing 154 by 2.2.

15. **A**

The nurse should administer half of the total needed fluid in the first 8 hours. Then the remainder should be administered over 16 hours. If 14,000 mL are required, 7,000 mL are administered in the first 8 hours and then 7,000 mL should be infused over 16 hours.

16. **B**

Hoarseness, stridor, audible airway, and sputum are indicative of the potential for a significant respiratory injury from inhalation. Upper airway edema is present in this patient because of the hoarse voice and the audible stridor. Racemic epinephrine every 2 to 4 hours is the needed physician order to treat this patient. Indications for intubation include an acute airway obstruction, copious secretions, or lower airway inhalation injury; this patient is presenting with an upper airway injury at this time, so intubation may not be necessary. There might be a need for this patient to have a laryngoscopy to assess the pharynx and vocal cords; however, the better choice is the racemic epinephrine because results of the medication will be faster acting to address the upper airway compromise. The nurse should keep the patient's head elevated at all times, but this is not as important as treating the bronchosconstriction. There is nothing in the scenario that would indicate the need for immediate intubation. Bronchoscopy is not indicated in this patient.

17. **D**

Early intubation for protection of airway would be indicated for a patient in respiratory distress from cyanide poisoning. Pulse oximetry is sometimes unreliable in carbon monoxide and cyanide poisoning so the saturation is probably less than 94% on a nonrebreather mask. Management would include using a cyanide kit, which contains amyl nitrate, sodium nitrate, and sodium thiosulfate, not sulfur nitrate.

18. **B**

Electrical burns may cause changes in the lenses within the eyes, resulting in complications such as cataracts. Electrical burn patients commonly experience associated neurological injuries and cardiac abnormalities as a result of the electrical current. Hearing loss is not frequently associated with electrical burns.

19. **A**

Urine output should be maintained between 50 and 100 mL/hr with electrical burn patients. If the pigment of the urine darkens as a result of the presence of myoglobin or hemoglobin, this can lead to renal dysfunction and possible failure. If the urine does turn dark, then the intravenous fluids are typically increased to increase the urine output and flush the toxins.

20. **C**

After initial stabilization, it is recommended that the urine output in an electrical burn patient, with absence of dark pigmentation, be maintained at 0.5 to 1 mL/kg/hr. For example, a patient who weighs 77 kg should have a urine output of 39 to 77 mL/hr.

21. C

Fluid resuscitation measurements cannot be calculated correctly in electrical burn patients because there is internal damage and equations using the total body surface area burned to calculate fluid administration volume are inaccurate. The fluids should be set at a rate that maintains urinary output of 75 to 100 mL/hr. Administering fluids at TKO (to keep open) rate would result in significant hypovolemia.

22. D

Burn-wound care should start with an antiseptic cleansing and debridement of loose nonviable skin. Topical antimicrobial agents are routinely applied to the site of the burn wound. Silvadene is the most commonly used antimicrobial and is well absorbed in burn wounds, it is painless but ineffectiveagainst deep burn infections. Sulfamylon provides good penetration of tissue and eschar and is routinely used with cartilage such as ears. Bursting blisters is not recommended unless a blister is very large and would increase the probability of infection.

23. B

Pulmonary edema is a complication of burns because of the inhalation injury and fluid resuscitation. Hyperkalemia (not hypokalemia) and hyponatremia (not hypernatremia) are common complications because of the fluid shift and capillary leakage. Hypothermia, not hyperthermia, commonly occurs because of the large portion of skin injured, resulting in loss of body heat.

24. B

The extent and speed of capillary refill is the most useful clinical method to assess the depth of the burn wound. With a gloved hand, blanch the site, if capillary refill is rapid, it usually indicates a superficial burn because of the increased blood supply to the area. The presence of capillary refill at the time of initial assessment does not mean that the burn will remain superficial, as time passes evolution of the burn may transform it into a deeper burn. Temperature of the wound can be useful because cooler wounds tend to be deeper wounds due to the decreased blood supply but is not as important as capillary refill. Palpation of the site is important because deeper burns have more damage to nocioceptors and will present with less pain than superficial burns, which are always painful due to the mixture of depths in burn wounds. Laser Doppler technique targets blood supply waves to assess wound depth, however, this technology is costly and sometimes not readily available.

25. A

An endotracheal tube is an appropriate airway management for burn patients with airway swelling; securing it with umbilical tape is the preferred method for this particular patient. Adhesive tape typically cannot adhere to the burns. Umbilical tape has cotton fibers that can ensure security of the endotracheal tube. Cricothyroidotomy is usually performed as a last resort in cases in which orotracheal intubation is impossible or contraindicated.

26. B

Infants and young children should receive crystalloid solution fluid resuscitation using the formula in addition to 5% dextrose at an infusion maintenance rate. Pediatric patients have limited glycogen storage, which is quickly exhausted during early post burn stages, therefore they require more blood sugar stability versus adult burn patients.

27. A

Setting the water heater at 120°F or below is recommended to avoid childhood burns. Instructing the parents to test the water before the child gets into the tub and placing a thermometer in the water are positive suggestions; but the water heater is a safety feature that can also prevent additional burns that could be acquired by other water sources in the home. The parents should aim for bath water at around 100°F for children. By prohibiting manipulation of the hot water, safety features for the faucet handles only mask the initial problem.

28. C

Burn patients typically develop poikliothermia in which they pickup the temperature of the environment. The skin injury results in the loss of heat so maintaining a room temperature of 86 degrees assists with the control of normal temperature for the patient. Applying ice to burn wounds is not recommended. Applying a cool dressing to the site within 10 minutes of the burn may be effective because it reduces the heat content and depth of the burn and relieves pain; but does not aid in the actual temperature regulation of the patient. Topical lidocaine is not recommended on burn wounds.

29. B

Patients with an alteration in capillary permeability have a fluid volume deficit so replacing their circulating volume with crystalloid solutions and blood products is warranted. The patient can be positioned with the legs elevated to determine responsiveness to fluid. Placing the patient in reverse Trendelenburg position will decrease venous return and may worsen the hemodynamic status.

30. B

Plasma colloid osmotic pressure is responsible for pulling fluid into the capillaries. Hydrostatic pressure forces the fluid out of the capillary at the arterial end. Interstitial free fluid pressure responds by pulling fluid out of the capillary when pressure is negative and forcing fluid back in when the pressure is positive. Interstitial fluid osmotic pressure pulls fluid out of the capillary.

31. C

Laryngospasm is more commonly associated with inhalation injuries than electrical burns. Spinal, long bone, and vertebral compression fractures are usually affiliated with electrical injuries because of violent skeletal muscle contractions during the electrocution.

32. B

Chemical exposure usually causes an inhalation injury below the level of the glottis as opposed to a thermal injury. Thermal injuries are usually limited to the upper airway. Superheated air causes laryngospasm, which closes the glottis and protects the lungs. Steam inhalation poses greater damage to the upper airway because steam has a greater heat-carrying capacity.

33. D

Histamine causes vasodilation and increased capillary permeability. Thromboxane A results in activation of platelets and prothrombotic properties, leukotrienes contribute to the inflammatory response, and bradykinin causes vasodilation but not necessarily an increase in capillary permeability.

34. B

The number of red blood cells is diminished because of hemolysis, but the blood viscosity increases because the percentage of red blood cells is higher, causing increased friction to the cells. There is an increase in peripheral resistance due to hypovolemia and increased blood viscosity.

35. B

Hypermetabolism occurs frequently in a burn patient and is evidenced by tachypnea, tachycardia, and a low-grade fever related to the increased sympathetic response. Hypometabolism will have the opposite physiological responses and does not commonly occur with burn patients. The patient with carbon monoxide poisoning and hypoxemia will have more problems with decreased oxygenation.

36. B

An alternating current is more dangerous because it does not travel in one straight direction but can periodically reverse direction, causing the victim's grip to tighten, strengthening the electrical source and lengthening the exposure to the current. This injury was caused by alternating current; so tetany caused by direct current is not the correct answer.

37. B

Nerves are the first structures that current can pass through, followed by blood vessels, muscles, skin, tendons, fat, and, lastly, bone because bone does not conduct electricity well.

38. B

Following an inhalation injury, the airway needs to be secured and respiration managed with mechanical ventilation. Positive-end expiratory pressure (PEEP) delivered with mechanical ventilation is the best was to assure adequate oxygenation by increasing end-expiratory pressure and recruiting alveoli. A nonrebreather mask is used initially for the administration of high-flow oxygen, but this does not secure the airway. Continuous positive airway pressure (CPAP) is used to maintain alveolar inflation and assist with oxygenation, but again does not secure the airway. Oxygen delivery should be humidified and warmed to reduce hypothermia but requires an airway, not just a face mask.

39. B

Cleansing burn wounds with mild soap and lukewarm water, applying a topical antimicrobial agent with silver such as silvadene, debridement of nonviable tissue, leaving blisters intact, and clipping hair around the wound are all proper techniques for burn victims with less than 15% total body surface area (TBSA) burn wounds. Shaving the eyebrows is not recommended because they may never grow back and they serve as landmarks.

40. D

Sodium thiosulfate is an intravenous substance administered to treat cyanide poisoning. Hyperbaric oxygen therapy delivers 100% oxygen under high pressure to patients with inhalation injuries from carbon monoxide, cyanide poisoning, carbon tetrachloride poisoning and hydrogen sulfide poisoning.

41. D

Cyanide poisoning should be suspected in this type of injury because of the type of substance that was burned. Textiles, polyurethane, and plastics can be a source of hydrogen cyanide. The inhalation of amyl nitrate and the intravenous administration of sodium nitrate will convert iron into methemoglobin, which attracts cyanide molecules, allowing the cyanide to free up cytochrome oxidase to participate in cellular production.

42. B

Patients with phenol contamination should be treated with copious amounts of irrigation to the site. Absorption of this substance can cause renal damage so blood urea nitrogen (BUN) and creatinine levels should be tested. Myoglobin and serum bicarbonate levels are usually monitored in patients with electrical burns. Serum calcium is depleted by hydrofluoric acid chemical burns and is monitored in those exposures.

43. D

Observing vital signs is part of the nurse's role in monitoring for anxiety but this is not a correct answer for reducing anxiety and fear. Facilitating family presence during care delivery, encouraging patients and families to openly express concerns and ask questions, and obtaining a referral for social services can aid in reducing fear and anxiety of the patient and family.

44. D

Avoiding unnecessary exposure and maintaining a warmer room temperature are appropriate interventions for the burn patient because this patient is at risk for hypothermia. Monitoring for signs and symptoms of compartment syndrome is appropriate because of the increased risk. Escharotomies are important for circumferential burns but the nurse would assist with the procedure, not perform it.

CHAPTER 10. PSYCHOSOCIAL ISSUES OF TRAUMA

1. B

The resuscitative phase occurs early following the trauma and the patient experiences fear of death or disability, loss of self-control, severe pain, avoidance behaviors, agitation, hostility, and overall negativity. The second phase is the critical care phase, which includes fear of altered function rather than fear of death, severe pain, sleep deprivation, and anxiety, which Mrs. Jack is currently experiencing. The last phase is the recovery phase and it includes the patient dealing with the losses, feeling "powerless," experiencing stages of grief, and relying on a support system. Community phase is not an identified phase of psychological progression in trauma care.

2. **D**

Although a trauma patient will frequently exhibit feelings of frustration, it is not identified as a part of the grieving process. The most widely accepted process of grieving includes denial, anger, bargaining, depression, and acceptance. Understanding the grieving process is important for nurses so they can recognize symptoms of grief and manage the behaviors of patients and their families during this time.

3. **C**

Promising the family that they "won't miss anything" is unreliable. The nurse should not "promise" that the patient's status will not change, or that a physician might not come in during time frame when they are gone. It is more effective to keep contact numbers visible and obtainable at bedside, call the family with updates, educate them about what to expect, encourage them to take a break and conserve energy for when the patient leaves the intensive care unit (ICU), and set up physician/family meetings to keep everyone on the same page with the plan of care.

4. **C**

Teach the family not to correct or argue with the traumatic brain-injured patient, especially when agitated. Teaching the family to communicate slowly, calmly, and in short sentences aids in lowering frustration and can help with agitation. Allow the patient to talk, but use distraction to change subjects to favorite hobbies or interests when the patient begins to become agitated. Encouraging the patient to talk about old memories provides comfort, especially with patients who are experiencing short-term memory loss.

5. **D**

Depression is a common psychosocial problem after a patient sustains a traumatic incident. The trauma patient needs to be assessed for coping mechanisms and current psychosocial state, especially if the patient sustained life-changing injuries. Protonix is a proton pump inhibitor that decreases the amount of acid produced in the stomach, which is common with an inpatient, but is not a common complication or medication after discharge. Vitamin B_{12} and vitamin D are not commonly prescribed at discharge.

6. **C**

Both posttraumatic stress disorder (PTSD) and depression can lead to suicide. The spouse should be instructed to call 911 or other emergency services if the patient with depression or PTSD expresses plans to harm self or others. This includes talking, writing, reading, or drawing about death. The patient should be following up with a primary and psychological physician, but this is a more serious event that needs immediate attention. Joining a trauma support group is beneficial and could help the patient; however, immediate help is warranted.

7. **C**

The patient with posttraumatic stress disorder (PTSD) commonly experiences anxiety and emotional arousal. PTSD may also present with difficulty concentrating, feeling jumpy, irritable, and hypervigilant. Reexperiencing the traumatic event commonly occurs and may include upsetting memories, flashbacks, and nightmares. Denial of the event is not typically a normal response with PTSD. Avoid reminders of the event by avoiding activities, places, or thoughts that remind the patient of the trauma.

8. **B**

Children can have extreme reactions to trauma and children younger than 6 years of age can develop bed-wetting habits after being potty-trained. Forgetting how to or being unable to talk, acting out the scary event during playtime, and being unusually clingy are other signs of posttraumatic stress disorder (PTSD). Older children and teens are more likely to develop disruptive, disrespectful, or destructive behaviors. Older children and teens may feel guilty for not preventing the injury or death.

9. **A**

The main treatments for people with posttraumatic stress disorder (PTSD) are medications coupled with psychotherapy. Prazosin is currently not Food and Drug Administration (FDA) approved although research has shown that Prazosin may be helpful with sleep disturbances and nightmares in PTSD patients. Fluoxetine, or Prozac, is a common antidepressant prescribed for PTSD patients. Cognitive restructuring helps make sense of the bad memories by aiding people with PTSD in looking at what happened in a realistic way. There is not an exposure therapy used in managing PTSD.

10. **A**

Allowing the patient to reconstruct the event in a trauma situation and to talk to multiple people about the event is part of the movement toward acceptance. Anger is a stage of grief, but it is not expressed in this manner. The reconstructing of the event and telling the story are done not to get empathy or to tell his or her side but to desensitize the event to allow acceptance. The patient may repeat the story or talk about the event repeatedly and the nurse should listen attentively each time.

11. **B**

The need for information is the number one identified need of the family following a trauma or hospitalization. Asking about labs and vital signs is frequent. The nurse should keep the family informed of the patient's status and what is "normal" for the injury. Learning comes with the family being well informed. Vigilance is also frequently experienced by the family but is not expressed as a need. They want to ensure that what is "said" is being done is "actually" what is being done. Hope is something that many families hold onto during a traumatic event, but the number one need remains the need for information.

12. **C**

The "hands off" phase is first. This is when the family is afraid of the environment, such as intravenous (IV) lines and monitors. The next phase is "pitching in" when the family feels comfortable with performing some tasks without the nurse, like applying lotion to skin. Lastly the "fitting in" stage happens when the family begins to know the nurse, they pick up on the culture of the unit, and assume some of the nurse's tasks, and bring the nurses food and treats. Suctioning may be more invasive and would not typically occur until long-term care is needed.

13. B

People who have ineffective coping frequently pace, talk fast, exemplify frustration, and are unable to make decisions. They may also have a difficult time using resources and become withdrawn. Stages of grief include denial, anger, bargaining, depression, and acceptance. Crisis intervention is emergency psychological care that occurs in a traumatic situation. The stress responses are the alarm, resistance, and exhaustion phases.

14. B

The nurse should inform the family that they will not be allowed to come and go freely during the resuscitation but can leave with the support staff if they feel the need to step out. The support person is responsible for communicating and providing updates to the rest of the family, limiting the visitors, and allowing the visitors to decide whether they want to be present in the trauma room during the resuscitation. This involves patient education and support of their decisions.

CHAPTER 11. SHOCK

1. B

The sympathetic nervous system, also known as the "flight or fight" response, when activated results in tachycardia, vasoconstriction, and increased myocardial contractility. The vasoconstriction shunts blood to vital organs such as the heart and brain. The parasympathetic nervous system would do the exact opposite; it causes vasodilation and bradycardia. The renin–angiotensin system is activated in a state of shock and releases angiotensin II and aldosterone. This also causes vasoconstriction but does not increase myocardial contractility or tachycardia but does decrease renal output.

2. A

In hemorrhagic shock, there is a shift of fluid from the extravascular to intravascular space in order to compensate for the low circulation. This results in both interstitial and intravascular depletion of fluid.

3. C

Class III hemorrhagic shock is experienced when a patient loses 30% to 40% of total blood volume, which is approximately 1,500 to 2,000 mL. This results in hypotension, a respiratory rate in the 30s, a heart rate greater than 120 beats per minute (bpm), urine output of 5 to 10 mL/hr, and the patient is usually confused and anxious. Class I is a 15% total blood volume (TBV) loss, approximately 800 mL; a respiratory rate in the 20s; heart rate is greater than 100 bpm; and the patient is slightly anxious. In class II, the patient loses 15% to 30% TBV, approximately 800 to 1,500 mL; respiratory rate is 20 to 30, heart rate is greater than 100 but less than 120 bpm, urine output is 20 to 30 mL/hr, with decreased capillary refill, and mild anxiety. Class IV hemorrhagic shock is when there is greater than 40% TBV loss, greater than 2,000 mL; respiratory rate is 30 to 40; heart rate is greater than 140 bpm, there is no urine output, hypotension, and lethargy.

4. A

Hypertonic solutions increase osmotic pressure intravascularly, not extravascularly, which draws fluid into the intravascular space. Hypertonic solutions improve myocardial activity; increase renal, splanchnic, and coronary blood flow, requiring a smaller fluid volume, and can be used in brain-injured patients to manage cerebral edema while replacing intravascular losses.

5. B

The universal blood donor type is O negative with a low anti-A titer. Male patients may receive O positive as uncross-matched blood, whereas women within child-bearing age require the negative. Massive transfusions are typically defined as infusions of 10 units of blood or more in a 24-hour period. A new cross-match is recommended after multiple uncross-matched blood transfusions to reduce error in the type and screen.

6. D

Hemodynamic instability is seen in patients requiring resuscitation efforts but is typically resolved following adequate resuscitation. The sequelae of resuscitation are hypothermia, coagulopathy, acidosis, and electrolyte abnormalities. Hypothermia happens following long extrication in cold climates, clothing removal, surgical exposure, alcohol usage, and large volumes of fluid administration. Coagulopathy is related to clot formation on lacerated vessels, dilution with volume replacement, platelet dysfunction resulting from hypothermia, or impaired hepatic function. Metabolic acidosis is a primary result of ischemic injury caused by hypoxia, hypoperfusion, decreased cardiac output, and fluid resuscitation. Hypocalcemia, hypomagnesemia, hypophosphatemia, hypo- or hyperkalemia are often seen following massive transfusions.

7. B

Administering vasopressin will increase vascular tone and blood pressure. It may be indicated following adequate resuscitation with fluids, blood, and blood products but is not the first-line choice. The prevention and treatment of acidosis in trauma patients should be by maximizing cardiac output, controlling the bleeding, and assuring adequate oxygenation. Fresh frozen plasma (FFP) contains normal levels of stable clotting factors, albumin, and immunoglobulins, which aid in stopping massive bleeding. Packed red blood cells (PRBCs) are used to replace blood loss.

CHAPTER 12. SYSTEMIC INFLAMMATORY RESPONSE SYNDROME/ MULTIPLE ORGAN DYSFUNCTION

1. A

Systemic inflammatory response syndrome (SIRS) is a condition of systemic inflammation, organ dysfunction, and organ failure. Proinflammatory cytokines initiate the inflammatory process such as elevation of white blood cells (WBC) and initiation of the complement system. Interleukins function directly on tissue or work by secondary mediators to activate the coagulation cascade and fever. Other cytokines stimulate the release of acute-phase reactants such as C-reactive protein and procalcitonin. Lactate elevates when SIRS is present, it is not a cellular response.

2. A

Gram-negative bacteria include *Escherichia coli*, *Klebsiella pneumonia*, *Pseudomonas aeruginosa*, *Enterobacter*, *Serratia*, and *Proteus*. *Pseudomonas* and *Klebsiella* have a higher mortality rate than other gram-negative organisms. *Pneumococcus* is a type of gram-positive bacteria. Both types of bacteria trigger an immune response and cause sepsis.

3. B

This is evidence that the patient is not demonstrating signs of infection (tachypnea, fever, tachycardia, altered mentation). In order for the patient to be free from injury, there needs to be an absence of injury signs such as bruises, broken teeth, and mucosal tears, and other signs of trauma. This scenario does not address these signs. A patient with optimal cerebral tissue perfusion will also have a urine output of 1 mL/kg/min and have a Glasgow Coma Scale (GCS) score of 15, and normal vital signs; more information is needed in the scenario to identify tissue perfusion (lactate levels, base deficit). A trauma patient with adequate gas exchange will be alert and oriented; have normal arterial blood gases (ABGs); normal skin color; skin will be warm and dry, the patient will have a regular respiratory rate, depth, and pattern of breathing. In order to determine adequate gas exchange the ABG values, a complete neurological assessment, and a skin assessment are needed, which is not provided in this scenario.

4. D

Normal pulmonary artery pressure is 20 to 30 mmHg systolic and 10 to 15 mmHg diastolic. Elevated pressures occur in pulmonary embolus and hypoxia because of pulmonary artery vasoconstriction. Mitral valve regurgitation causes an increase in resistance blood backing up in the pulmonary artery during systole, elevating pulmonary artery pressures. Low arterial pressures are also reflected in the pulmonary artery.

5. B

The normal lactate level is 0.5 to 1.0 mEq/L and is considered elevated if greater than 2.0 mEq/L. The average initial lactate level for survivors is 2.8 mEq/L versus nonsurvivors' initial lactate level of 4.0 mEq/L. The lactate level has been shown to predict survivability following sepsis. There is a significantly increased chance of survival if lactate levels normalize within 24 hours. The survival rate is improved if lactate levels normalize within 48 hours but if greater than 48 hours the risk of mortality significantly increases.

6. D

Even though an endpoint to sepsis resuscitation efforts is debatable, each endpoint needs to be taken into account in combination with clinical assessment. The central venous pressure (CVP) needs to be greater than 8 to 10 mmHg in a spontaneous breathing patient, $ScvO_2$ greater than 70%, with stable mean arterial pressure (MAP), adequate urine output, adequate skin perfusion, improved level of consciousness, and normalization of lactate levels. The major goal of resuscitation is organ perfusion to prevent cellular dysfunction and cell death.

7. B

Sepsis management bundle includes low-dose steroids in patients with septic shock. Recommendation for glucose control is to keep glucose less than 150 mg/dL, but maintain the glucose level between 80 and 110 mg/dL increases the risk of hypoglycemia, which can negatively affect outcomes. Patients in septic shock are at increased risk for pulmonary injury and acute respiratory distress syndrome (ARDS). High plateau pressures need to be avoided. Recommended inspiratory plateau pressure is less than 30 cm H_2O. Monitoring plateau pressure is more important than the peak inspiratory pressure for ventilation management.

CHAPTER 13. INJURY PREVENTION AND PUBLIC EDUCATION

1. **C**

Enhancing awareness of biological warfare is not a part of research but is considered public education. All of the other choices are methods that would enhance research to achieve the common trauma-prevention goal of reducing injuries.

2. **D**

Direct mortality is not a part of the cost evaluation because it is the actual loss of life. But indirect mortality reflects the loss of productivity because of years of life lost. Indirect morbidity is a factor because of the lost productivity; medical care costs account for a large portion, and include all of the costs for the care received.

3. **A**

Injury-prevention programs may use one of these four Es: education, enforcement, engineering, or economic incentives. Education in injury prevention should be targeted toward high-risk groups. Enforcement of injury-prevention programs can be accomplished through the passing of laws and legislation. Engineering is the design and development of better protective gear. Economic incentives involve the use of money to change behavior. Elective is not a part of injury-prevention programs.

4. **A**

A mandatory seat belt law is an example of injury prevention by enforcement. Enforcement includes the passing of laws and legislation. The fine for infractions of the law is an example of an economic incentive. The development of air bags in vehicles is an example of engineering, which is the designing of protective vehicles or gear. A class provided in high school regarding drunk driving is education for trauma prevention.

5. **B**

A pediatric patient in the emergency department is suspected of being abused. Notifying child protective services is a type of secondary prevention. Primary prevention would have been an intervention to prevent the initial occurrence of abuse. Secondary prevention is an intervention to decrease the injury or prevent it from occurring again. Educational trauma prevention involves education to the public regarding prevention of trauma. Engineering trauma prevention is the change of the design of a product or vehicle that will decrease injury.

6. **C**

Tertiary prevention involves efforts following the incident that will optimize the outcome from injury, regardless of the severity of injury (after the event). This includes utilizing best practices and guidelines to improve the outcomes of trauma patients. Educational prevention is the use of public intervention with education in prevention of trauma. Secondary prevention does not prevent trauma but is an intervention that may lessen its injuries. Enforcement involves fines or fees that are used to enforce changes, which will prevent trauma.

7. B

Education is the least effective injury-prevention strategy and requires the most amount of time to produce the desired effect. Engineering is the most effective because the change in design can provide primary prevention without involvement from the person. Enforcement can be more effective in some situations but still requires decision making from the individual. Ergonomics is not a type of trauma prevention.

CHAPTER 14. PREHOSPITAL CARE

1. C

The prevalence of injury is defined as the number of affected persons with a particular injury present in a population at a specified time divided by the number of persons in the population at that time. Incidence of injury is defined as the number of new cases of an injury that occur during a specified period of time in a population at risk for that injury. Mechanism of injury is the way an injury occurs during a trauma. Morbidity following an injury is the death rate for a specific injury.

2. B

The "scoop and run" concept is defined as rapid transport to the nearest appropriate trauma center with minimal interventions except basic ABCs (airway, breathing, circulation) performed in the prehospital setting. If the transport time to the nearest trauma center is short, limited time should be spent at the scene. Delays at the scene to "stabilize" a patient beyond airway and breathing can increase morbidity and mortality. The nearest hospital may not actually be the most appropriate trauma center for definitive care of a trauma patient. Not all trauma patients though require a level 1 trauma center for quality care.

3. C

Prehospital personnel should instruct families not to try to follow the ambulance during transport because of the need to obey traffic laws.

4. C

Optimal time on the scene for major trauma patients is 10 minutes. Performing interventions too long delays the transport of the patient to definitive care. A primary survey should be completed, which includes securing an airway and stopping blood loss. The primary survey typically takes longer than 2 minutes. Obtaining intravenous fluids (IVs) and initiating fluid resuscitation can occur during transport and should not delay transport.

5. A

Rapid assessment of the pulse rate (fast, slow, or normal) and quality is included in the primary survey; obtaining the actual heart rate is part of the secondary survey. Heart rate and blood pressure are important for assessing the hemodynamics but are considered part of the secondary survey.

CHAPTER 15. PATIENT SAFETY AND PATIENT TRANSFERS

1. **C**

    Burns, amputations, brain injuries, spinal cord injuries, and specialty populations such as pediatrics or pregnant patients would all be appropriate categories of injuries or situations for which transfer agreement would be beneficial. Fractures can usually be treated at any facility and should not require transfer.

2. **C**

    Stabilization of the patient in the initial receiving center is required. Inhalation injuries or large body surface area burns need to be transferred to a burn center. Transfers are usually for full-thickness burns greater than 5% total body surface area (TBSA) and greater than 20% TBSA for partial-thickness burns. Partial- or full-thickness burns to hands, feet, face, genitalia, or major joints should be transferred to a burn center.

3. **D**

    Have the patient's family remain until the patient departs to be available for further questions and to update them on the plan of care. Providing a nursing report to the receiving facility is a requirement of the nurse to facilitate continuity of care. The nurse should copy the medical record along with radiographic studies to accompany the patient. Bedside provides reports to the transporting service of the referring hospital and then the transporting service delivers them to the receiving facility. The transferring nurse will also need to call the report to the receiving facility.

4. **D**

    Discharge planning involves an evaluation of the patient, discussing options with the patient and/or family, planning the actual transfer and arranging any tests or procedures required before leaving. Not all patients are candidates for rehabilitation and depends upon the patient's ability to participate in the rehabilitation. Discharges and transfers are frequently delayed because the accommodation or transportation is either unavailable or late; there should not be any delay in the final step of transfer.

5. **B**

    During intrafacility transfer, if the receiving location is to assume care of the patient, then a nurse-to-nurse communication and report are required before transfer. This communication between nurses is important to prevent errors in management of the trauma patient. A transport team is not necessarily required when transferring a patient within the facility. Providing extra fluid with the patient when transferring between facilities is not typically necessary within the facility. It is not always required to complete all tests before transferring the patient within the facility.

6. **B**

    Interfacility transfers include those transfers in which the patient is moved from one facility to another. So hospital to hospital, hospital to rehabilitation or long-term care facility are considered interfacility transfers. Hospital to dialysis department is intrafacility transfer. The patient remains within the hospital.

7. **D**

The nurse providing discharge instruction to a Spanish-speaking patient should use an official hospital-approved translator. It is not recommended to use family members for interpretation even if they are bilingual. The patient may not understand enough English so a translator is recommended. The patient should have both verbal and written discharge instructions.

8. **D**

Placement of chest tube for a pneumothorax, initiating intravenous fluids for resuscitation, and intubation to secure an airway are all interventions used to stabilize the trauma patient and should be initiated before transfer. A full set of radiographs and trauma workup are best performed at the trauma center and should not delay the transfer.

CHAPTER 16. FORENSIC ISSUES

1. **C**

Preparing the family beforehand minimizes the shock of the situation and also prepares them to make the decision whether to actually see the patient or not at that time. The nurse should make the patient and the room as presentable as possible without tampering with possible evidence. The nurse should not wash the body or remove any invasive lines because they could contain forensic evidence. Comforting the family is a therapeutic nursing process; the clothes should not be packaged and sent with the family but should be kept for evidence.

2. **A**

The trauma nurse should get an order for a toxicology screen on the patient and collect the sample. The toxicology screen is an objective measure that would prove suspected assessment without passing judgment or inflicting incrimination. The behavior is documented correctly, but the nurse should not document *alleged* and subjective accusations such as smell of alcohol on his breath. Do not let personal judgment affect professionalism. Reorienting the patient, explaining treatment, and providing resources for a patient would be proper care. Making the assumption that the patient is an "alcoholic" is passing judgment and the emergency room is not the right time or place for making assumptions.

3. **D**

Biological evidence that is collected from victims of violent crimes includes hair, semen, saliva, skin, and blood. Scrapings under the victim's nails may need to be collected but the actual nails do not need to be removed and collected as evidence.

4. **A**

Emergency medical care should never be delayed to collect forensic data from a trauma patient. Patient care should come first. The goal is to collect evidence concurrent with the management of the patient. It does not necessarily need to be collected as soon as the patient arrives. Even if the clothing is soiled, it is still considered forensic evidence and should be packaged accordingly. The police do not need to remain in the resuscitation room.

5. **C**

The majority of forensic evidence collection typically occurs within the emergency room, but forensic evidence may continue to be found in the operating room and inpatient units as well. Data collection can occur concurrent with the care of the patient and does not have to occur only after stabilization and in the intensive care unit.

6. **A**

Gunshot residue appears as dark powder, soot, particles, or small-punctuated hemorrhages. If the gunshot wound is suspected to be self-inflicted, the hands should be placed in paper bags to preserve the evidence. Plastic bags will cause moisture that will destroy the evidence. Patient care does come first but the hands can be covered while still providing care to the patient. Do not wash the hands because that will destroy evidence.

7. **B**

When removing the trauma victim's clothing, do not cut through the bullet holes or tears in the clothing. This preserves it for forensics. The shirt can be cut off but avoid cutting areas of potential evidence. Do not circle the hole or tear in the shirt because that may damage some of the residue, which may be forensic evidence. Do not document "entrance" or "exit" wounds.

CHAPTER 17. END-OF-LIFE ISSUES

1. **B**

A do not resuscitate (DNR) order does not mean that health care providers do not treat the patient. Blood transfusions may stabilize the patient and provide relief from symptoms. The degree and the amount of interventions initiated to "save" the patient should be a separate decision from the DNR status. The DNR status tells health care providers what to do in case of cardiac or respiratory arrest. The nurse's next step is to discuss the treatment and obtain a blood transfusion consent form, but the first steps of notifying the physician and obtaining the order are initiated.

2. **D**

Providing supplemental oxygen may decrease the feeling of dyspnea without prolonging life. Lateral positioning of the patient can decrease that "rattling" sound because it will reduce the fluids that are collecting in the back of the throat. Dryness of the face and mouth can be a common discomfort near death and providing lip balm to the lips or wetting the mouth routinely with swabs may provide comfort. Temperature sensitivity should be considered during the end of life and providing comfort measures by warming or cooling the patient is not considered treatment.

3. **A**

Encourage the family to talk to the patient even though the patient is unresponsive and sedated, it is possible that even if a patient is unconscious, he or she may still be able to hear. It is also therapeutic for the spouse to talk to the patient so that a feeling of fulfillment can be achieved. Saying that "he won't be able to hear what you are saying" is incorrect and the nurse should always encourage communication even if the patient is unresponsive or sedated, it is never too late for the family to say how they feel. The last response is not a therapeutic response, there is no proven evidence that talking to the patient is unbeneficial.

4. A

A child cannot give consent for organ donation unless he or she is an adult older than the age of 18. The spouse, legal guardian, adult sibling, adult child, or parents are all acceptable individuals to consent for organ donation.

5. C

An apnea test is performed during brain death testing to determine the absence of the drive to breathe using CO_2 challenge. Cerebral blood flow scan may be used in determining brain death but is not required and is not performed at the bedside. Meningeal testing is used if the patient is suspected of meningitis. The Babinski reflex is not a component of brain death determination.

6. C

Hypothermia mimics brain death and should be reversed before death is declared. Warming the patient externally and internally is recommended before brain death testing occurs. Metabolic acidosis is a greater concern than metabolic alkalosis in determining brain death. Apnea is actually a required criterion for brain death determination.

7. B

Spontaneous motor movement and false triggering of the ventilator can occur in brain-dead patients. One of the determinants of brain death is a loss of papillary reaction and reflexes. Initiation of conversation regarding organ donation should be done by the organ procurement agency. An EEG cannot replace a bedside examination of the patient when declaring brain death.

8. C

A dead brain does not produce antidiuretic hormone (ADH), which results in diabetes insipidus (DI), an excessive diuresis resulting from a lack of ADH. Patients with the syndrome of inappropriate antidiuretic hormone (SIADH) actually produce too much ADH. Cerebral salt-wasting syndrome (CSWS) is more common in patients with subarachnoid hemorrhage. Cushing's syndrome results in overproduction of corticosteroids or ACTH, which would not be produced by the brain after brain death.

9. C

Dyspnea in a dying patient can be managed with oxygen therapy, elevating the head of the bed, and administering opioids and anxiolytics. Oxygen would be administered to alleviate discomfort but is not applied to prolong life. Intubation is primarily used to prolong life and is not recommended at the end of life.

CHAPTER 18. TRAUMA QUALITY MANAGEMENT

1. B

Quality improvement is a method of evaluation and improving processes of patient care that emphasizes a multidisciplinary approach to problem solving that focuses on the system. Improving quality of the system includes implementing corrective actions where and when needed. The goal of quality-improvement programs is to shift the focus away from individual errors to system-wide errors. Quality improvement does not focus only on mortality like morbidity and mortality conferences do.

2. **A**

A common problem with the quality-improvement program in trauma centers is that problems may be identified but there is failure to correct the problem. The lack of adherence to a developed protocol is considered a quality-improvement problem that should be addressed but is not as significant a barrier as inability to close the loop. Most of the time, the problem can be identified and a decision can be reached on preventable versus nonpreventable deaths.

3. **B**

The primary goal of morbidity and mortality conferences is to identify opportunities for improvement in outcomes. The deaths are reviewed to determine preventable (not nonpreventable) deaths and to identify the problems to be able make changes to improve outcomes. Quality improvement is not intended identify personnel issues as much as to look at systemic problems. Sentinel events are tracked but are not the primary focus for morbidity and mortality conferences.

4. **D**

Quality improvement involves identifying problems, developing reasonable corrective action plans, following through on implementing these plans, and evaluating whether the corrective action has had its intended consequences, which is the "closing the loop" component of the quality-improvement plan. Just implementing an action does not necessarily mean the action had the intended outcomes.

5. **C**

Audit filters are identified variables that are routinely tracked to determine whether pre-determined acceptable standards are being met. Adverse events or complications are examples of audit filters, which may be tracked in trauma systems. Audits should identify "near misses" in patient care that do not result in a poor outcome but might indicate a patient care process that can be improved.

CHAPTER 19. STAFF SAFETY AND CRITICAL INCIDENT STRESS MANAGEMENT

1. **B**

The nurse is exemplifying crisis intervention strategies for the family of the trauma patient. Therapeutic communication is part of crisis intervention, but the whole picture involves more than communication; it also incorporates facilitation of care. A crisis is a sudden unexpected threat to life, whereas stress is the actual arousal of the body in response to a situation; therefore, the strategies are geared differently. Stress interventions are not harmonious with crisis interventions. The nurse is incorporating the concepts of psychosocial needs by informing the family, but the compassion and maintenance of hope develops with the rapport and delivery of care.

2. **D**

Reflective verbalized content can confront their thought process in a nonthreatening way. The nurse should allow the defense, which may be needed at that time. The nurse should not confront the patient and should always be honest.

3. **D**

Debriefings and defusings provide staff the opportunity to express feelings, anger, frustration, grief, and facilitate closure of the incident by using special techniques sensitive to these stressful situations. This is not a critiquing time and criticizing of anyone's performance is not tolerated.

4. **C**

The definition of *workplace violence* is an act of aggression directed toward persons at work or on duty and ranges from offensive language to homicide. Violence reported by hospitals includes assault and battery, hostage situations, homicide, kidnapping, armed robbery, theft, vandalism, and bomb threats. Violence can range from verbal abuse all the way to homicide.

5. **D**

The trauma nurse should use extreme caution when working with a patient in police custody. To avoid personal injury, the trauma nurse should not let the offender (person in custody) distract or manipulate him or her during the course of an assessment or treatment. Allow police officers to remain in the room during assessment and treatments when patients are in custody to maintain safety of health care providers. The trauma nurse should never leave a patient in custody go unattended, even with bathroom privileges.

6. **B**

Prevention of violence is the best management. The training of hospital employees needs to include how to recognize potential violence, defuse the violence, and deal with the aftermath of the violence. Deescalating techniques are recommended but are used more to prevent violence than when it actually occurs. When working with an aggressive patient use the least amount of physical force necessary, remain focused and centered, and attempt to redirect the patient's behavior. Crisis management is taught but the best way to manage violence is to prevent it.

7. **A**

Do not attempt to touch a violent patient without assistance and use security staff for a show of strength. Touching a violent person may escalate the situation. Maintain a distance from the aggressive patient and do not approach the patient alone. Body language can either escalate or deescalate the crisis with a violent patient. Continuous talking to deescalate the situation is recommended when a potentially violent patient is involved. Avoid punitive or judgmental statements and use good listening skills to deescalate a potentially violent situation.

8. **A**

Once the situation permits, it is advisable to restrain a violent or agitated patient to ensure safety. A chest restraint is not recommended because of the increased risk of injury to the patient. If necessary, use three stabilization techniques to get control of the potentially violent patient: physical restraint, sedation, or chemical restraint. The trauma nurse should document indications for restraint and record safety checks on all restrained patients.

CHAPTER 20. DISASTER MANAGEMENT

1. **B**

   This is considered a multiple casualty incident because there are greater than 10 but less than 100 casualties. A multiple patient incident is categorized as fewer than 10 casualties and a mass casualty incident results in greater than 100 casualties and involves responses from multiple hospitals.

2. **A**

   Nerve agents are the most toxic of all chemical agents and affect the cardiovascular, respiratory, gastrointestinal, musculoskeletal, and central nervous systems, with inhibition of acetylcholinesterase the main mechanism of action. Vesicants are also known as *blister agents* and are contracted by inhalation or topical exposure, damaging the cardiovascular and central nervous systems. Pulmonary agents are contracted by inhalation and primarily affect the respiratory system. Blood agents interfere with oxygenation and are inhaled or ingested.

3. **C**

   Atropine and 2-PAM Cl are the only antidotes for nerve agents such as Tabun, Sarin, or VX (venemous agent X). Dimercaprol is the antidote for lewisite, which is a type of vesicant. Hydroxocobolamin, amyl nitrate, sodium thiosulfate, and sodium nitrate are antidotes for blood agents such as cyanide. Moreover, there are no antidote pulmonary agents. These patients should receive aggressive airway/breathing management.

4. **C**

   Incapacitating agents such as BZ (a glycolate anticholinergic compound) cause hallucinations and illusions; riot-control agents, such as Mace cause lacrimation, and both are only treated by decontamination. Pulmonary agents are treated with decontamination, and breathing/airway management. Blister agents are treated with decontamination, airway/breathing management, and possibly dimercaprol.

5. **A**

   A hallmark sign of cyanide exposure is the report of smelling almonds. Cyanide places patients into metabolic acidosis; hence, the patient's lethargy and tachypnea. Carbon monoxide is another type of blood agent, but does not present these distinct features. Chlorine is a type of pulmonary agent and mustard is a vesicant agent.

6. **C**

   Category C biological agents are the third highest priority level because they refer to future agents that could possibly emerge because of availability and ease of production. High-priority biological agents that can be transmitted from one person to another, such as anthrax, are considered risks to national security and part of category A biological agents. Category A agents also have a high mortality rate and tend to cause public alarm. Category B agents are the second highest priority agents, such as brucellosis, and result in moderate to low mortality rates.

7. A

Although these are both pulmonary agents, phosgene exposure can have delayed effects for up to 48 hours after exposure and present with difficulty breathing, productive cough, and hypotension. Pulmonary edema, a burning sensation reported in the nares, and chest tightness are all features of chlorine exposure that phosgene does not share.

8. D

Symptom clusters suggest that there could be a possibility of infectious agent exposure. The symptoms that the patients are presenting with do display evidence of the plague. Smallpox, botulism, and anthrax are all other examples of infectious agents that spread throughout the community and may create a symptom cluster pattern.

9. B

All of the following are true regarding smallpox: There is no cure for smallpox, but administration of immune globulin and the smallpox vaccine (up to 4 days after exposure and before the rash appears) could protect, prevent, or limit the severity of the virus.

10. C

The smallpox virus remains contagious until all of the scabs fall off; the healing skin will have a "pitted" appearance where the scabs once were. After 2 weeks, most of the pustules begin to scab over, but the patient remains contagious. A patient with smallpox experiences high fevers that last about 2 to 4 days, but after the rash completely spreads throughout the body the patient begins to feel better and becomes afebrile; the patient will experience a return of fevers until the scabs form.

11. C

Clostridium botulinum is the bacterium that produces botulinum. Ricin is a toxic poison formed from the by-products of castor bean and causes pulmonary and systemic effects such as hypotension. *Yersinia pestis* is also known as the plague and is one of the most potent biological warfare agents. *Variola* is the virus that causes smallpox.

12. B

This is categorized as a radiological dispersal device. A simple radiological device spreads radioactive material without an explosive device. A reactor would be an attack at a nuclear plant. Improvised nuclear devices are any nuclear weapons that are not associated with the military.

13. C

If gastrointestinal symptoms start to occur within the first 2 hours of radiation exposure, this is a sign that fatality is probable and that the level of radiation is elevated greater than 800 rads. With exposure to less than 100 rads, survival is probable and with exposure to 200 to 800 yards survival is possible. The Geiger–Muller survey meter measures external contamination. In order to decontaminate radioactive patients, clothing should be removed and double-bagged, the receiving area should be divided into clean and dirty areas to limit the materials exposed to radiation.

14. A

This is the role of the Hospital Emergency Incident Command System or HEICS. The Emergency Medical Treatment and Labor Act or EMTALA is a federal law that requires anyone coming to an emergency department to be stabilized and treated, regardless of insurance status or ability to pay. Emergency Disaster Command Station and Hospital Emergency Medical Disaster System are not actual terms in disaster management.

15. C

Level C equipment includes an air-purifying respirator or face cartridge mask and a splash-proof chemical-resistant suit. Level A is a self-contained breathing apparatus and a chemical-resistant suit. Level B would be a self-contained breathing apparatus or positive pressure-supplied air respirator and a chemical-resistant suit. Level D protects against nothing and skin protection is minimal.

16. C

Decontamination of potentially contaminated victims should be a priority before care can be initiated, even though this may delay interventions.

17. B

Disaster management should include plans to care for unusually high volumes of patients in the event of an unexpected surge of volume. Crisis planning is typically more directed toward individual patient management. Community planning is not related to disaster management. Hurricanes are one type of disaster for which a relief center is put up after the disaster to care for those without home, food, or water.

18. A

People injured from an explosion or mass casualty event will rapidly seek care at the nearest hospital and may not present to facilities designated by existing response plans. Optimally, victims of a mass casualty incident should be tracked from the scene to the hospital for easier identification and location by family. The emergency department is the entry point of victims following a disaster or mass casualty event and becomes the initial communication center regarding the disaster. The knowledge of the magnitude of injuries and numbers of casualties will determine the appropriate facility's response.

19. B

The three areas that are critical to clear beds to allow room for incoming survivors of a large event are the emergency department, operating room, and intensive care units. In attempt to free up areas and beds to receive incoming survivors, the emergency department may need to transfer patients to noncritical beds in the hospital.

20. B

There are four levels of triage during a disaster: black (deceased), red (immediate), yellow (delayed) and green (nonurgent). A red tag is considered salvageable but in need of immediate intervention. A black tag would indicate the person is either deceased or is likely to die from the injuries. A person triaged as red during a disaster will be the first transported to the highest level of care followed by those identified by a yellow tag. A patient who is considered most likely to survive despite lack of medical treatment is considered *walking wounded* and are triaged green or nonurgent during a disaster.

CHAPTER 21. REGULATIONS AND STANDARDS

1. **B**

   The Consolidated Omnibus Budget Reduction Act (COBRA)/Emergency Medical Treatment and Labor Act (EMTALA) requires that an individual seeking medical care be provided a medical screening exam by a qualified medical professional. The START system is known as simple triage and rapid treatment. In START, victims are grouped into four categories, depending on the urgency of their need for evacuation. Health Insurance Portability and Accountability Act (HIPAA) has the primary goal of making it easier for people to keep health insurance, protect the confidentiality and security of health care information, and help the health care industry control administrative costs. Trauma designation is the certification of hospitals that specialize in trauma.

2. **B**

   The Trauma and Injury and Severity Score (TRISS) is used to calculate the probability of survival, the lower score predicts greater survival. A trauma patient with a high TRISS who expires does not require performance improvement because the risk of death is great. A trauma patient with a low TRISS who experiences a bad outcome should be reviewed for performance improvement as the risk of death is low.

3. **A**

   The Consolidated Omnibus Budget Reconciliation Act (COBRA) applies to all patients who come to the emergency department requesting examination or treatment for a medical condition. COBRA requires that once a person has a medical screening exam, the decision may be to treat and discharge the patient, transfer the patient to a qualified facility after stabilizing treatment, or admit the patient. COBRA requires that to transfer a patient after stabilizing treatment to another qualified facility, the receiving facility must have an accepting physician, and have available beds and services. When transferring a patient, COBRA requires that the transferring hospital must have either the patient or a legal representative sign a certificate stating the physician has reviewed risks and benefits of the transfer. COBRA requires that the transferring hospital arranges appropriate transportation to the receiving facility and is responsible for any complications that occur during transport; it does not require a nurse to accompany all patients.

4. **C**

   The Health Information Portability and Accountability Act (HIPAA) defines *protected health information (PHI)* as information related to the provision of health care. This includes past, present, or future physical or mental health conditions of an individual. HIPAA ensures that patients have access to their own medical records but a nurse cannot access the records of family members. Information regarding patient's medical records may be shared between one or more health care provider involved in the care without a patient's consent. HIPAA allows information regarding patient's medical records to be shared to obtain reimbursement for health care delivered to the patient. HIPAA allows health care professionals involved in quality assessment and improvement to have access to patient's medical records without the patient's consent.

5. **B**

The receiving trauma center must be notified before the transfer to ensure that a physician will accept the patient and there is an appropriate bed available for the patient. The transferring hospital should stabilize the patient but not delay the transfer until all diagnostic tests are done. The sending hospital is responsible for the transportation, type and level of care, as well as any complications that may occur during the transport.

CHAPTER 22. ETHICAL ISSUES

1. **B**

Moral distress is caused when the ethically appropriate action is known but cannot be acted upon by the person. To act against one's own conscience causes feelings of shame or guilt and violates one's sense of wholeness and integrity. Empathy is the capacity to understand or feel what another person is experiencing. Beneficence is an ethical principle used in ethical dilemmas. A moral agent is a person able to make right and wrong decisions.

2. **C**

Ethic committees should be consulted when an ethical dilemma is not readily resolved. Common causes and scenarios for ethical dilemmas include contradictory beliefs, competing duties, conflicting principles, lack of clear clinical or legal guidelines. The physician can make a recommendation but cannot make the decision for the family. The nurse should not support one family's opinion but should facilitate decision making among the family members.

3. **D**

The ethical principal of beneficence considers the balance between benefit and harm in which action maximizes the benefit and minimizes the harm. This is the principle frequently used to analyze futile care and withdrawal of life support. Autonomy means *self-governing* and is the freedom to make choices that affect one's life. Nonmaleficence is an ethical principle that requires actions do not inflict harm. Paternalism is based on the belief that health care professionals have the duty to benefit the patient.

4. **A**

The ethical principle of beneficence refers to the responsibility of health care providers to benefit the patient, usually through acts of kindness, compassion, and mercy. Nonmaleficience is an ethical principle that requires actions not inflict harm. The definition of *harm* becomes crucial when applying this principle and includes deliberate harm, risk of harm, and harm that occurs during beneficial acts. Veracity is the requirement to provide patient's and decision makers with all the information needed to make an autonomous decision. Fidelity relates to the concept of faithfulness and the practice of keeping promises. It is the loyalty that exits in a nurse–patient relationship.

5. **D**

According to the Emergency Medical Treatment and Labor Act (EMTALA), all patients require emergency care to stabilize injuries whether they are able to pay for the services or not. Blood transfusions may be against certain people's religious beliefs, emergency interventions may be determined by the trauma surgeon without a signed consent, and decisions regarding futile care commonly occur without consent in emergency situations.

TCRN® Practice Test Answers and Rationales

1. **C**

   A normal central venous pressure (CVP) reading is 3 to 8 mmHg. A low CVP, especially following a liver repair, indicates hypovolemia. The first-line treatment is to administer intravenous fluids. Sometimes antibiotics, such as Zosyn are given when there is a low CVP and an infection, or sepsis involvement, but the first-line treatment is fluid hydration. The same is true for vasoconstricting medications; they are ordered for hypotensive patients, but if "the tank is dry" we need to "fill" it before we can "squeeze" it. When the CVP reading is high diuretics are given to extract the extra fluid load.

2. **B**

   Positioning the pregnant patient 15 to 20 degrees on the left side while remaining on the backboard will reduce the risk of aspiration in the patient and increase blood return and circulation to the fetus by reducing the cord compromise that occurs when lying supine for a long period of time.

3. **B**

   The salmon-colored aspirate is very likely indicative of blood from the oral facial trauma that was swallowed following the trauma. Fresh red blood is indicative of a stomach injury and would require surgery. The patient can also have stomach pain from other sources such as peritonitis, which is a common injury in trauma patients resulting from the spillage of intestinal contents into the peritoneal cavity.

4. **A**

   A left-sided diaphragmatic rupture is more common than a right-sided diaphragmatic rupture because the liver acts as a protective barrier to the right diaphragm. Right-sided ruptures do happen, but are not as likely as a left-sided diaphragmatic rupture. Bilateral diaphragm injuries are not common. The diaphragm will not have a penetrating injury in a blunt mechanism.

5. **B**

   A degloving injury is associated with an avulsion. It is a full-thickness injury that is caused by ripping; the skin is pulled away from the soft tissue and the edges cannot be approximated. A laceration is an open wound caused by a sharp object or the rupture of skin from a blunt object. A contusion is a closed wound and an abrasion is only a partial-thickness injury; the wound described is full thickness and open.

6. **C**

Common symptoms of posttraumatic stress disorder (PTSD) include substance abuse, depression, and suicidal thoughts or actions. This patient recently experienced a traumatic event, which is likely to produce symptoms of PTSD. Symptoms of PTSD can sometimes take weeks, months, or even years before they appear. Psychosis and manic-depressive states may lead to a suicide attempt but there is nothing in this scenario indicating the presence of a psychiatric disorder. Addiction is often a result of the PTSD.

7. **D**

An axial loading injury involves the direct force being transmitted along the vertebral column, this causes a burst pattern of injury for vertebral fractures and frequently involves multiple levels of injury. A rotational injury is a combination of forward flexion and lateral displacement of the cervical spine, such as a victim in a spinning motor vehicle collision. Hyperextension injuries occur with a backward thrust of the head such as in a rear-end collision in which whiplash is experienced. Hyperflexion injuries happen when there is a forceful flexion of the cervical spine and can be caused by a front-impact in motor vehicle collision.

8. **D**

Nasoorbitalethmoid (NOE) injury presents with the depressed nose "pug" profile and a widened, flattened, frontal view of the nose. *Telecanthus* is the term used for the illusion of the eyes being further apart. This is typically seen with an NOE injury but it is a symptom, not an actual type of injury. Nasal fractures will usually present with a deformity, but not as distinguished as in an NOE injury. An ethmoid fracture is part of this injury but the symptoms this patient presented with demonstrate the involvement of the nasal and orbital bones as well.

9. **A**

A positive Saegesser's sign presents with left upper quadrant abdominal pain and radiation to the neck caused by irritation of the phrenic nerve commonly found following splenic injury. This is a serious finding and can indicate a life-threatening hemorrhage. A positive Kehr's sign is pain in the left shoulder while in the supine position after a splenic injury. *Cervicalgia* is a term for neck pain but here the pain is originating in the abdomen and the nurse should take into consideration the diagnosis of the patient. Kernig's sign is severe stiffness of the hamstrings and an inability to straighten the leg when the hip is flexed to 90 degrees. This is usually seen in patients with meningeal irritation and meningitis.

10. **A**

A positive bulbocavernosus reflex would be an anal contraction in response to squeezing the glans penis or clitoris, or tugging on an indwelling Foley catheter. The Achilles reflex is dependent on the S1 and S2 nerve roots and is performed while the ankle is in dorsiflexion. Brudzinski's sign tests for meningitis. The hips and knees will flex upon flexion of the neck. A positive Babinski response is when the great toe dorsiflexes and the remainder of the toes fan out.

11. **A**

Embolization is particularly beneficial in splenic injuries grade III or higher, which previously would have required laparotomy with possible splenectomy. CT criteria can be used effectively to triage patients among simple observation, embolization, or surgery but there has been a change in hemodynamic stability so a repeat scan would not be necessary at this time. The CT scan is able to diagnose an injury to the splenic parenchyma but does not demonstrate possible splenic vascular injury. Vascular injury can be seen on angiography and, if injury is present, should proceed to embolization.

12. B

The Emergency Medical Treatment and Labor Act (EMTALA) states that the receiving facility must provide a medical screening and stabilization within its capabilities if a medical emergency condition is present. The Consolidated Omnibus Budget Reconciliation Act (COBRA) has to require group health plans to provide temporary group health coverage that otherwise might be terminated. Consolidated Origin of Budget Reconciliation Act and the Emergency Medical Treatment Act are both not recognized laws.

13. A

Oxygenation holds the highest priority of care, followed by controlling areas of hemorrhage, then circulatory volume. Securing the airway will achieve proper oxygenation, controlling the bleeding would be next, and then administering intravenous fluids to promote adequate cerebral circulation. The overall goal would be for the patient to be normovolemic; once normovolemia is achieved, further elevation of mean arterial pressure and cerebral perfusion pressure is usually accomplished with vasopressor administration. Blood transfusions are usually not indicated if the patient is only bleeding in the head.

14. A

Postoperative management will include wound care, ostomy care, and drainage maintenance. Complications include infection, fistulas, abscesses, peritonitis, and bowel obstruction. Colostomy closure is usually 6 to 8 weeks after surgery. Wounds left open for significant spillage are delayed with a primary closure of 4 to 5 days after surgery.

15. C

Posterior pelvic fractures are more likely to result in bleeding complications than an anterior pelvic fracture. Medial fractures are not recognized as a pelvic fracture. Anterioposterior compression may cause hemorrhage but posterior–anterior is not a pelvic fracture location.

16. B

Burn shock occurs when the capillary permeability causes sodium shifts intracellularly, drawing fluid from the vascular space into the cellular space. This results in hypovolemia and cellular edema. If managed appropriately with fluid resuscitation, hypotension and tachycardia may not occur. Burn shock occurs early within hours of the burn injury and can be prevented or treated with fluids. It does not resolve spontaneously. Burn shock can cause vaodilation but if hypovolemia occurs it will result in tachycardia, not bradycardia.

17. C

Central herniation is a downward displacement of the brainstem that affects respiratory pattern and level of consciousness. Bilateral pupils will enlarge and become nonreactive. Uncal herniation would include ipsilateral dilation of the pupil. Patients with subfalcine herniation complain of a headache and contralateral leg weakness. Tonsillar herniation patients present with headache, stiff neck, and flaccid paralysis.

18. **B**

Developing a critical incident stress management (CISM) team, may be beneficial in aiding trauma staff in job-related stress, providing assistance to staff feeling the negative effects of working in a trauma environment, and providing education and prevention strategies. This team is usually composed of a mental health professional and peer support personnel. The CISM is better than a support group or just turning to other peers for support. This team is readily available at the time of the event, whereas consulting a mental health professional would not be an immediate intervention.

19. **C**

CT scans have replaced plain films as the "gold standard" because they are capable of three-dimensional reconstruction capabilities of axial sections. Angiography is considered with evaluation of massive facial trauma if there is suspicion of an injury to a major vessel at the base of the skull, lateral pharyngeal space, and cavernous sinus. It is not a gold standard for all facial injuries. Contrast studies are used to identify injuries to the pharynx and the esophagus, not facial fractures and injuries.

20. **A**

It is most important to ensure an adequate airway and provide definitive airway control if required before transporting the patient. This is the responsibility of the transferring hospital. The diagnostic studies can be done by the receiving trauma center and should not delay the transfer. A central line is not recommended before transport but a patient peripheral intravenous (IV) should be in place. Consults should not be obtained until the patient is in the receiving trauma facility.

21. **B**

CT is the preferred method because it provides the most comprehensive diagnosis of traumatic pancreatic injury with a low complication rate. Endoscopic retrograde cholangiopancreatography (ERCP) is increasingly being used to help in both early and delayed diagnosis of pancreatic ductal injuries in patients with strong clinical evidence of pancreatic injury and an equivocal CT scan. An ERCP is the most *accurate* investigation for diagnosing the site and extent of ductal injury but is invasive and is associated with higher rate of complications. Although ultrasound (US) is easy to perform, portable, and cost-effective, pancreatic injuries are difficult to diagnose but US can be useful in the follow-up of complications such as pseudocysts. X-ray of the abdomen in patients with pancreatic trauma is nonspecific and is not beneficial to diagnose pancreatic injuries.

22. **C**

A teardrop fracture of the anterior vertebral body and posterior dislocation is commonly caused by hyperflexion mechanism of injury. A simple fracture is caused by acceleration or deceleration forces spinal cord compression usually occurs as a linear fracture of the spinous or transverse process. Compression fractures occur because of anterior or lateral flexion, hyperflexion, or vertebral body compression. A burst fracture occurs with axial loading and will result in a comminuted fracture of the vertebral body, which can result in a spinal cord injury.

23. **B**

Making sure that the wrench is taped to the halo vest is most important to ensure that it can be removed in case of an emergency. Weights should be hanging freely at all times when traction is applied, not when wearing a halo device. Hair should be kept short to reduce the risk of hair getting caught in the pin sites. The liner is an important piece; make sure it is on before application in order to reduce skin breakdown and irritability against the vest. The wrench is most important because it will be needed to loosen and remove the vest for emergencies and adjustments.

24. **A**

A diffuse axonal injury has a shearing effect on the axons and can result in permanent injury to the brain. About 90% of survivors with severe diffuse axonal injury remain unconscious or in a vegetative state. The 10% who regain consciousness are usually severely neurologically impaired. Acquired brain injuries result from damage to the brain caused by strokes, tumors, anoxia, hypoxia, toxins, degenerative diseases, near drowning, or other conditions not necessarily caused by an external force. Hypoxic brain injuries are caused by oxygen deprivation and prolongation of this state leads to cell death. A closed head injury occurs when the brain is injured as a result of a blow to the head or sudden motion that causes the brain to collide against the skull.

25. **B**

Pulselessness is the late sign of compartment syndrome and indicates the loss of the extremity. Pulses and capillary refill remain intact even with elevated intracompartmental pressures. It requires extremely high pressures to collapse the major arteries, causing a loss of pulse. Pain, parasthesia, and paralysis are the early findings of compartment syndrome, which involve the nerve structures.

26. **C**

Halo immobilization is the expected treatment modality to promote healing of the odontoid fracture by limiting C1–C2 rotation. Soft collar application is not used for an unstable fracture, and would not assist in stabilizing a C1–C2 fracture. C1–C2 surgical fusion is necessary in some cases in which nonunion occurs, but halo is the first-line treatment. Paralysis and, in some cases, death occurs in unstable dens fractures with cord involvement, although a type II is considered "unstable" there is no cord involvement.

27. **B**

Trauma center designation is outlined by the state and can vary from state to state. Requirements for a trauma designation in the state are determined by the legislation or regulatory governing bodies within the state. Trauma center verification is overseen by the American College of Surgeons. The American College of Surgeons, during trauma center verification, determines the facility's commitment, readiness, resources, policies, and performance improvement. It is not a federally mandated criteria or a self-designation by the hospital.

28. **D**

The nurse should be concerned about any feelings of depression or thoughts of harming one's self and the nurse should also inquire about the patient's living situation and safety measures at home, especially because this population is at high risk for falls.

However, this vulnerable population is especially at risk for battery, spousal abuse, and domestic violence. The health care provider needs to consistently inquire about the possibility of domestic violence in the pregnant patient, especially with bruising that may not fit the presented mechanism of injury.

29. C

Tachycardia, hypoxemia, pallor/cyanotic skin, tachypnea, decreased lung compliance, increased work of breathing, crackles, wheezes around the injured site, and blood-tinged sputum are all symptoms of pulmonary contusions. Hemothorax symptoms are very similar except for the crackles being present and the alarming peek pressure, which reflects the decreased lung compliance. Myocardial contusions will have tachycardia and hypoxia, but are more likely to present with cardiac changes such as arrhythmias and decreased cardiac output. Diaphragmatic injuries may present with rhonchi and decreased breath sounds if bowel is herniated into the thoracic cavity.

30. C

A cerebral contusion is caused by damage to parenchymal blood vessels, resulting in hemorrhage or bruising of the brain tissue. A concussion is a type of diffuse brain injury. It is a temporary change in neurological function that occurs in a minor brain trauma. A subdural hematoma is a hemorrhage within the subdural space. Like contusions they usually occur in the frontal and temporal lobes and can produce a mass effect, leading to neurological deterioration. Diffuse axonal injury (DAI) is a type of brain injury, but is widespread rather than localized. DAI causes microscopic damage to axons within the brain and severe DAI is associated with significant morbidity and mortality.

31. C

Zygomatic fracture cerebrospinal fluid leaks are uncommon in this injury. Cribriform, ethmoid, and temporal bone fractures can involve dural injuries and cerebral spinal fluid (CSF) leaks. Clear or blood-tinged nasal drainage should be a high suspicion for a CSF leak and should be assessed for a halo sign.

32. A

In the presence of an increased capillary permeability, colloid solutions can leak protein into interstitial and intrapulmonary spaces, with fluid following. Colloids may also cause coagulopathy and worsen bleeding complications. Hyperglycemia needs to be monitored in solutions that contain dextrose but not necessarily with colloids. Colloids do not have metabolic acidosis as a common complication.

33. D

Adaptation is not a recognized stage of stress. The alarm stage includes any physical, emotional, or mental upset that causes an instant reaction by the body to combat the stressor, also known as the "fight-or-flight" reaction. In the resistance stage, the body tries to become balanced, or returns to homeostasis. The last stage is exhaustion. After combating stress for days to weeks, the body shuts down completely, leaving the immune system compromised and vulnerable to illness.

34. C

Patients who have a tracheal rupture present with respiratory distress and radiographic studies that suggest an injury to the right mainstem bronchus. The mechanism of injury for a tracheal rupture is a blunt or penetrating trauma to the neck or chest. A pneumothorax results from air introduced into the pleural space and presents with dyspnea, tachypnea, tachycardia, decreased breath sounds, and chest pain. A tension pneumothorax occurs when air enters the pleural space on inspiration but cannot escape upon expiration, causing a rise in intrathoracic pressure that collapses the lung, and results in a mediastinal shift. These patients have severe respiratory distress, tracheal deviation, distended neck veins, and absent breath sounds on the affected side. Rib fractures are the most common injury from blunt injuries to the chest or sternum but they display dyspnea, chest pain, chest wall ecchymosis, and bony crepitus.

35. **B**

An orbital blowout fracture is the fracture of the orbital walls without associated fractures of the orbital rims; this can cause entrapment of the inferior or medial rectus muscle, thereby restricting extraocular movements. A zygomatic fracture will have periorbital ecchymosis, but extraocular eye movements are not usually affected. A LeFort I fracture is a horizontal fracture through the maxillary body and does not affect extraocular movements.

36. **D**

Brown–Sequard cord syndrome explains the presentation because of the transverse hemisection of the cord. Central cord injury presents with a loss of motor/sensation below the level of the lesion, notably greater motor losses occur in the arms and bladder dysfunction occurs as well. Anterior cord–injured patients would have loss of pain, temperature, loss of motor function below the level of injury, but touch and vibration will be intact. Posterior cord injuries would reveal intact motor and temperature sensing.

37. **C**

A hemothorax is caused by lung parenchymal lacerations, injuries to intercostal vessels, and injuries to the internal mammary artery. A pneumothorax occurs when air is introduced into the pleural space, causing the lung to collapse. Open pneumothorax is usually caused by penetrating trauma with air flowing freely in and out of the site of injury with each breath. Tension pneumothorax occurs when air enters the pleural space and becomes trapped, building pressure and shifting the mediastinal structures.

38. **A**

Assessing for extraocular eye movements should be avoided in an open-globe injury. Motility of the eye and any pressure applied to the globe can result in the loss of vision. These injuries are serious and frequently require emergency ocular surgery. Hyphema (accumulation of blood in the eye), chemical burns to the eye, and orbital fractures all require a full ocular assessment, which frequently includes visual inspection of the eye for uncontrolled bleeding or lacerations, pupillary assessment—including consensual response—a visual acuity examination, assessment of quality of vision, and extraocular eye movements.

39. **C**

Diffuse axonal injury is not typically the result of a direct blow to the head. This injury results from the brain moving back and forth in the skull as a result of acceleration or deceleration or a rotational mechanism. Automobile accidents, sports-related accidents, falls, and shaken baby syndrome are common causes of diffuse axonal injury. When rotational mechanism causes the brain to move within the skull, axons are sheared. As tissue slides over tissue, a shearing injury occurs, this causes lesions that are responsible for making the patient unconscious.

40. C

The best method to treat a tar burn is to remove loose skin and leave the tar intact. Peeling off the tar will cause more damage to the skin that is stuck under the tar. Slowly dissolve the tar with repeated applications of a liquefying agent such as Neomycin cream. It may take days for all of the tar to be removed. A reflex reaction is to immerse the injured area in water to immediately cool and harden the tar, but then it is difficult to remove from the skin. Neosporin cream is an antibiotic combination that also has an emulsifier as a base and is useful for tar burns but is not the first-choice cream. Antibiotic creams are effective in dissolving tar because of their emulsifying properties and petrolatum base.

41. A

It is important to place the family in a private, safe environment is recommended before delivering the news. However, the nurse should not go alone to deliver this news. Getting security to accompany the team may be indicated in some situations but can be overpowering too. If the situation escalates, escorting the aggressive family members out is suggested but would not be an initial response. Using words like *expired* or *passed* does not enforce the reality of the situation that the patient is dead and should not be used.

42. A

This patient is experiencing strong symptoms of posttraumatic stress disorder (PTSD). It is common to experience some degree of PTSD after a trauma and extensive stay in an intensive care unit. Patients with PTSD may have trouble sleeping, keeping their mind focused, and have increased irritability or angry outbursts. With bipolar disorder, there are significant mood swings, risky behavior, grandiose beliefs, and extreme depression and sometimes suicidal ideations. This patient had a significant trauma event and that is most likely triggering the change in behavior and not the new development of psychosis. Delirium symptoms are similar to PTSD, but this patient is not experiencing altered mentation or hallucinations.

43. C

When the pelvic ring is fractured in more than one place it is labeled an *unstable pelvic fracture*. A stable pelvic fracture can withstand forces without deformation and would not involve a bilateral fracture. Pelvic fractures are commonly classified by the force that caused the injury, but are not classified as displaced or dislodged.

44. A

Vitrous hemorrhage, hyphema, and optic nerve injury can occur with orbital fractures. Opacification of the globe is commonly a result of an alkali chemical injury to the eye and is not associated with ocular fractures. Opacification can occur with traumatic exposure but is not associated with orbital fractures. Vitreous hemorrhage is the extravasation of blood into the areas in and around the clear gel that fills the space between the lens and the retina of the eye, the vitreous. A hyphema is a pooling or collection of blood inside the anterior chamber of the eye. The blood may cover most or all of the iris and the pupil, blocking vision partially or completely and is usually painful.

45. A

Fat embolism is a common complication from pelvic fractures or long bone fractures. The patient is complaining of pelvic pain and there is blood noted at the urinary meatus, making the assessment suspicious of a pelvic fracture. The patient is hypotensive, hypoxic, tachypniec, tachycardic, and has petechiae on the chest, which is the presentation of a patient with fat emboli. Pulmonary embolism would present with hypotension, tachycardia, and hypoxia, but would not have the petechiae upon the chest. Hypovolemic shock and hemorrhagic shock could present similar with the hypotension and the tachycardia, but the key was tying the assessment to the injury. Pelvic fractures can be associated with large blood volume losses, but the evaluation indicated the presence of fat emboli according to the injury and the presentation.

46. C

The nurse should always use the names of all visitors and document their demeanor and appearance objectively. Avoid using forensic statements such as "exit" "entry" wound. Use direct quotes when possible.

47. D

Physical therapy (PT) works with gait and ambulation, whereas occupational therapy (OT) works with upper extremities, fine motor control, and activities of daily living. Both therapies work as a team but that response does not answer the family's question. They are both very important to the rehabilitation of the patient.

48. B

These are all disasters that occur in the community and not at a health care facility, which makes them community-based incidents. These typically are the least common types of disasters and are frequently categorized as mass casualty incidents. There is no distinction of rural-based mass casualties.

49. B

Once the diagnosis of a traumatic aortic aneurysm is made, the systolic blood pressure (SBP) should be maintained at 130 mmHg or below. Most trauma patients have low blood pressure but the patient should still be monitored closely for increases in blood pressure (BP). The higher BPs can increase the risk of aneurysm rupture.

50. C

The family should not take personal items except for valuables because all trauma patients are potential forensic cases until completely ruled out. Items, such as personal clothing, need to be carefully packed and kept with the body as potential evidence. The term *accident* indicates nonintentional versus intentional events and should not be used unless the investigation is complete. Trauma-death patients need to be handled with special consideration for forensic evidence. Nurses need to be aware of the environment around them and the belongings that came with the patient because they can be used as potential evidence.

51. C

The five Ps in the neurovascular assessment are used to evaluate extremity trauma and assess for complicatons. The five Ps include pain, paresthesia, pallor, paralysis, and pulslessness. Pain, paresthesia, and paralysis correlate with the nerve injury and pallor and pulselessness are used to assess vascular perfusion.

52. C

The initial technique recommended to stop the bleeding would be to apply pressure and a pressure dressing. Most complete amputations result in vessel spasm and occlusion of bleeding. Elevating the extremity would help by decreasing bleeding, edema, and pain. A tourniquet may be used if the pressure does not control the bleeding and is placed closely above the level of amputation. Clamping of the vessels might make reanastomosis of the vessel impossible and is not recommended. Local digital nerve block causes direct trauma by the needle and is not recommended.

53. C

Ringer's lactate is the fluid of choice in massive fluid resuscitation; it is a balanced salt solution, which is isotonic. Normal saline can lead to hypernatremia and hyperchloremic acidosis. Saline 0.45% is a hypotonic solution and does not resuscitate the intravascular space. Dextrose should be avoided as it may cause hyperglycemia, cerebral edema, and osmotic diuresis.

54. A

The subarachnoid hemorrhage score used is the Hunt Hess Scale but it is used for cerebral hemorrhagic strokes and not trauma. The revised trauma score, Apache II, and emergency trauma score are all used to determine the severity of the trauma and predict mortality.

55. B

This patient is presenting with a complication of venous congestion following reimplantation of the extremity. The reimplanted exremity appears blue, cool to touch with brisk capillary refill, and skin turgor is tense. The nurse should maintain the extremity level. Lowering the extremity may increase edema but placing it above the level can decrease perfusion. Betadine scrub does not affect venous congestion and is not a type of treatment. Antiplatelet medication is the treatment used to decrease arterial blood not venous congestion.

56. C

The mechanism of injury indicates a high risk for liver injury; this patient is presenting with symptoms of a hepatic injury. Splenic injuries also present with involuntary guarding but the hallmark sign is reported pain in the left shoulder when lying supine, known as *Kehr's sign,* and the patient will have tenderness in the left upper quadrant. Large-bowel injuries will present with involuntary guarding and rebound tenderness but not pain in the right upper quadrant. It also typically presents with associated signs of hypovolemic shock and rectal bleeding. Gastric injury patients have abdominal pain and peritoneal irritation with gross blood can be seen in gastric aspirate with this injury.

57. A

The Certification of Transfer was violated. Violation of this law includes sending no certificate or sending an unsigned certificate, failing to weigh the benefits versus risks, using improper reasons for transfer, or misstating or lying about the benefits of transfer. The Emergency Medical Treatment and Labor Act (EMTALA) is the federal law that requires anyone coming into the emergency room to receive treatment regardless of his or her insurance or ability to pay. Trauma Transfer Guidelines are available in most states and trauma centers have these guidelines to assist in the appropriate transfer of trauma patients between nontrauma centers and trauma centers. The Consolidated Omnibus Budget Reconciliation Act (COBRA) requires that group health plans provide temporary continuation of insurance coverage that otherwise might be terminated.

58. D

Administering labetalol to address hypertension is incorrect for the initial management of autonomic dysreflexia (AD). It can result in significant hypotension when the source is identified and removed. Removing the causative agent is the initial goal. Assessing the skin for pressure ulcers and repositioning to take the pressure off the area can help relieve the pain from the pressure ulcer site. Bladder and bowel issues are the most common causes of AD, so relieving the bladder and removing a fecal impaction will aid in relieving AD symptoms. Remember, relieving the source of pain will resolve the hypertensive state.

59. B

Obstructive shock results from inadequate circulating blood volume directly related to an obstruction of outflow or compression of great vessels. Spinal cord injuries do not cause obstructions to outflow from the ventricles but will present more as distributive shock because of the disruption of the sympathetic nervous system, resulting in vasodilation. Cardiac tamponade compresses the heart during cardiac filling, which does not allow the heart to fill the heart chambers adequately. Having a tension pneumothorax decreases stroke volume by obstructing venous return to the right atrium. Air emboli can lead to pulmonary artery obstruction, which will affect cardiac emptying.

60. B

Patients taking beta-blockers, calcium-channel blockers, or those who have pacemakers may not have a tachycardic response to hypovolemia. This lack of response may lead to a delay in the diagnosis of hypovolemic shock. When obtaining the history, medications should always be included for this reason. The examiner should also rely on signs of decreased peripheral perfusion other than tachycardia or blood pressure for an accurate diagnosis of hypovolemia. Elderly patients may not be able to tolerate hypovolemia but that does not explain the question's statement. Patients with pacemakers may not be able to become tachycardic, but can still become hypotensive.

61. A

Fluids should be warmed to avoid hypothermia when the capillary leak has been stabilized. Peripheral access is the route preferred over central-line access because of the increased risk of bleeding caused by coagulopathy of a burn patient and time requirements. Burn patients require fluid resuscitation and should not have limited fluids.

62. B

All of these complications are associated with facial injuries and can negatively affect outcome, but airway always comes first. The actual facial trauma is usually a lower priority than other traumatic injuries in multisystem trauma patients unless there is presence of an airway obstruction.

63. **B**

A 2-L fluid challenge is commonly used in resuscitation to assist with determining the amount of blood loss. If the vital signs stabilize after the fluid administration without further deterioration in status, the patient probably has had a blood loss less than 20%. If the vital signs stabilize after the bolus, but deteriorate when the infusion is stopped, the patient probably has blood loss greater than 30%. If the vital signs fail to stabilize with the fluid bolus, then the blood loss is probably greater than 40% and may require immediate surgery to control the hemorrhage.

64. **C**

Fungal infections have increased significantly through the years. They are more difficult to treat and are harder to diagnose. Treatment of fungal infections is frequently a presumptive therapy with negative blood cultures. It is more difficult to culture fungus from blood cultures so the provider needs a higher suspicion of a fungal infection. Fungal infections are usually opportunistic infections and are frequently caused by the use of antibiotics altering the normal flora or present in immunosuppressed patients. Fungal sepsis has a higher mortality rate than bacteremia. There are more than 750,000 cases of fungus-related sepsis each year.

65. **A**

The primary goal of all trauma patients is to regain independence and to meet maximal recovery. Following a traumatic injury, the patient may not always return to his or her prior level of function or become productive; so is not a primary goal of rehabilitation, which is not to lengthen life but to improve the quality of life.

66. **C**

MRI has the capability of revealing ligamentous injury, spinal cord injury, and instability, and provides prognostic information regarding long-term neurological outcome in patients with spinal cord injury without radiological abnormalities (SCIWORA). CT is a poor choice because it would reveal bony abnormalities that are usually not present and limited spinal cord involvement results. Myelography and angiography have no defined role in the evaluation of SCIWORA.

67. **D**

Transfusion-related acute lung injury (TRALI) is a "two hit" insult to the patient's lungs. The first hit is the stressful situation, in this case the trauma, which causes neutrophils to adhere to the pulmonary endothelial bed. The second hit is the actual blood transfusion, which contains donor antibodies that activate the neutrophils, resulting in increased capillary permeability and noncardiogenic pulmonary edema. This causes a sudden onset of fever, cough, and hypoxia. Most patients require intubation, but will usually recover within 96 hours. The patient did not present with any signs of hemolytic blood transfusion reaction, including shock state and disseminated intravascular coagulation. The patient has no identified risks or presence of chronic obstructive pulmonary disease (COPD). Pneumothorax presents with dyspnea, tracheal shift, and diminished or absent breath sounds on the affected side.

68. D

Typically, a level 1 trauma center is the comprehensive regional center capable of providing total care for every aspect of trauma injury. Level 1 trauma centers provide care from prevention through rehabilitation for trauma patients. Research and formal teaching in trauma centers are efforts to direct innovation in trauma care and improve outcomes. Trauma centers provide a comprehensive quality-assessment program and continuing education. Level 2 trauma centers typically have immediate coverage by general surgeons, whereas level 3 may only have prompt availability.

69. A

Ecchymosis of the flank area is called Grey–Turners sign, and is indicative of retroperitoneal bleeding. The sign may not be present on initial presentation and can take hours or even days to appear. Esophageal injuries will present with subcutaneous emphysema, peritoneal irritation and pain referred to the neck, chest, shoulders, and abdomen. Splenic injuries will have positive Kehr's sign, which is pain in the left shoulder when lying supine or in the Trendelenburg position. The liver is located in the peritoneal space; so would not present with signs of retroperitoneal hemorrhage.

70. C

Hyperventilation resulting in hypocapania causes cerebral vasoconstriction, which decreases cerebral blood flow. This can result in brain ischemia and is not recommended. Hyperventilation does lower intracranial pressure (ICP) but also lowers oxygenation and cerebral perfusion (not increases). Hypocapnia decreases blood flow and cerebral perfusion. A patient's CO_2 level should be greater than 35.

71. A

If a laceration is on the cheek, assessment of the cranial nerve VII (facial nerve) should be performed by the trauma nurse. The temporal branch of the facial nerve innervates the frontalis muscle of the forehead. The facial nerve and the parotid duct may require anastomosis before suturing. The parotid duct routes saliva from the major salivary gland to the parotid gland and into the mouth. Temporal, eyebrow, and forehead injuries would not be at risk for injuring the facial nerve or parotid ducts.

72. D

Although life-saving measures take precedence over the preservation of possible evidence, the nurse should take care in removing clothing of trauma patients. Patient's clothing needs to be removed carefully to maintain its integrity as much as possible. Laying a white sheet under the bed allows the nurse to place the clothing on the sheet. Never throw clothes on the floor to avoid gross contamination of critical evidence. Placing a clean white sheet on the floor and emptying all items onto it preserves all evidence so that it can be packed, handled properly, and given to the authorities without accidently misplacing items.

73. A

Patients with joint injuries usually experience significant pain; if there is a decrease in sensation or an absence of pain, this could presumedly be nerve injury involvement. Popliteal vein and artery involvement is most likely present and that increases the risk of avascular necrosis; however, the question asks what is the best reason for the patient not feeling pain at the site, and that would be associated with the peroneal nerve being damaged. If nerves are involved, the relay of nerve impulses is blocked or diminished, which decreases pain sensation.

74. C

The simple triage and rapid treatment (START) method begins with assessment and, once a color is established, the nurse should move on to assess another patient. Remember: STOP-TAG-MOVE ON.

75. A

The patient needs an emergent thoracotomy. Intrathoracic hemorrhage, evidence of pericardial tamponade, systemic air emboli, and severe intrathoracic hemorrhage are all indications for the need of an emergent thoracotomy in patients with penetrating trauma to the chest. After the emergency thoracotomy and resuscitation to a perfusing rhythm, then the patient can be transported to the operating room. A chest tube placement would not be part of effective resuscitation efforts in this patient as the patient is presenting more like a pericardial tamponade than a hemothorax. A pericardial window is indicated in managing pericardial tamponade but in this patient the underlying injury has caused the pulseless electrical activity (PEA) and the patient requires emergency thoracotomy for rapid correction.

76. D

Administering vasopressor medication, such as Levophed, vasopressin, and dopamine, could worsen organ perfusion in situations of continued hypovolemia without adequate fluid resuscitation. Using the vasopressor to increase the blood pressure can decrease perfusion to the kidneys and gastrointestinal tract, resulting in hypoperfusion and organ dysfunction. Excessive use of vasopressors in order to target a higher blood pressure will increase cardiac workload and worsen cardiac output and perfusion and is not recommended.

77. A

The psychological criteria is not included in the Centers for Disease Control and Prevention (CDC) triage system. The four steps are physiologic criteria such as Glasgow Coma Scale score less than or equal to 13, anatomic criteria such as the presence of a flail chest, mechanism of injury such as adult falls from greater than 20 feet, and special considerations that include burn patients.

78. C

Carboxyhemoglobin levels of 0% to 13% are normal, 14% to 24% is an elevated level, toxic level is 25% to 35%, and a lethal level is above 60%. Treatment with inhaled oxygen helps to reduce the carbon monoxide from the hemoglobin and decreases the half-life of carboxyhemoglobin. It is recommended that oxygen therapy should be continued until the carboxyhemoglobin levels have decreased below 15% and any neurological symptoms have resolved.

79. B

The triad of complications following a trauma includes hypothermia (not hyperthermia), coagulopathy, and metabolic acidosis. Hypotension and decreased hemoglobin are commonly experienced with blood loss, however, it is not considered a component of the triad.

80. C

Increased circulating blood volume has been associated with the development of elevated pressures and compartment syndrome in the abdomen, chest, cranium, and extremities. Too much or too rapid resuscitation can worsen the bleeding by dislodging clots. Dilution lowers the blood viscosity and decreases the ability to carry oxygen leading to tissue hypoperfusion. Fluid resuscitation should be with 250-mL fluid boluses to reach a systolic blood pressure goal of 80 mmHg or a palpable radial pulse.

81. B

An arteriogram should be considered when there is a fracture sustained at ribs 1 to 3 because the amount of force required to break those ribs can result in further thoracic injuries such as aortic injuries, vascular injuries, and tracheobronchial injuries. The secondary findings related to rib fractures include a hemothorax, pneumothorax, and lung contusion. These findings are more easily seen on chest CT scans than on chest x-rays, but chest x-ray may be a screening tool. An ultrasound of the kidneys or carotids does not diagnose potential inuries associated with rib 2 fractures.

82. A

This patient is exhibiting signs of sepsis. The nurse should obtain blood cultures before administering any antibiotics. Antibiotics should be administered as soon possible to improve outcomes and are recommended within 1 hour of onset of sepsis; cultures need to be drawn very quickly. Lactate level should also be drawn initially to assess for tissue perfusion. Antipyretics may be indicated but are not a priority over blood cultures and antibiotics. Measuring central venous pressure and central venous oxygen saturation is recommended to be completed within 6 hours but is not the initial action in sepsis.

83. C

This is the 1998 law passed called the Routine Referral Law and requires hospitals to notify the associated organ procurement organization of deaths or impending death. The Uniform Anatomical Gift Act was passed in 1968; this ensured a national method was used to obtain organs for transplant and allows for organ donation. The Consolidated Omnibus Budget Reconciliation Act required hospitals receiving Medicare and Medicaid reimbursement to have written protocols for identifying donors and providing families with the option. In 2004, the Organ Donation and Recovery Improvement Act provided grant money to further increase organ-donation awareness.

84. A

The correct method of calculation would be 4 × 80 kg × 27% total body surface area (TBSA) = 8,640 mL of crystalloid solution, usually lactated Ringer's. The patient's weight needs to be converted to kg. The fluid of choice is usually Ringer's lactate. Normal saline is an isotonic crystalloid but can cause hypernatremia and hyperchloremia with large volumes of resuscitation. Dextrose fluids are not indicated in burn trauma resuscitation.

85. A

Disseminated intravascular coagulation (DIC) is a frequent complication of many obstetrical diseases. It presents with abnormal bleeding, bruising, petechiae, and organ dysfunction. The treatment is urgent. Lab values would reveal an elevated

PT/PTT (prothrombin time/partial thromboplastin time), decreased fibrinogen, decreased platelets, and a positive D-dimer. Abruptio placentae occurs when the placenta separates from the uterine wall, resulting in disruption of maternal–fetal circulation, which is what the patient presented with, but is now showing signs of a coagulopathy. Antigen–antibody reaction occurs when the fetus is Rh positive and the mother is Rh negative; the mixing of blood causes a thrombolytic reaction. Amnioitis is an infection that includes an elevated white blood cell (WBC) count, maternal and fetal tachycardia, tender uterus, and a fever greater than 101°F.

86. A

Contraindications for autotransfusion include blood that is potentially contaminated from a bowel injury with fecal spillage. Bright-red blood indicates fresh blood and is not a contraindication. If the drainage is purulent or bile-colored then the autotransfusion would be contraindicated because it indicates the presence of infection or contamination of bowel contents. A patient with a suspected tracheobronchial injury would have an airleak with bubbling in the water-seal chamber of the chest tube system and would require surgical intervention, but would not require autotransfusion. Chest tube output greater than 500 mL is a definitive candidate for autotransfusion.

87. B

Epidural hematomas (EDHs) are commonly arterial and expand rapidly. EDHs can be venous at times but usually are only seen with a depressed skull fracture or in pediatric patients. Increased mortality with epidural bleeds usually occur in patients younger than 5 years or older than 55 years. These patients can rapidly deteriorate and need close monitoring. Not all EDH injuries require surgery, a few can be observed for neurological changes and blood expansion upon imaging.

88. A

Neurogenic shock occurs with injury at T6 or above. Neurogenic shock symptoms usually are temporary and often last less than 72 hours; spinal shock is variable and can last from hours to weeks. Neurogenic shock presents with loss of ability to sweat below level of injury, hypotension, and bradycardia. Neurogenic shock is a form of distributive shock that results in a temporary loss of sympathetic tone. Spinal shock presents with flaccidity and loss of reflexes and includes a marked reduction or loss of somatic and/or reflex functions of the spinal cord below the level of the injury. Autonomic dysreflexia occurs after spinal shock has resolved and causes hypertension above the level of injury. Hypovolemic shock presents with hypotension and tachycardia (not bradycardia).

89. C

Organ donor network staff trained to approach families about organ procurement should be the only ones to discuss organ donation with the family. The person who tells the family that their loved one is dead should not be the person who approaches them to discuss organ donation, nor should the attending physician. The nurse who comforts the family should also not discuss this topic even if a close rapport has been established.

90. D

If clear fluid is leaking from the nose or ears, this is considered a medical emergency because it is indicative of a cerebral spinal leak. Nausea, vomiting, and being harder to wake than normal may indicate an increase in intracranial pressure (ICP) and requires a return to the emergency room (ER). Persistent headache may require follow-up care but does not necessarily require a return to the ER. This is called postconcussion syndrome.

91. C

A pericardiocentesis is performed by a physician to treat patients who are experiencing cardiac tamponade. The symptoms include hypotensin, tachycardia, elevated jugular distension, and muffled heart sounds. The excessive blood in the pericardial sac is aspirated from the pericardial sac. A thoracotomy is an incision into the chest wall and typically is a necessity for patients who sustain a penetrating injury involving the anterior or precordial thoracic area, such as a gunshot wound to the chest. Chest tubes for autotransfusion are placed to treat patients who have a hemothroax in order to decompress the lung and transfuse the blood. A needle thoracentesis will require insertion of a 14-gauge needle into the second intercostal space midclavicular line in order to treat a tension pneumothorax. This patient does not exhibit signs of hemothorax or tension.

92. C

This description of the burn wound describes a deep partial thickness (second-degree burn). A superficial partial-thickness (second-degree) burn would be different than what is described because it involves the epidermis and part of the dermal layer. This burn appears red to pale ivory and is moist. A superficial (first-degree) burn involving the dermis results in erythema without blisters. A full-thickness (third-degree) burn involves epidermis, dermis, and subcutaneous tissue. These burns appear white, cherry red, brown, or black, and are dry, hard, and leathery.

93. B

Tachycardia is the first and most indicative sign of shock for pediatric patients. The heart rate increases to maintain cardiac output. Blood pressure is an unreliable indicator of shock in these patients. Tachypnea may be present in the pediatric shock patient, but sustained tachycardia is the most reliable sign. Fever does not indicate presence of shock.

94. D

Making major life decisions during periods of depression is not recommended. It is recommended for patients to keep their usual daily routine while going through a period of depression. Volunteering time or joining a charity to occupy time keeps them active but also gives a sense of self-worth. If the trauma is prominent in the news media, have the patient limit exposure to the news.

95. C

Although encouraging the patient to eat by bringing in favorite foods to stimulate appetite is therapeutic, *forcing* the patient to eat is not recommended. Going without food and water is generally not painful, unless the patient is complaining of being hungry or thirsty. Losing one's appetite is common and is considered normal in the dying process because the body is beginning to shut down unnecessary organs to sustain life and provide essential needs to the vital organs.

96. D

A physiatrist specializes in rehabilitation. A podiatrist specializes in foot care. Psychologists and psychiatrists specialize in the psychological and mental adaptation to injuries.

97. A

Patients who have an altered mental status and are unable to follow commands should be tagged red for immediate treatment. Other patients who should be tagged red present with respirations over 30 breaths per minute, capillary refill greater than 2 seconds or absence of radial pulse, and unconscious patients who are still breathing. Black tag indicates the patient has expired or death is imminent. Yellow is stable for the moment and treatment can be delayed. A green tag represents the "walking wounded"—those with minor injuries who will require treatment at some time but is not critical.

98. A

Pelvic fractures are the second most common cause of death in multisystem trauma patients. Mortality is caused by hemorrhagic shock. Pelvic fractures can result in up to 3 L of blood loss or more from injured vessels. Cranial fractures may or may not be associated with brain injury. Hip and extremity fractures can result in immobility but are not as high a risk of mortality as pelvic fractures.

99. A

The focused assessment with sonography for trauma (FAST) is a portable and rapid examination that detects fluid in the abdomen. It is considered positive if 200 to 500 mL of fluid is detected. CT scan is the primary diagnostic modality for intra-abdominal injuries but requires transport out of the emergency room and can miss the diaphragm, bowel, and some pancreatic injuries. Diagnostic peritoneal lavage (DPL) is frequently unreliable because of the high incidence of false-negative rates. It is invasive and can miss injury to the diaphragm and retroperitoneum. Intravenous pyelogram (IVP) is used to evaluate the kidneys, ureters, or bladder.

100. B

Generally, it is not appropriate to inform the family of a death over the phone unless the family lives far away. In this case, the nurse should inform the family of the death and provide them with an accurate time of death to reduce the amount of guilt that might be felt for not being present. Waiting for the physician is not necessary and having the family come to the facility is inappropriate because the patient will not be in the emergency department anymore by the time they arrive.

101. D

The spleen, liver, small bowel, duodenum, and pancreas are the most commonly injured organs in blunt abdominal trauma. A solid organ is more commonly injured in blunt trauma than a penetrating injury. The liver is usually involved because of the large size, location, and its being a solid organ. The small bowel is frequently injured because of its quantity and mobility within the abdomen. A duodenal injury is frequently seen because of a deceleration mechanism of injury causing tearing of the duodenum at the point of ligament fixation. The large bowel is a hollow organ that collapses and is less likely to be injured with a blunt mechanism.

102. **A**

The primary phase is the elimination of trauma-related injuries. An example is installing a stoplight at a dangerous intersection to lower the risk of collisions. Secondary prevention is the reduction of injury severity during the incident. An example is an airbag, which can reduce the injury that occurs during impact. Tertiary prevention is the efforts to improve the outcome after trauma. The example of tertiary prevention is the utilization of best practice to improve outcomes. Intermediate phase is not a recognized type of trauma prevention.

103. **B**

Hip dislocation left untreated can lead to avascular necrosis. The patient is displaying symptoms of impaired circulation to the extremity from the injury. An angiography is used to diagnose vascular trauma, but an immediate reduction is warranted to minimize the risk for permanent disability. Early hip reduction is recommended, especially within 6 to 24 hours of the initial injury. Traction might be used postoperatively if alignment is needed. A cast is not indicated in a hip fracture.

104. **D**

Following a splenectomy the patient needs to have preventative vaccinations to decrease certain infections. The pneumococcal vaccine is highly recommended because of the increased risk of pneumococcal pneumonia infections postsplenectomy. The meningococcal conjugate vaccine is recommended for people without a functional spleen because getting meningitis could be deadly in an immunocompromised patient. Influenza is a highly contagious viral infection and is a common cause of pneumonia as well as other bacterial infections. Therefore, once-yearly influenza vaccination is recommended for people without a functional spleen. Most adults do not need the polio vaccine because they have already been vaccinated as children. The polio vaccine is recommended if traveling outside the country or if you are exposed to others infected with the poliovirus.

105. **B**

Intravenous pyelogram (IVP) includes contrast dye administered intravenously with consecutive x-rays obtained. The test is able to view kidneys, ureters, and the bladder. After the dye is injected, the patient is evaluated for renal function, extravasation from ureters and bladder, and devitalized segments of the kidney or ureteral deviation.

106. **D**

CT scan of the abdomen and pelvis can be performed in situations in which the trauma physician suspects abdominal or thoracic trauma but should be avoided from routine diagnostics because the fetal dose of radiation is high at 2.60 rads. Cardiotocography monitors fetal heart rate and uterine contractions and is very useful in detecting fetal distress. Peritoneal lavage is not contraindicated in the pregnant patient because it is an open technique isolated to only the peritoneum and can be inserted above the umbilical site. The focused assessment with sonography for trauma (FAST) examination uses ultrasound waves so the exposure to radiation is minimized.

107. **C**

Comfort care typically involves discontinuing therapeutic interventions and diagnostic testing, such as MRI care, which do not contribute to comfort care. The focus of comfort care is relieving any pain, this includes administering analgesics, sedatives, and using alternative pain-relieving measures. The goal is to relieve or prevent any further suffering, so administration of morphine is indicated and should not be discontinued. Hospice or palliative care teams may be consulted for further evaluation of proper end-of-life/comfort care.

108. B

The need for information includes accurate information delivered in a timely manner that the family fully understand and comprehend; this develops a trusting relationship between caregiver and patient/family. Maintaining hope is so important even when the situation is grim because it is the only positive emotion that can be maintained to gain recovery. The need for compassion by the nurse providing the care is important but independent decision making is not necessarily an initial need by patients and their families. Nourishment and sleep are important but are not typically the initial psychosocial need of trauma patients and family members.

109. A

This patient is showing signs of a pulmonary embolism (PE). PE symptoms include respiratory distress, chest pain on inspiration, low blood oxygen saturation, tachypnea, and tachycardia. When a patient in the intensive care unit (ICU) requires sedation and mechanical ventilation, PE clinical manifestations usually present with hypotension and oxygen desaturations. The risk for deep vein thrombosis and pulmonary embolism are high in trauma patients and these patients should be treated prophylactically. Cardiogenic shock presents with tachycardia and tachypnea but is also associated with weak pulses, pale skin, diaphoresis, and a decreased urine output. Hypovolemic shock may present with these symptoms as well but there is no hint of suspected bleeding and the patient has been in the ICU the past 3 days. Acute respiratory distress syndrome presents with shortness of breath with rapid, shallow breathing, mottled/cyanotic skin, whited-out chest x-rays, and increased airway resistance.

110. C

The process of rehabilitation should begin on admission. The immediate initiation of recuperation promotes recovery and results in decreased length of stay in the hospital. Even in hemodynamically unstable patients, rehabilitation can begin with performing tasks of pulmonary toileting. Waiting for a patient to be ready to interact with a physical therapist may never happen, according to the individuals' diagnosis. Activities, such as passive range-of-motion exercises, do not require reciprocated interaction with physical therapists. Waiting until discharge to initiate rehabilitation is doing a disservice to the patient by not working toward recovery from day 1.

111. B

Research has shown that when the death of a child is traumatic, especially if witnessed, the parents are likely to be more traumatized by the experience, become obsessed with the death, and replay the events over and over in their heads. However, allowing the parents to stay with the child after death can assist with some of the healing and acceptance. Conversely, if the parents do not see the body of the deceased they are likely to stay in a state of denial and disbelief for a longer period of time.

112. B

This patient's wound location is an important key to the answer being a diaphragm injury. Penetrating injuries below the nipple line, stab wounds to the anterior chest wall and flank areas should be considered high risk for a possible diaphragm injury because of the large surface area of the diaphragm. Sharp epigastric pain, dyspnea, bowel sounds present in the lower to midchest, and decreased breath sounds on the injured side are all signs of a ruptured diaphragm and the diaphragm defect may allow for the stomach, small intestine, and spleen to enter the thorax. Hemothorax will have dyspnea and decreased breath sounds to the injured side, but will also have chest pain, signs of hypovolemia/shock, and dullness to percussion. Flail chest-injured patients have dyspnea, chest wall pain, and the hallmark sign of paradoxical chest wall movements. Pulmonary contusions have dyspnea, hemoptysis, chest wall contusions/abrasions, chest pain, and hypoxia.

113. C

Angiography is considered the "gold standard" diagnostic for an aortic injury. Chest x-ray is a screening test and can increase suspicion if it detects a widened or abnormal mediastinum. CT scans do not reveal the presence of aortic injuries. The focused assessment with sonography for trauma (FAST) examination is useful in detecting whether there are areas of hemorrhage in the abdomen or pericardial space but is not used to diagnose an aortic injury.

114. B

The key word in this example is *allocating*. In a disaster setting, it is not as important to use optimum resources but to allocate available resources to achieve the greatest good for the greatest number of patients, not an individual patient.

115. B

Respiratory dysfunction would be medically based treatment in the acute care setting, not rehabilitation based. Physical therapy in a respiratory patient might be of benefit to the patient as early mobility, but this would be a secondary benefit to the rehabilitation service, not a primary service. Behavioral dysfunction includes the assessment for irritability, aggression, increased emotional lability, or restlessness. The patient would benefit from psychological support, occupational therapy for reinforcement of autonomy in activities of daily living (ADL), physical therapy to promote mobility and create a change in scenery, social work, and family encouragement. A collaborated approach in a behavioral patient could recognize the reasoning behind the behavior. Patients with motor dysfunction, such as paresis, spasticity, or ataxia, are appropriate for physical therapy rehabilitation but occupational therapy could be used for ADL support as well.

116. C

Floods are the most common type of natural disasters and flooding and can cause infectious and vendor-borne diseases to spread through the water and contaminate the public. Hurricanes can cause flooding but usually result in drownings, electrocutions, and debris injuries. Tornados cause injuries with flying debris and falling objects without a prolonged effect on public health. Fires are considered a natural disaster but can frequently be man-made and also have less residual effect on public health.

117. D

Premature labor is the most frequent complication in a pregnant trauma patient. Premature labor is dangerous because it can go unnoticed by the patient, so the nurse should always assess for contractions, back pain, fetal heart tones, vaginal discharge, and cervical dilation. Fetal demise can occur with trauma but premature labor is more common. Abruptio placentae is the most common cause of fetal death after motor vehicle collision and uterine rupture is rare but usually will occur with compression injuries or in patients who have had cesarean sections in the past.

118. B

The hot zone is where only basic care is provided such as opening an airway or applying a simple dressing. The warm zone is where decontamination actually occurs. The parking area is in the hot zone in this particular example. Patients should not be transferred to the emergency department until after the patient is clean and decontaminated.

119. C

The Lund and Browder chart is a more accurate assessment that takes into account the changes in body surface area related to individual growth and different depths of burns within the burn wound. The rule of ones or hand rule is also used to determine the size of irregular burns and is more accurate than the rule of nines but not as accurate as Lund and Browder chart. This method uses the individual's hand as a guideline to determine the extent of the burn. The hand is approximately 1% of the total body surface area. The rule of nines is the universal determinate of extent; it is easy to determine the surface area but is not as accurate as Lund and Browder.

120. C

The goal of restoration in rehabilitation is to return the patient to the pretraumatic level of functioning. The goal of compensation in rehabilitation is to replace pretraumatic functioning with other strategies. The goal of adaptation in rehabilitation is to change life-style roles and expectations to adapt to any disabilities that occur because of the traumatic event. Recovery to the level before the injury is not always possible.

121. A

Although carbon monoxide inhalation is probable, the patient is suffering from hypoxemia/asphyxia. This causes a lack of oxygen and is associated with an increase in the amount of toxic substances being inhaled from the closed compartment. Adult respiratory distress syndrome presents typically 48 hours or more after the initial injury. Hypermetabolism occurs following burn injuries but is not a cause of early respiratory failure.

122. A

Septic shock is hypoperfusion and hypotension despite resuscitation efforts, including fluid resuscitation and vasopressors. A patient in severe sepsis exhibits hypoperfusion and/or hypotension but has not been managed yet with fluids and vasopressors. Organ dysfunction frequently includes signs of altered mental status, ileus and acute oliguria, which were not identified in this scenario. Sepsis is the systematic response to infection, white blood cell count is greater than 12,000, respiratory rate is greater than 20 breaths per minute, heart rate is greater than 90 beats per minute, and temperature elevation, or hypothermia, is present.

123. C

The nurse should attempt to stabilize and treat the patient until time for transfer. When a hemodynamically unstable patient has to transfer, the transfer should not be held as long as the risk analysis is in favor of transferring to benefit the patient. Intubation should occur before transfer, if needed, but the patient should still be transferred to the facility more capable of caring for the patient. A team of qualified personnel needs to accompany the patient with resuscitative measures at the ready. The nurse can call for a reference on initial wound care for the patient, but it is not the best response to address the question of transferring an unstable patient.

124. C

Airway is the first assessment and should be completed before any other task. A possible cervical spine injury requires maintaining spinal precautions until cleared, but ensuring an airway is the first priority. Although assessing the level of consciousness is a high priority because brain injury is commonly associated with facial trauma, securing an airway is a first priority. Cleansing facial wounds is important to prevent scarring but is not the priority of care.

125. B

The goal of a trauma registry is to compile data that can show trends that may be useful in improving trauma care and developing injury-prevention programs. Trauma registries have been used to serve a number of purposes, including quality improvement, epidemiology, clinical and outcomes research, and policy development. Trauma registries are not used to identify individual practice issues.

126. C

Rhabdomyolysis occurs when there is a disruption in the muscle cell membrane, thus releasing myoglobin into the bloodstream, which is not easily filtered by the kidneys. It leaves tubular deposits of pigment to obstruct the renal tubules, leading to acute kidney injury. These patients are usually in a significant amount of pain and the myoglobin released gives the urine a very dark reddish brown color. Hypovolemic patients will have decreased urine output and may be concentrated, but the color would not be this reddish brown. Some antibiotics, such as Flagyl, may darken the color of the urine, but antibiotics were not discussed in the question nor would this be an adverse reaction. Urinary tract infections (UTIs) will also cause urine to change color and become cloudy but not dark.

127. B

A spinal cord injury is the most common injury associated with near-drowning events. Diving and associated cervical spine injuries most commonly occur at the C5–C6 level and/or as a burst fracture. Seizure activity can be seen, especially in patient with epilepsy, but is usually witnessed after near-drowning accidents. Hypothermia, not hyperthermia, is common with submersion in water less than 70°F for about 4 to 6 minutes. Carbon monoxide poisoning is usually suspected in boating facilities, not near-drownings.

128. B

The disaster nurse should place a black tag on the patient. Expired patients, or patients for whom death is imminent, should be labeled with a black tag. The nurse should not leave the patient untagged because that impedes others who are also assessing the population, visualizing a black tag frees up health care personnel to go assess other viable patients and not waste time. Immediate resuscitation efforts are contraindicated in an agonal, unresponsive patient during a disaster because the patient is less likely to survive. Labeling the patient with a red tag would be inappropriate because red-tagged patients have life-threatening injuries that are often issues such as airway maintenance or surgical issues and immediate correction increases survival.

129. C

Palliative care is a useful tool because it provides interventional care that affirms life and neither accelerates nor postpones death. It can be initiated at any stage of treatment, not just end of life. Hospice is considered end-of-life care when patients are thought to be terminal or within 6 months of death. Psychosocial-centered care is a concept that meets the needs of the patient/family by providing information, compassionate care, and facilitating hope. Rehabilitation is the act of restoring something to its original state.

130. B

Arterial lactate levels have no advantage over venous lactate levels. When obtaining a lactate level by venipuncture, using a tourniquet can increase the lactate levels because of increased lactate at the site of the puncture. The sepsis resuscitation bundle includes a lactate level being obtained within 6 hours of onset of sepsis. Hyperlactatemia is typically present in patients with severe sepsis and septic shock resulting from hypoperfusion with the conversion to an anaerobic metabolism so is used to recognize an occult hypoperfusion before the onset of organ dysfunction.

131. C

The nurse should brush off dry chemicals, such as lime, with a dry towel before irrigating with water. The combination of water and the dry chemical can produce a corrosive substance that can cause further damage. Identifying a neutralizing agent is not necessary for this type of dry chemical injury. Petroleum products are applied to patients with tar or asphalt burns.

132. B

The responsibility for arranging transfer belongs to the referring institution, not the receiving institution. The receiving hospital must be notified before initiation of transport and cannot refuse to accept the patient unless physically unable to care for the patient. The transferring facility must provide the proper level of trained personnel to accompany the patient.

133. D

Rehabilitation begins at the time of admission with actions such as recognizing and treating complications. The longer the time between injury and rehabilitation, the less likely the patient will be able to rehabilitate fully. Rehabilitation interventions should be initiated in the intensive care unit before transfer to the progressive care unit or discharge to an acute care in-house rehabilitation center.

134. A

Extra drainage systems are not recommended during transport, and would not be an intervention that supports circulatory maintenance. Providing extra fluids to the team gives the transport team fluids that may be required during transport. Extension tubing will aid in reducing the incidence of disconnection and discontinuation of intravenous lines upon transferring and moving the patient but is not as important for circulation as fluids. Keeping an uninflated shock garment under the patient is not recommended for patients being transferred to a trauma facility.

135. C

The American College of Surgeons Trauma Quality Improvement Program (TQIP) works to elevate the quality of care for trauma patients. The goal is to improve the quality of trauma care. TQIP accomplishes its work by collecting data from trauma centers, providing feedback, and identifying opportunities for improvement. The program provides education and training, establishes national comparisons, and facilitates the sharing of best practice.

136. D

Recently extubated patients may need speech therapy because the vocal cords may still be recovering from having a tube passed between them, compressing them to the walls of the larynx, resulting edema. Consults come from the emergency department for traumatic cases with injury or aspiration. Psychiatric patients may benefit from speech therapy with refusal to eat being a common finding with a need to rule out dysphagia.

137. B

Abdominal compartment syndrome (ACS) patients may present with difficulty breathing, decreased urine output, syncope, nausea and vomiting, and an increased abdominal girth. ACS syndrome is primarily seen in abdominal surgical and trauma patients. A patient with hypovolemia could present similarly, but would most likely not have the abdominal distention. Infection is possible with all injuries, but for only being in the emergency room for that length of time, the severity of symptoms makes it less likely. Cholangitis is a bacterial infection that can occur when the bile duct is blocked. It is not commonly associated with pelvic fractures and treatment should include fluid resuscitation, paracentesis, and possible decompressive laparotomy.

138. A

A cystogram requires a Foley catheter insertion and contrast-filled bladder to evaluate with x-rays. It can reveal peritoneal extravasation following bladder rupture. A retrograde urethrogram also requires a Foley catheter, injection of contrast dye and x-rays but is used to diagnose ureteral rupture. Intravenous pyelogram (IVP) includes contrast dye administered intravenously and consecutive x-rays are obtained. The diagnostic test includes views of the kidneys, ureters, and bladder. A voiding urethrogram is an x-ray study of the bladder and urethra.

139. A

Touch is effective in some situations but may not always be effective in all situations and actually may worsen the situation. Some people may perceive touch as "threatening" during this stage of crisis. Maintaining good eye contact establishes honesty and reflects active listening. The nurse should remain calm and emotionally available in order to connect during this sensitive time.

140. A

The right kidney is more frequently injured because of its lower positon because of the large space that the liver occupies in the abdomen. The left kidney is more protected by the rib cage. The injury is seen more commonly in a deceleration mechanism and is associated with rib fractures or injuries.

141. C

Body temperature more than 101°F or less than 96.8°F, heart rate greater than 90 beats per minute, and a respiratory rate greater than 20 beats per minute are signs of sepsis. In severe sepsis, the patient may also exhibit a change in mental status, decreased urine output, decreased platelet count, abdominal pain, or respiratory distress indicating presence of hypoperfusion. This can advance to septic shock and multiple organ dysfunction.

142. B

The most common mechanism of injury in colon injuries is penetration, especially from gunshot wounds. Surgical procedures may include closure, resection with anastomosis, or closure with proximal colostomy. Right-colon colostomies are avoided because of their difficulty, loop colostomies are easily constructed but may not fully contain fecal material distally, and the Hartmann's procedure is a complete diversion with a double-barrel colostomy.

143. A

A cystogram takes views of the bladder and urethra. This would be the correct answer because bladder injuries are commonly associated with pelvic fractures. It is the most sensitive test that can detect a bladder tear. A Foley catheter would be contraindicated because of the possible bladder injury. CT and sonography are inadequate tests when assessing for a bladder injury.

144. B

An aortic transection is the disruption of the intimal, medial, and adventitial layers. The most common site for a traumatic aortic injury is the level of the isthmus, which is the level of the arch just distal to the great vessels. A ligament secures the aorta at this level so when there is a sudden deceleration mechanism, the aorta tears at the ligament.

145. B

Level 2 responders are hospitals, receiving facilities, and trauma centers. Level 1 responders are emergency medical services, including general public responders, and law enforcement. Level 3 responders are government agencies; there is no fourth-level responder.

146. A

Speech therapy aids motor speech disorders, such as problems saying sounds, syllables, and words. This speech abnormality occurs not because of muscle weakness or paralysis. The brain has problems in planning to move body parts, such as the lips, jaw, and tongue, needed for speech. The patient knows what he or she wants to say, but his or her brain has difficulty coordinating the muscle movements necessary to say those words; so the patient fabricates in order to achieve desired outcomes.

Occupational therapy (OT), physical therapy (PT), and a psychologist are not the specialists needed to improve this speech apraxia.

147. B

When the shaft of the radius and ulna is fractured this means that enough force was applied to fracture the shaft, and the force could be transmitted to the affiliated joints such as the wrist, elbow, and shoulder. The clavicle could be fractured in this type of injury; however, it would not be from the impact of the initial injury to the shaft.

148. B

It is rare that an irradiated patient would infect a health care provider and spread the contamination to other patients, so all resuscitation and lifesaving efforts should be initiated before any decontamination begins. Wounds can be covered with water-proof drapes before decontamination to prevent further contamination.

149. A

The rule of nines is calculated with each body part totaling a value of nine. The head = 9%, chest (anterior) = 9%, abdomen (anterior) = 9%, upper/mid/low back and buttocks = 18%, each arm = 9%, each palm = 1%, groin = 1%, each leg = 18% total (front = 9%, back = 9%). In this scenario, the bilateral lower extremities wound accounts for 36% (18% × 2), the groin 1%, the anterior chest 9%, and abdomen 9%. This adds up to 55% of the total body surface area burned.

150. D

Administering steroids has not been revealed to improve outcomes and is currently not recommended in traumatic brain injury (TBI) treatment. Analgesics decrease intracranial pressure (ICP) by decreasing pain, agitation, and metabolic demands. Administration of 3% saline infusion decreases cerebral edema, aiding in decreasing ICP. This hypertonic solution increases vascular osmolality and increases perfusion to vital organs. Maintaining CPP greater than 60 increases cerebral blood flow.

151. C

Burn patients are treated just like any other trauma patient; the priority is the airway. Patients who suffer from burns to the face, neck, or have obvious inhalation injury should have their airway assessed first and will mostly likely require intubation. This should be assessed before history is obtained, intravenous catheters are placed for fluid resuscitation, or wound care is provided.

152. C

Complications of cardiac contusions include arrhythmias, cardiogenic shock, depressed ventricular wall motion, congestive heart failure, and thrombus formation/embolism. Hypovolemic shock is not a complication of a cardiac contusion. Hypovolemic shock occurs with large blood loss.

153. B

The purpose of the trauma registry is to obtain, code, and sort information on trauma events for analysis, and reporting individual and aggregate results. Registry data is used for performance improvement, medical research, statistical analysis, critical pathways, care coordination, epidemiology, and injury prevention. Registry data then goes to the National Trauma Data Bank and is compiled annually and disseminated in the form of hospital benchmark reports, data-quality reports, and research data sets. Action Registry is a quality-improvement program that focuses on high-risk STEMI (ST-elevation myocardial infarction)/NSTEMI (non-ST segment elevation myocardial infarction) patients for clinical guideline recommendations. Impact Registry assesses the prevalence, demographics, management and outcomes of pediatric and adult congenital heart disease patients who undergo diagnostic catheterizations and catheter-based interventions.

154. A

Central cord syndrome is caused by injuries that result in swelling at the center of the cord. The mechanism includes hyperextension injuries and interruption of blood supply to the spinal cord. Anterior cord syndrome is usually from anterior cord compression or disruption of the anterior spinal artery. Posterior cord syndrome also occurs with hyperextension but this is the rarest of the syndromes. Brown–Sequard syndrome occurs with transverse hemisection of the cord and usually is caused by a penetrating injury.

155. C

Abdominal compartment compression results in altered cellular oxygenation and initiates cellular injury leading to hypoperfusion and cellular death. Abdominal compartment syndrome (ACS) is recognized with growing frequency as the cause of increased morbidity related to metabolic acidosis, decreased urine output, respiratory failure, and decreased cardiac output. The cause of these events might easily be mistaken for other pathologic events, such as hypovolemia, if the clinician is not alert to the morbidity associated with ACS.

156. B

The fetal presenting part should be elevated to relieve pressure off the cord because cord compression cuts off the oxygen supply to the fetus. Arrangements should be made for urgent cesarean delivery. Never attempt to push the cord back in or cover with sterile gauze. Placing the patient in the Trendelenburg position is not completely contraindicated but relieving the direct pressure off of the cord is most effective.

157. D

A patient with a full-thickness burn will usually not feel pain on the actual site because of damage to the nerve endings, but the patient will feel pain in the surrounding tissue in first- and second-degree burns. Temperature assessment of the skin is important because burn tissue may feel cold as a result of hypoperfusion and fluid loss. Palpation for pulses on circumferential burn is important because there may be direct injury to vessels and vascular compromise. A decreased or loss of pulse is an abnormal finding.

Bibliography

CLINICAL PRACTICE: HEAD AND NECK

Barbosa, R., Jawa, R., Watters, J. M., Knight, J. C., Kerwin, A., Winston, E. S.,...Rowell, S. (2012). Evaluation and management of mild traumatic brain injury: An Eastern Association for the Surgery of Trauma practice management guideline. *Journal of Trauma & Acute Care Surgery, 73*(5, Suppl. 4), S307–S314.

Brywczynski, J. J., Barrett, T. W., Lyon, J. A., & Cotton B. A. (2008). Management of penetrating neck injury in the emergency department: A structured literature review. *Emergency Medicine Journal, 25*(11), 711–715.

Bullock, M. R., & Povlishock, J. T. (2007). Guidelines for management of severe traumatic brain injury. *Journal of Trauma, 24*(Suppl. 1), vii–viii.

Cecil, S., Chen, P., Callaway, S., Rowland, S., Adler, D., & Chen, J. (2010). Traumatic brain injury: Advanced multimodal neuromonitoring from theory to clinical practice. *Critical Care Nursing, 31*(2), 25–37.

Delpachitra, S. N., & Rahmel, B. B. (2015, September 10). Orbital fractures in the emergency department: A review of early assessment and management. *Emergency Medicine Journal, 33*(10), 727–731.

Geyer, K., Meller, K., Kulpan, C., & Mowery, B. (2013). Traumatic brain injury in children: Acute care management. *Pediatric Nursing, 39*(6), 283–289.

Hadley, M., & Walters, B. (2003). Guidelines for the management of acute cervical spine and spinal cord injuries. *American Association of Neurological Surgeons, 72*(Suppl. 2), 1–259.

Hadley, M., Walters, B., Grabb, P., Oyesiku, N., Przybylski, G., Resnick, D., & Ryken, T. (2013). Guidelines for for the management of acute cervical spine and spinal cord injuries. *Neurosurgery, 72*(Suppl. 2), 1–259.

Papadopoulos, H., & Salib, N. K. (2009). Management of naso-orbital-ethmoidal fractures. *Oral Maxillofacial Surgery Clinics of North America, 21*(2), 221–225.

Rundquist, J., Gassaway, J., Bailey, J., Lingefelt, P., Reyes, I., & Thomas, J. (2011). Nursing bedside education and care management time during inpatient spinal cord injury rehabilitation. *Journal of Spinal Cord Medicine, 34*(2), 205–215.

Schroll, R., Fontenot, T., Lipcsey, M., Heaney, J. B., Marr, A., Meade, P.,...Duchsne, J. (2015, August 28). Role of computed tomography angiography in the management of Zone II penetrating neck trauma in patients with clinical hard signs. *Journal of Trauma & Acute Care Surgery, 79*(6), 943–950.

Thompson, H., & Mauk, K. (2011). Care of the mild traumatic brain injured patient. *AANN and ARN Clinical Practice Guideline Series*. Retrieved from www.AANN.org

Weitzel, N., Kendall, J., & Pons, P. (2004). Blind nasotracheal intubation for patients with penetrating neck trauma. *Journal of Trauma: Injury, Infection, & Critical Care, 56*(5), 1097–1101.

Wisniewski, P., Semon, G., & Liu, Xi (2014). Surgical critical care evidence-based medicine guidelines. Retrieved from www.Surgicalcriticalcare.net

Yew, C. C., Shaari, R, Rahman, S. A., & Alam, M. K. (2015). White-eyed blowout fracture: Diagnostic pitfalls and review of literature. *Injury, 46*(9), 1856–1859.

Ziccardi, V. B., & Braidy, H. (2009). Management of nasal fractures. *Oral & Maxillofacial Surgery Clinics of North America, 21*(2), 203–208.

CLINICAL PRACTICE: TRUNK

Akoglu, H., Akoglu, E. U., Evman, S., Akoglu, T., Denizbasi, A., Guneysel, O.,…Onur, E. (2012). Utility of cervical spinal and abdominal computed tomography in diagnosing occult pneumothorax in patients with blunt trauma: Computed tomographic imaging protocol matters. *Journal of Trauma & Acute Care Surgery, 73*(4), 874–879.

Al-Qudah, H. S., & Santucci, R. A. (2006). Complications of renal trauma. *Urologic Clinics of North America, 33*, 41–53.

Bělohlávek, J., Dytrych, V., & Linhart, A. (2013). Pulmonary embolism, part I: Epidemiology, risk factors and risk stratification, pathophysiology, clinical presentation, diagnosis and nonthrombotic pulmonary embolism. *Experimental & Clinical Cardiology, 18*(2), 129–138.

Campbell, M. R. (2007). Abdominal and urological trauma. In L. Newberry & L. M. Criddle (Eds.), *Sheehey's manual of emergency care* (6th ed., pp. 301–313). St. Louis, MO: Elsevier Mosby.

Clancy, K., Velopulos, C., Bilaniuk, J. W., Collier, B., Crowley, W., Kurek, S.,…Haut, E. R. (2012). Screening for blunt cardiac injury: An Eastern Association for the Surgery of Trauma practice management guideline. *Journal of Trauma & Acute Care Surgery, 73*(5 Suppl. 4), S301–S306.

The EAST Practice Management Guidelines Work Group, Holevar, M., DiGiacomo, C., Ebert, J., Luchette, F., Nagy, K.,…Yowler, C. (2003). Practice management guidelines for the evaluation of genitourinary trauma. *Eastern Association for the Surgery of Trauma.*

Hoff, W., Holevar, M., Nagy, K., Patterson, L., Young, J., Arrillaga, A., Najarian, M., & Valenziano, C. (2002). Evaluation of blunt abdominal trauma. East Practice Management Council. *Journal of Trauma, 53*(3), 602–615.

Kornezos, I., Chatziioannou, A., Kokkonouzis, I., Nebotakis, P., Moschouris, H., Yiarmenitis, S.,…Matsaidonis, D. (2010). Findings and limitations of focused ultrasound as a possible screening test in stable adult patients with blunt abdominal trauma: A Greek study. *European Radiology, 20*(1), 234–238.

Pryor, J. P., Pryor, R. J., & Stafford, P. W. (2002). Initial phase of trauma management and fluid resuscitation. *Trauma Reports, 3*(3), 1–12.

Romano, F., Garancini, M., Uggeri, L., Degrate, L., Maternini, M., & Uggeri, F. (2011, August 29). The implications of patients undergoing splenectomy: Postsurgery risk management. *Open Access Surgery, 4*, 21–34.

Seamon, M. J., Haut, E. R., Van Arendonk, K., Barbosa, R. R., Chiu, W. C., Dente, C. J.,…Rhee, P. (2015). An evidence-based approach to patient selection for emergency department thoracotomy: A practice management guideline from the Eastern Association for the Surgery of Trauma. *Journal of Trauma & Acute Care Surgery, 79*(1), 159–173.

Shariat, S. F., Roehrborn, C. G., Karakiewicz, P. I., Dhami, G., & Stage, K. H. (2007). Evidence-based validation of the predictive value of the American Association for the Surgery of Trauma Kidney Injury Scale. *Journal of Trauma: Injury, Infection, and Critical Care, 62*, 933–939.

Simon, B., Ebert, J., Bokhari, F., Capella, J., Emhoff, T., Hayward, T., Rodriguez, A. & Smith, L. (2012). Management of pulmonary contusion and flail chest: An Eastern Association for the Surgery of Trauma practice management guideline. *Journal of Trauma & Acute Care Surgery, 73*(5, Suppl. 4), S351–S361.

CLINICAL PRACTICE: EXTREMITY AND WOUND

Bittner, E. A., Shank, E., Woodson, L., & Martyn, J. A. (2015). Acute and perioperative care of the burn-injured patient. *Anesthesiology, 122*(2), 448–464.

Butz, D. R., Collier, Z., O'Connor, A., Magdziak, M., & Gottlieb, L. J. (2015). Is palmar surface area a reliable tool to estimate burn surface areas in obese patients? *Journal of Burn Care & Research, 36*(1), 87–91.

Clamp, J. A., & Moran, C. (2011). Hemorrhagic control in pelvic trauma. *Trauma, 13*(4), 300–316.

Dechert, T. A., Duane, T. M., Frykberg, B. P., Aboutanos, M. B., Malhotra, A. K., & Ivatury, R. R. (2009). Elderly patients with pelvic fracture: Interventions and outcomes. *American Surgeon, 75*(4), 291–295.

Fox, N., Rajani, R., Bokhari, F., Chiu, W., Kerwin, A., Seamon, M., . . . Frykberg, E. (2012). Evaluation and management of penetrating lower extremity arterial trauma. *Journal of Trauma & Acute Care Surgery, 73*(5), S315–S320.

Friese, R. S., Malekzadeh, S., Shafi, S., Gentlello, L. M., & Starr, A. (2007). Abdominal ultrasound is an unreliable modality for the detection of hemoperitoneum in patients with pelvic fracture. *Journal of Trauma: Injury, Infection, and Critical Care, 63*(1), 97–102.

Furey, A. J., O'Toole, R. V., Nascone, J. W., Sciadini, M. F., Copeland, C. E., & Turen, C. (2009). Classification of pelvic fractures: Analysis of inter- and intraobserver variability using the Young-Burgess and Tile classification systems. *Orthopedics, 32*(6), 401.

Papini, R. (2004). Management of burn injuries of various depths. *British Medical Journal, 329*(7458), 158–160.

Sheridan, R. L. (2003). Burn care: Results of technical and organizational progress. *Journal of the American Medical Association, 290*(6), 719–722.

Shlamovitz, G. Z., Mower, W. R., Bergman, J., Chuang, K. R., Crisp, J., Hardy, D., . . . Morgan, M. T. (2009). How (un)useful is the pelvic ring stability examination in diagnosing mechanically unstable pelvic fractures in blunt trauma patients? *Journal of Trauma: Injury, Infection, and Critical Care, 66*(3), 815–820.

Silver, G. M., Freiburg, C., Halerz, M., Tojong, J., Supple, K., & Gamelli, R. L. (2004). A survey of airway and ventilator management strategies in North American pediatric burn units. *Journal of Burn Care & Rehabilitation, 25*(5), 435–440.

Stander, M., & Wallis, L. A. (2011). The emergency management and treatment of severe burns. *Emergency Medicine International, 2011*, 161375.

Su, W. T., & James, H. (2014). Management of traumatic amputations of the upper limb. *British Medical Journal, 348*, g255.

Swithick, D. N., Benjamin, J. B., & Ruth, J. T. (2003). Timing of vascular and orthopedic repair in mangled extremities: Does it really matter? *Journal of Trauma: Injury, Infection, and Critical Care, 54*, 211.

Theron, A., Bodger, O., & Williams, D. (2014). Comparison of three techniques using the Parkland Formula to aid fluid resuscitation in adult burns. *Emergency Medicine Journal, 31*(9), 730–735.

Yuxiang, L., Lingjun, Z., Lu, T., Mengjie, L., Xing, M., Fengping, S., . . . Jijun, Z. (2011, November 11). Burn patients' experience of pain management: A qualitative study. *Burns, 38*(2), 180–186.

CLINICAL PRACTICE: SPECIAL SITUATIONS

Boschert, S. (2010). Massive transfusion protocol ups RBCs, plasma. *American College of Emergency Physicians.* Retrieved from www.acep.org

Brown, J. B., Cohen, M. J., Minei, J. P., Maier, R. V., West, M. A., Billiar, T. R., . . . Sperry, J. L. (2013). Goal directed resuscitation in the prehospital setting: A propensity-adjusted analysis. *Journal of Trauma and Acute Care Surgery, 74*(5), 1207–1214.

Collins, T. (2011). Packed red blood cell transfusion in critically ill patients. *Critical Care Nurse, 31*(1), 25–33.

Geoghegan, J., Dennis, A., & Manji, M (2010). Hypotensive resuscitation. *Trauma, 12*(3), 149–153.

Institute for Healthcare Improvement. (2012). *How-to-guide: Prevent catheter related urinary tract infections.* Cambridge, MA: Author.

Institute for Healthcare Improvement. (2012). *How-to-guide: Prevent central line-associated bloodstream infections.* Cambridge, MA: Author.

Institute for Healthcare Improvement. (2012). *How-to-guide: Prevent surgical site infections.* Cambridge, MA: Author.

CONTINUUM OF CARE

American Trauma Society. (2004). Trauma system: Agenda for the future. Retrieved from www.ems.org.

Centers for Disease Control and Prevention. (2001). Motor vehicle occupant injury: Strategies for increasing use of child safety seats, increasing use of safety belts, and reducing alcohol-impaired driving. A report on recommendations of the Task Force on Community Preventive Services. *Morbidity and Mortality Weekly Report*, 50(No. RR-7).

Cotton, B. A., Jerome, R., Collier, B. R., Khetarpal, S., Holevar, M., Tucker, B., ... Riordan, Jr., W. P. (2009). Guidelines for prehospital fluid resuscitation in the injured patient. *Journal of Trauma, 67*(2), 389–402.

Lockey, D., & Deakin, C. (2005). Prehospital trauma care: Systems and delivery. Continuing education in anesthesia. *Critical Care and Pain, 5*(6), 191–194.

Nathans, A., et al. (2008). *Regional trauma systems: Optimal elements, integration, and assessment, American College of Surgeons Committee on Trauma: Systems consultation guide*. Chicago, IL: American College of Surgeons.

National Center for Injury Prevention and Control. (2006). *CDC injury fact book*. Atlanta, GA: Centers for Disease Control and Prevention.

Petersen, S. R., & The Ad Hoc Committee on Rural Trauma, ACS Committee on Trauma. (2002). *Interfacility transfer of injured patients: Guidelines for rural communities*. American College of Surgeons. Retrieved from www.facs.org

Sasser, S., Hunt, R., Faul, M., Sugarman, D., Pearson, W., Dulski, T., ... Gali, R. (2012). Guidelines for field triage of injured patients: Recommendations of the National Expert Panel on field triage. Centers for Disease Control and Prevention. *Morbidity and Mortality Weekly Reports, 61*(1), 1–20.

Tom, C., & Gallagher, S. S. (2005). *Injury prevention and public health* (2nd ed.). Burlington, MA: Jones & Bartlett.

Warren, J., Fromm, R., Orr, R., Rotello, L., & Horst, M. (2004). Guidelines for the inter- and intrahospital transport of critically ill patients. *Critical Care Medicine, 32*(1), 256–262.

World Health Organization. (2007). *Preventing injuries: A guide for ministries of health*. Geneva, Switzerland: WHO Publications.

World Health Organization. (2008). *Violence, injuries, and disability biennial report, 2006–2007*. Geneva, Switzerland: WHO Publications.

PROFESSIONAL ISSUES

Campfield, K., & Hills, A. (2001). Effect of timing of critical incident stress debriefing (CISD) on post-traumatic symptoms. *Journal of Traumatic Stress, 14*, 327–340.

Flannery, R. B. (2005, February). *Assaulted Staff Action Program (ASAP): Fifteen years of empirical findings*. Paper presented at the Eighth World Congress on Stress Trauma and Coping: Crisis Intervention: Best Practices in Prevention, Preparedness and Response, Baltimore, Maryland.

Higginson, J., Walters, R., & Fulop, N. (2012, May 3). Mortality and morbidity meetings: An untapped resource for improving the governance of patient safety? *BMJ Quality and Safety, 21*, 576–585.

Kaczmarek, D. (2007). *Disaster preparedness: Manual for healthcare*. Chicago, IL: Materials Management Professional.

The Joint Commission on Accreditation of Healthcare Organizations. (2003). Health care at the crossroads: strategies for creating and sustaining community-wide emergency preparedness systems. Retrieved from www.jointcommission.org

The Joint Commission on Accreditation of Healthcare Organizations. (2007). Hospital accreditation standards for emergency management planning. Retrieved from www.jointcommission.org

Mock, C. Juillard, C., Brundage, S., Goosen, J., & Joshipura, J. (2009). Guidelines for trauma quality improvement programmes. *World Health Organization*. Retrieved from www.who.int

Index